OPTIMAL

EYESIGHT

ALSO BY ESTHER JOY VAN DER WERF:

Available in paperback and e-book:

Read Without Glasses at Any Age – The Natural Method to Near Vision Clarity. (2013) Practical advice to prevent or overcome farsightedness and presbyopia so reading glasses can be avoided or thrown out.

Bates Method Nuggets – The Fundamentals of Natural Vision Improvement by William H. Bates, M.D. (2010). A compilation of the best of Dr. Bates' writings; clear and practical advice covering all aspects of his method.

Available as e-books:

Better Eyesight – The original magazines as published by Dr. William H. Bates. The complete, unedited, and searchable collection of all of Dr. Bates' monthly magazines which were originally published from July 1919 to June 1930.

The Bates Method View-series. A series of e-books on various visual challenges:
- *The Bates Method View of Cataracts*
- *The Bates Method View of Conical Cornea*
- *The Bates Method View of Floating Specks*
- *The Bates Method View of Glaucoma*
- *The Bates Method View of Nystagmus*
- *The Bates Method View of Presbyopia*
- *The Bates Method View of Retinitis Pigmentosa*
- *The Bates Method View of Strabismus / Squint*
- *The Bates Method View of Eye Education in Our Schools*

Medical Articles by William H. Bates, M.D, 1886-1923. The complete collection of 30 medical articles written by Dr. Bates and published in various medical journals during 1886-1923.

All are available from www.visionsofjoy.org

OPTIMAL EYESIGHT

How to Restore and Retain Great Vision

How eyestrain leads to myopia, astigmatism, dry eyes, light sensitivity, night blindness, computer vision syndrome, amblyopia and strabismus, and what you can do about it.

Esther Joy van der Werf

Foreword by Amelia Salvador, M.D.

Published by Visions of Joy

Optimal Eyesight
Copyright © 2019 by Esther Joy van der Werf

The author of this book does not dispense medical advice or prescribe the use of any technique as a form of treatment for physical, emotional, or medical problems without the advice of a physician, either directly or indirectly. The educational services that are provided by Esther van der Werf are not licensed by the State of California. The intent of the author is only to offer information of a general nature to help you in your quest for visual and emotional well-being. In the event you use any of the information in this book for yourself, which is your constitutional right, the author, the publisher, and any third party involved in the creation of this book assume no responsibility for your actions.

Library of Congress Cataloging-in-Publication Data

Van der Werf, Esther.
  Optimal Eyesight : How to Restore and Retain Great Vision / Esther van der Werf. – 1st ed.
  ISBN 978-1-935894-24-7 (hardcover with color illustrations)
  ISBN 978-1-935894-21-6 (paperback with color illustrations)
  ISBN 978-1-935894-17-9 (paperback with grayscale illustrations)
  ISBN 978-1-935894-22-3 (ebook PDF)
  Library of Congress Control Number: 2019909092
  1. Van der Werf, Esther, 1966 – Health--Vision. 2. Health--Self-help. I. Title.
  TXu 2-144-059 2019

First Edition, September 2019
Second Printing, June 2020

Published by Visions of Joy, Ojai, California. Contact information at: www.visionsofjoy.org

Editors: Jean-Noel Bassior and Emma Ellis
Illustrations and cover design by Jane Shanahan
Author photograph on cover by Aubrie Woods

I dedicate this book to my dear friend and colleague

Robert M. Lichtman

4 September 1969 – 11 February 2015

With deep gratitude for his friendship and his inspiration to dig deeper into truth.

Bobby and I met in the summer of 2000 when we both studied eyesight improvement at the Natural Vision Center of San Francisco. After completion of our course, through many conversations, Bobby led me to become a dedicated student of the traditional Bates Method. His brilliant mind was much faster than mine at understanding Dr. Bates' truly effective relaxation techniques to release eyestrain and improve vision. Together we evaluated the differences between Bates' work and the typical misunderstandings of it that are prevalent nowadays. The more we learned, the more we returned to and applied Dr. Bates' sound advice.

This book is the result of that in-depth study and more than a decade of putting it into practice. Without Bobby, I might never have figured it out. Thank you, dear friend; I still miss our brain-storming sessions! I'm pretty sure your sojourn in heaven includes some in-depth conversations with Dr. Bates himself... ♥

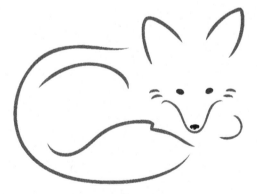

Bobby's dog *Snuggles*

Contents

Part IV – How to Apply the Relaxation Methods

Foreword

First of all, I would like to thank Esther for asking me to write these lines. I consider it a great honor.

It was at the 2002 International Holistic Vision Conference in Paris that I first met Esther. Since then, I have been intrigued to observe the dedicated path she has taken in studying the Bates Method to improve eyesight the natural way.

I have seen her again at every International Conference thereafter, and each time she has presented another interesting angle of her work. What has impressed me most is the deep understanding she has gained of Dr. Bates' original writing, and how that has enabled her to make available to us all the simple yet powerful path the method offers towards visual recovery.

As you read this book, you will find yourself immersed in the desire to improve your way of seeing. Your interest will grow in wanting to experience each of Esther's suggestions. You will discover different ways of looking, of thinking. and of imagining. And, best of all, you will be inspired to put the natural solutions offered into practice.

This book provides the opportunity and motivation to take back the reins of our visual and our general health. It is my opinion that society is greatly in need of this, having left them for too long only in the hands of medical professionals and optical and pharmaceutical companies.

During my years of work as an ophthalmologist, I have become convinced that the use of glasses is not the solution for visual problems. They are like a band-aid that can only momentarily alleviate a situation. In the long run, they do nothing to resolve the underlying issue and, instead, perpetuate it.

Esther's clear and simple language will appeal to all audiences. She describes the steps, one by one, that you can take to reach your goal of visual clarity. What makes this book especially effective is her holistic approach to how we use our eyes, from breathing, posture and eating habits to our exposure to natural light, and even our emotions. Of course, too, she does not neglect the life-changing effect that the new technology of computer and smartphone screens has had on us all.

Esther's great strength is in presenting simple activities to change your habits and use your eyes differently. And with her writing, you will feel accompanied every step of the way on the path to complete visual health.

Thank you, Esther, for all your work and dedication.

Amelia Salvador, M.D.
Denia (Alicante), Spain, February 2019

Who this Book is For and How to Use It

Who this book is for

If you have mild vision problems (whether eyestrain, myopia, astigmatism, dry eyes, light sensitivity, night blindness, computer vision syndrome, or eye suppression), this book is absolutely ideal for you. It is written with you in mind. You are likely to get to clarity without needing personal help from a Bates Method teacher, although with a good teacher you may progress faster. You are likely to make steady improvements on your own if your myopia level is below 3 diopters, or your astigmatism level is less than 2 diopters.

If you have moderate vision challenges (3 to 6 diopters of myopia, 2 to 4 diopters of astigmatism, amblyopia, strabismus or mild stages of eye diseases), this book will likely help you a lot, yet you may want some personal guidance from an experienced Bates Method teacher[1] to get the most from what you learn here.

Beyond those levels of myopia and astigmatism, this book will still be very valuable to you, yet I highly recommend you also take lessons from a qualified teacher to guide you along. Can you still make progress on your own following the advice in this book? Of course, and I encourage you to get started as soon as you can, because you are at higher risk of further vision challenges if you don't learn to relax your eyestrain now. Can you get to clarity if you have more than 6 diopters of myopia? Yes, absolutely; you won't be the first to do so.

If you see clearly and have no vision issues, this book is a great resource on how to keep your vision at its optimal level or how to improve it even further.

If you are farsighted or presbyopic and see better at distance than you do close up, I expect you will enjoy and get value from this book, yet you will get more specific advice for your visual challenges in my book *Read Without Glasses at Any Age.*[2]

How to use this book for optimal results

This is a highly practical book. To get the most out of it, you need to know a few things about your own vision. I suggest you do the first three steps below before you read the whole book.

1. Establish your Optimal Practice Distance from the chart (see Appendix A).

2. Measure your current far point for each eye and make a note of those distances (see Appendix B).

3. Write down your starting visual acuity (see Appendix C). This book uses the imperial system, in which "normal acuity" is 20/20, i.e. the ability to read the 20-line on the letter chart from 20 feet distance. A table is provided in Appendix D for easy comparison of various ways to record visual acuity.

4. Find and learn to recognize your strain patterns (see Chapter 4).

5. Apply relaxation techniques from Chapters 5 to 15 and mainly use the ones that give you the best results (these may change).

6. Establish your personal path to clarity with help from Chapters 16 and 17. Chapters 18 to 24 can be used or skipped depending on your needs.

7. Look for this eye image which marks all practical suggestions in the book. It will help you find practices relevant to the chapter topic.

8. Check your visual acuity regularly, especially if you use reduced prescription glasses or contact lenses.

9. Step down to lower diopter lenses as soon as you can read the 20-line on a letter chart from 20 feet with your current lenses.

Applying the knowledge you gain from this book will not take much time; it's essentially a matter of awareness and choice. Once you recognize your eyestrain and you know how to use your eyes without that strain, you simply can choose in every moment of the day to either continue to strain your eyes, or to use them as nature intended: effortlessly. This book will show you how – you'll see!

Notes
- Names of some students mentioned in this book have been changed.
- If medical terms such as amblyopia, astigmatism and diopters are mysterious new words to you, please see the Glossary in the back of this book for an explanation.

Preface

This book is largely based on the Bates Method, which many people have never heard about, and many others completely misjudge as a method of eye exercises. That's a shame, but this book will clarify this method both for those who are new to it and those who erroneously consider it to be just another system of eye exercises.

The Bates Method is named after a famous ophthalmologist, Dr. William Horatio Bates (1860-1931). In 1885 Bates received his medical degree from the College of Physicians and Surgeons at Columbia University in New York and became a successful eye surgeon and instructor of ophthalmology at the New York Postgraduate Medical School and Hospital.

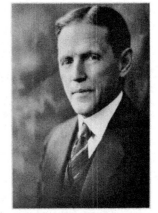

Dr. William H. Bates

Most eye doctors have had patients tell them that their vision improved after a period without using glasses,[1] and Bates was no exception. He observed that some of his patients recovered normal vision despite having been diagnosed with myopia and prescribed glasses. Myopia, or nearsightedness, was (and still is) considered incurable. Not satisfied with chalking these unusual cases up to an error in his measurements, Bates set out to learn why these patients had regained their sight. Thus began his independent study of the eyes at Columbia University.

Bates found that the refractive state of human eyes is not static; it fluctuates. He discovered that stress worsens sight and relaxation improves it; that people with good eyesight have different visual habits than people without; and that wearing glasses always causes vision to deteriorate.

Publications

Between 1886 and 1923, Bates published his findings in medical journals such as the New York Medical Journal. A total of 30 articles were published.[2] His efforts were mostly ignored and rejected by his peers; it was too much of a challenge to the established doctrine. During that period, Bates' first book, *Better Eyesight Without Glasses*, was published in 1918 by Henry Holt & Co. Inc.[3] but was apparently deemed to be so much of a threat by his colleagues that it was taken out of distribution. In the same year, Bernarr MacFadden, a leader in the physical culture movement at that time who ran his own Physical Culture Publishing Company, convinced Bates to co-author *Strengthening the Eyes – A New Course in Scientific Eye Training in 28 Lessons.*[4] However, this turned Bates' methods toward an exercise regimen. Perhaps for this reason, or again due to pressure from his colleagues, Bates had his name removed from all subsequent publications by MacFadden. In July of 1919, Bates started his own Central Fixation Publishing Company and launched *Better Eyesight; A Monthly Magazine Devoted to the Prevention and Cure of Imperfect Sight Without Glasses*.[5] This magazine was aimed at educating his patients and the general public about his methods. It ran for eleven years.

In 1920, Bates self-published his own book and called it: *Perfect Sight Without Glasses*. It was also known as *The Cure of Imperfect Sight by Treatment Without Glasses*.[6] This became popular and used copies can still be found for sale. After his death, edited versions of this book were again published by Henry Holt & Co in 1943, titled: *Better Eyesight Without Glasses*.

The method gets a name

As many success stories were published in the magazines and word of this maverick eye surgeon's methods spread, people began to ask Bates if his treatment had a name. His response:

> Many people have asked me what I call my treatment. The question was a very embarrassing one because I really have no name to give it unless I can say that my methods are the methods employed by the normal eye. When a person has normal sight, the eye is at rest, and when the eye is at rest, strange to say, it is always moving to avoid the stare.[7]

That same issue of *Better Eyesight* includes the very first mention of the term "Bates Method." Despite Bates' own hesitance at calling it that, it stuck.

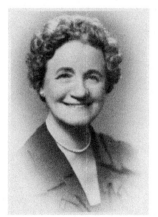

Emily (Lierman) Bates

Retirement plans

In the January 1930 issue of his magazine, Bates announced that the monthly publication would be discontinued after the June 1930 issue so he and his wife Emily could devote more time to the writing of new books on his treatments. For personal help he referred people to "authorized representatives": doctors, nurses, teachers and others who had been trained in his methods. Unfortunately, Dr. Bates became ill in 1930 and he died in the summer of 1931. In 1940 Emily re-published his 1920 book with a new chapter added at the end,[8] but that was the only new material printed.

Carrying the torch

Some of those taught by Bates himself were doctors, yet many were not medically trained. Among the latter group was Margaret Corbett from Los Angeles. Corbett (1889-1962) became one of the most well-known teachers to carry the method forward. She established a school, published three books of her own,[9-11] had many famous people among her clientele, and trained other teachers.

Taken to court

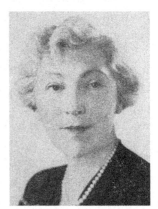

In 1940, Corbett was taken to court for practicing medicine without a license, yet she won her case, thanks in part to many testimonials from students who had benefited greatly from her teachings, including the famous author Aldous Huxley. A bill was then introduced into the Californian State Legislature to make vision education illegal without an optometric or medical license. After a lively campaign in the media and a strong fight from Corbett, the bill was defeated. Today, the Bates Method continues to be passed on by people like myself who benefited from it and wish to help others.

Margaret D. Corbett

Beyond Bates

Much of this book is based on Dr. Bates' method, yet I have diverged from it in some areas (such as astigmatism, breathing, nutrition, night vision, use of light-emitting screens) where the work of others surpasses Bates' knowledge. This brings the method forward into the 21st century and adds to its effectiveness.

Whether you are new to the Bates Method or have some experience with it already, I trust you will benefit from what you find in the following pages.

Introduction

I was astonished and delighted when I first learned to relax my eyes and returned to 20/20 acuity in only two weeks after 16 years of blurry vision. Two months later I regained the crisp clarity of my teenage years – an even better 20/15 visual acuity. Yet, besides the joy I felt at regaining my clear vision at age thirty-three, I also felt some anger. Why had nobody told me that there was a natural option for improving my sight?! I could have saved myself all those years of nearsightedness, had I simply known this easy method existed!

I had not actually expected to improve my vision. I had tried eye exercises in my mid-twenties, for longer than a mere two weeks, with only frustration and disappointment as a result. So I was skeptical of vision improvement methods, no longer believing it was possible – and yet, I still hated glasses. The glasses I was prescribed in my late teens made me feel separate from the world, turning me into a spectator rather than a participant, and I could not get used to that. I cunningly "lost" my glasses a few months after I got them, to the dismay of my parents who'd paid for them. I was more comfortable in my blurry world than I was trapped behind those crutches. Really, all I hoped for when I started this second attempt in my early thirties was for my vision to not get any worse. If I could remain at my mildly blurry level (about -1.25 diopters), I figured I could manage squinting through life and avoid ever needing glasses. That would be fine with me. So I was surprised that the Bates Method of relaxation was clearly different and obviously far more effective than eye exercises.

As soon as I had 20/20 vision, I tested the method on my friend Ted, who had been using glasses for many years and was more nearsighted than I'd been. When I placed him in front of a letter chart at 20 feet without his glasses and asked him what he could read, he peered straight ahead for a while then responded: "Did you hang something on the wall?" I had no idea his vision was that bad, and, thankfully, my ignorance of how "impossible" it would be to improve from worse than 4 diopters of myopia allowed me to proceed with an unwarranted level of optimism.

I challenged Ted to not use his glasses for one whole week. He was hesitant (not surprisingly), but I offered to do any and all driving and got him to agree. He handed me his glasses, and I hid them to make sure he wouldn't cheat. For that week we practiced daily together what I had learned from the book *Relearning to See*[1] by Tom Quackenbush and, amazingly, at the end Ted did not ask for his glasses back! I didn't remind him the week was up; we simply continued, slowly changing his old, strained habits of seeing into seeing with more ease. One month into it, I decided that Ted should probably check his visual acuity with the letter chart again. Same chart, same distance. This time, however, he read all the way down to the 50 line, where he began to make some mistakes. Wow! We were both astonished. From not being able to see the chart at all to being merely one line away from 20/40 acuity, which means one line away from passing the driver's test without glasses, in just one month... This was an incredible improvement!

I sent a "thank you" letter to Tom Quackenbush, who promptly invited me to his teacher training program in the summer of 2000. I had already quit my previous job and didn't have anything better or more interesting to do, so I accepted.

I became passionate about anything to do with eyesight improvement after taking Tom's course. For a few years, I would talk about it to anyone willing to listen and tried my new skills out on various friends, but rarely had the success I was hoping for. In 2003, I moved to New Paltz, New York, to train with Dr. Marc Grossman, a behavioral optometrist whom I had met at a vision educators' conference in Oregon. Marc was familiar with the Bates Method and willing to let me try it on his patients. I had some nice successes there, but still failed to help everyone the way I wanted to. I knew I had to keep looking for better answers.

Bobby's brilliance
Living in New York State had put me back in touch with Bobby Lichtman in New York City, one of the other trainees who took Tom's course with me. Bobby had experienced similar frustrations with applying what we had been taught. Like me, he was a ferocious reader who read many books on the Bates Method. By then we had both acquired copies of all 132 issues of Dr. Bates' *Better Eyesight* magazine, which described in practical detail how Bates worked with his patients to improve their vision. During our teacher training, we had helped Tom proofread his second book, *Better Eyesight*,[2] an edited version of this magazine collection, but now that we had the originals, we realized how much editing Tom had done. So we favored the originals, despite the poorly photocopied digital format, instead of Tom's nicely printed book.

Bobby was the first to find inconsistencies between what we'd read in the original magazines and what we'd been taught by Tom. Bobby called one day and asked me to read a certain paragraph in one original issue of *Better Eyesight* and compare it to a paragraph on the same topic in *Relearning to See*. The two seemed to say opposite things. We wondered why, but were mainly interested in testing Bates' way. More phone calls like this followed from Bobby, who became increasingly excited about the treasures he was finding in the old magazines. He pulled me along, while I scrambled to keep up with his rapid pace.

As we delved deeper into Bates' original advice and compared it to that of past and present teachers, we were astounded to find some major differences. We learned that almost all Bates vision improvement books contain errors and misunderstandings that have been passed on from one teacher to the next since Dr. Bates' death. Like a game of "telephone," the clear message that Dr. Bates gave in the 1920s had become so distorted eight decades later that the effectiveness of his techniques had drastically diminished. No wonder the method was viewed as "quackery" by so many eye doctors! Although Bates was a highly respected eye surgeon, he had struggled with acceptance of his work by his colleagues; his controversial methods were considered a threat to the established doctrine. These effective methods were therefore rejected, rather than properly investigated. With this dilution over time, the medical profession was even less likely to give the method any due consideration, and this time, rightly so.

In 2004, Bobby and I began to adapt our approach to what we'd learned from Bates himself. Two years later, I converted the photocopied magazines into 770 pages of searchable Word text that allowed for even easier research. Now we could pick Dr. Bates' brain on any topic we wanted at the speed of modern technology. The results were a return to the traditional Bates Method: effective and easy-to-apply techniques to reduce eyestrain and restore optimal eyesight. We finally started getting the results we hoped for with our students.

> **The real voyage of discovery
> consists not in seeking new landscapes
> but in having new eyes.**
> Marcel Proust[3]

I secretly hoped Bobby would write this book. His brilliant mind would have created a masterpiece. Bobby did start writing, yet sadly he became ill with a brain tumor. Our lengthy phone calls became shorter and less frequent as his cognitive powers diminished. With his passing in 2015, the obligation to finish and publish this book landed squarely on my shoulders.

Not rocket science
I do not claim to know everything there is to know about how human eyes work. There is always more to learn. But I do know this: reducing eyestrain is possible, and it is not rocket science. Anybody can learn how to see with more ease and less effort. And when you do, chances are very good that you will experience delightful side effects when you release the effort (and the glasses or contact lenses) that you have been using to see. Blurry vision begins to retreat, the world magically clears up around you, color perception improves, self-confidence rises and your dependency on those nuisance lenses becomes less and less. That is worth knowing about. That is worth many hours of me writing so you too can benefit from what I have learned over the past 19 years as a Bates Method teacher.

I am glad to accompany you on your vision journey, regardless of whether this is new to you or you've tried different methods before and have not yet reached your desired clarity. I expect this book will help you understand where you are on your path to clarity, what you can do, and what you may want to avoid doing, to reach your vision goals.

My wish for you is to find what I did: the sheer joy of seeing with natural clarity!

Love & Light,
Esther Joy van der Werf
Ojai, California, August 2019

Part I

–

What Causes Blurry Vision?

1. Your Eyes Are Not Weak

As a reader of this book, I assume you are dealing with some blurry vision, mainly at a distance. If your distance vision is fine and your blur is at the near point, you will likely benefit most from my previous book, *Read Without Glasses at Any Age*.

This book, *Optimal Eyesight,* is for the multitude of myopic eyes among us, as well as for the astigmatic eyes, dry eyes, strabismic eyes, amblyopic eyes, light-sensitive eyes, computer-strained eyes, or any combination of these. You are dealing with blurry vision at a distance, while your near vision is generally good, or even perfectly fine. You have a clear zone that extends perhaps only a few inches from your eyes, while for many readers it probably extends a foot or more. This is known as your far point, and I'll show you how to measure it and keep track of your progress.

Your main reason for reading these pages is to find out if you can reduce that blurriness or perhaps, like I did years ago, you've given up on the thought of improving your eyesight, but hope to find something that will stop it from getting worse. Perhaps the idea of laser surgery scares you and you'd rather give nature one more chance before subjecting yourself to the risks and side effects that surgery could bring to your eyes and life. Perhaps you already had refractive surgery years ago, and the crisp clarity it gave you for a while is slipping away. You may have had a diagnosis from an eye doctor of "incipient cataract" or "at risk for glaucoma," or similar early stages of common eye diseases, and you wonder if you can halt or slow the progression down that slippery slope.

Or, you may be fed up with glasses and contact lenses, and you'd really like a better solution. Perhaps you have not used lenses yet but are on the verge of needing them, and you really would rather not ruin your good looks with glasses. Or you hated your glasses, switched to contact lenses, and now have dry eyes that reject the contacts and you wonder what to do next. These are some of the typical problems people have when they first contact me.

Somewhere inside of you there is a nagging feeling that says there must be a better way; a way for your eyes to work well, or better than they do now, at least. Even though your eye doctor doesn't believe in it, you've been searching for an answer and you're willing to "do whatever it takes" to find a solution that works for you. Now you have found your way to this book, and you've come to the right place.

In this book you will find answers to all those nagging questions. Answers that will make sense to you; answers that truly help you reach your goals for your eyes. Less eyestrain, less blurriness, more ease in seeing, more clarity. By the time you're done reading, you will have a clear understanding of what causes blurry vision and what helps it go away. You'll be able to take good care of your eyes and avoid glasses for life if you have not used them yet, or reduce the power of your lenses over time instead of the ever-increasing powers that may have been your reality until now.

Credentials

Who am I to make these promises? An eye doctor? Nope, not at all. I am just an ex-myope, who tried unsuccessfully to improve my eyesight with eye exercises, then stumbled upon some truths and returned to clear vision in such a short time that I wondered why nobody ever told me this simple method existed! That led me to study anything to do with eyesight. I became a certified Natural Vision Educator; worked with an optometrist for two years; followed an eye surgeon around for two weeks of additional training; attended many natural vision conferences; became a regular speaker at these conferences and even organized a professional conference myself. I am an active Board Member of the North American Association of Vision Educators.[1] After nearly two decades on this vision journey, it has brought me to the point of being considered the foremost expert in the world on the Bates Method of natural vision improvement.

You may have heard of the Bates Method, and you may have tried it, with or without success. A lot of what is taught as the Bates Method today has little or nothing at all to do with what Dr. William H. Bates, the originator of the method, taught. So, if you tried it and failed before, don't be discouraged. This book is going to surprise you with truly effective methods, not futile eye exercises.

When my colleague Bobby and I started figuring out the traditional Bates Method – the way it was before the modern misinterpretations – I wished there was a guidebook for it. Bates had intended to write another book but died before he could do so. Bobby died too before he could write his book. That left me to write this book – for myself, for Bobby, and for our students. During the ten years this book has been "in progress," it has evolved as my own understanding of Bates' methods increased. In another ten years it may evolve even further, but I am not taking for granted I'll still be around, so this is what I know right now, and what I think you ought to know. I am passionate about getting this information out. I cannot visualize myself leaving this earth without first doing my job of passing this knowledge on to you. You need it, you deserve the truth, and I trust you will love the simplicity of this method and will pass it on like I did.

No crutches and no exercises

Imagine what your life will be like when you are not dependent on crutches for your eyes! You'll experience the joy of seeing clearly with your own eyes, right from the moment you wake up in the morning to the time when you happily close them at night, with gratitude for another day of clarity and joy. And then there are the happy side effects to enjoy: more vivid color perception; increased depth perception; greater self-confidence; higher energy levels; less eyestrain; fewer headaches; looking more relaxed and younger; no more fear of going blind – just to name a few. Yes, I promise you are going to like the "new you" that comes along with your "new vision" when you apply what you learn in this book. And I promise it is not difficult, nor boring, nor does it resemble eye exercises. Nope: NO eye exercises. This method is all about ease, and about nature's way. You'll understand that your eyes are not weak at all, and likely not "incapable" in some way. They are very capable little beings that have been waiting for the opportunity to get a vacation from the chronic stress they have suffered, possibly for years! You will learn how to give them that break, and how to keep them happy and functioning at their best.

Proof
Now some of you will be asking for "proof" that I'm telling the truth. And preferably "scientific proof" to back me up. I can come up with that (see References, page 291), but I believe that nothing will convince you more than your very own experience. Nothing beats personal proof. Everything else is hearsay. I want you to have that personal proof, and not take anything less as evidence.

A myopic Dutch chemist contacted me some years ago, asking why he had never heard of the Bates Method, nor had his eye doctor who proclaimed that eye exercises do not work, so why should he trust the testimonials and claims I make on my website? I wrote a polite reply that he should not trust me or anyone else's testimonial, only his own experience, and I briefly added that the Bates Method is based on relaxation, not effort or eye exercises. A few weeks later he wrote back – and his tone had changed from critical skepticism to sheer surprise and delight. He had gone without his glasses for those few weeks, practiced looking at things without effort, and his vision had been clearing up more and more each day! He was stunned and happy, wished me all the best, and told me to keep doing what I was doing.

In a lecture I gave at a holistic vision conference in Madrid on the topic of sunlight, a similar issue came up: Why trust what I say (in this case that eyes need sunlight for health) over what is so widely proclaimed by doctors these days: that sunlight is harmful to your eyes? There was a fair amount of fear in my audience that day, and I knew I had to deal with it before I could expect them to truly listen to any advice I had about gradual and safe exposure of the eyes to sunlight for better vision. So I gave the following example, which vision educators are familiar with. Eye doctors used to say that binocular vision could never be achieved if it wasn't established by age eight. They instilled fear in parents that their child would likely go blind in the amblyopic eye if the problem wasn't addressed by that age. The brain would be unable to use the eye later in life, they proclaimed. Well, I was 36 when I first experienced stereoscopic vision.

My amblyopic left eye wasn't actually discovered until my teacher training course with Tom Quackenbush at age thirty-three. But it did explain my inability to see in 3-D as a child; I just never knew how to express it because I didn't know what I was missing or what "space" in this world was supposed to look like! Neuroscientist Susan Barry had a similar experience of developing depth perception as an adult. She was in her late 40s when she experienced the world in 3-D for the first time. She wrote a best-selling book about it: *Fixing my Gaze.*[2] Susan and I are not "exceptions to the rule." The "rule" was never correct to begin with, yet doctors proclaimed it for many, many years, and lots of them still do! So, does that make it impossible for you to have depth perception if you've never had it before? Nope, it only means you have not yet been shown how to train your eyes and brain to develop that ability. All that fear that was created unnecessarily is still being created today – on the same topic, and on many other topics. That's why it's worthwhile to question your doctors and rely more on your own experience. Don't buy into fear mongering; check for truth first. Chances are that there is a better way.

In general, science is great, when it is done right. Medical science, however, depends on whose research you believe, and these days is often so blatantly influenced by the profit margins of big pharmaceutical industries, that you are far better off making up your own mind than trusting what you read in medical journals. I'm not kidding; even the editor-in-chief of *The Lancet*, a well-respected medical journal, claims that: "much of the scientific literature, perhaps half, may simply be untrue."[3] He's not a lone voice, as evidenced by articles such as: "America's other drug problem: how the drug industry distorts medicine and politics,"[4] "Why Most Published Research Findings Are False,"[5] and "Neuroscientist shows what fasting does to your brain & why big pharma won't study it."[6]

No effort

I promise that you will benefit from this book once you understand the basic concept of releasing the effort you've probably put into improving your sight until now. Effort will never improve your sight. Relaxation will. It's easy, simple, natural and common sense, but it can take a bit of time, understanding, and recognition of ingrained strain patterns before they let go, so you can have your optimal eyesight.

Expect results!

Remember how long it took for your eyes to reach their current point of blurry vision? I predict it will not take anywhere near that long for the journey back to clarity. The sooner you take the first step, the sooner you'll reach your optimal eyesight. Come along; let me show you how to achieve it.

2.   The Old View Turns a Blind Eye

The old view (which, unfortunately, is still the current paradigm) says that eyes that don't see clearly have "grown" out of their healthy, round shape into a distorted shape, which causes blurry vision. According to this view, there is nothing that can be done about wrongly-shaped eyes; you unfortunately inherited a "bad-eyes-gene" from your parents.

The typical solutions offered are to wear glasses or contact lenses that compensate for the distortion (cumbersome crutches at best), or to have laser surgery (which basically etches the present prescription onto your cornea and comes with risky and at times painful side effects), or, for children, to use eye drops that slow the progression of myopia (but don't halt or reverse it). In this old view, acuity is considered to be fairly static; the presumption is that the prescription measured by the eye doctor will hold steady throughout the day. Thus, lenses that are also static in their prescription are considered the "perfect answer."

Yet vision is not static – almost everyone has noticed that their sight fluctuates. Tiredness, tension and poor light usually cause worse vision, while being rested, relaxed and under good light generally allows better vision. Sitting in an artificially-lit, windowless room with your head stuck behind a phoropter so a doctor can test your vision with small black letters is typically a stress-inducing moment that produces a temporary, negative result. This does *not* accurately reflect how well you see under normal circumstances.

In addition, the old view does not tolerate the concept that vision can improve; the assumption is that it can only get worse. And it does get worse, because the "solutions" offered – glasses, contact lenses, surgery or drugs – do not address the cause of the problem; they only add to it. In fact, they intensify poor vision over time, leading to possible eye diseases and even blindness.

Glasses and contact lenses
When vision "fails" and an eye doctor prescribes compensating lenses, he or she gives you a tool that restores your acuity for the letter chart. At first glance this may seem like a good idea, but take another look and you'll find some problems with this option...

Glasses have an optical center. This is the thinnest point of a concave (minus) lens and the thickest point of a convex (plus) lens. Vision is best when looking directly through that central point of the lens, but other lines of sight are distorted. This distortion affects your peripheral vision and leads to a reduction in eye motion.

One vision student wrote: "When looking through the glasses, my vision is sharp, however, the image as a whole seems warped, especially in my peripheral vision." Many people have a hard time getting used to these distortions when they first get glasses. They may find it tricky to walk down stairs because their depth perception is skewed when looking through the lower part of the glasses. To adapt, they may bend the head unnaturally far down when they descend stairs, unless they briefly remove their glasses.

Polycarbonate lenses have a worse reputation for distortion than others, and large frames are more problematic than small, but all lenses create some distortion despite the sharper vision that they provide centrally.

In the 1950s, corneal contact lenses became an alternative to glasses, followed by the appearance of the more comfortable soft lenses in the 1970s. Many people prefer contacts over glasses because the artificial lens moves with the eyes, which eliminates the optical center problem and its peripheral distortion. However, as the eyes were not designed to have an extra layer on the cornea, turning the eyes far to one side or even just blinking may push a contact lens out of place. This obviously displaces the optical center and distorts vision until you push the lens back in place. An out-of-place contact lens is an uncomfortable experience, so the contact lens wearer learns to blink less and, like a person wearing glasses, learns to restrict eye motion. Contact lenses also carry the risk of damage to the cornea each time they are put in and taken out, and the liquid used to store contacts in their case can harbor bacteria, which may lead to infections.

The reduction in motion freedom of the eyes when using glasses or contacts, the static prescription covering a fluctuating acuity, and the lack of blinking when wearing contacts all contribute to eyestrain. As the eyes move less, you compensate for this restriction by adopting more ways of moving the head and body. This causes imbalances and chronic strain in the body. Neck tension is the most common problem by far. People with bifocal lenses or those with astigmatism are especially prone to tight neck muscles due to head-tilt adaptations for bifocals and increased peripheral distortions from astigmatism cylinders.

Also, research has shown a link between retinal dopamine and myopia. Dopamine appears to protect against nearsightedness, and its release is regulated by light intensity. Interestingly, when you wear glasses or contacts, dopamine release is reduced within hours, thus contributing to an increase in myopia.[1]

Using lenses to help you see has some additional side-effects as well. Wearing glasses may make you feel nerdy, or like you're hiding behind them and wish you could come out to join everyone else on the other side of that barrier. They can feel heavy on the nose, tight at the ears, fog up in cold weather, scratch and break easily. Contacts allow you to hide the "deficiency" that you are dealing with, but your eyes can only tolerate them for so long. Did you know contact lenses are a class II medical device, as are the fluids required to be used with them, due to their risk of causing injuries?![2,3] I get squeamish just thinking about that...

Laser surgery

LASIK, the most common laser surgery, involves cutting the edges of the cornea so it can be flapped open, allowing a laser to alter the tissue underneath. The cornea is a highly sensitive part of your eye; it is full of nerves that will be destroyed in the process, which may leave you with incredible pain afterwards. For some people, this pain does not go away and has even led a few to commit suicide.

Laser surgery does *not* give you great vision for life. Your eyestrain did not get cut out in the process, and therefore your vision is still subject to decline. A pair of glasses does not guarantee you are set for life with that prescription, and, similarly, the corneal modification caused by laser surgery (whether LASIK, LASEK or PRK) is not a guaranteed correct prescription for your eyes. Chances are high that you will end up with glasses again, sooner or later.

The side effects of refractive surgeries are often swept under the rug, especially in your orientation talk. When the eye doctor tells you that the risks are tiny and the worst you'll experience is some dry eye, which will go away, you probably feel reassured. They may tell you that less than 1% of patients have trouble, yet this "fact" is based on a flawed study done by one man, with unverifiable results. That is not science. Reality is very different! A shocking 41% of patients still have side effects six months after LASIK and experience visual problems or pain they did not have before the surgery. A worrisome 4% have extreme debilitating problems.[4]

Laser surgery is an *industry*! They are essentially cutting into a healthy eye and damaging it for life! And they first need your "informed consent" to do so. Read this consent form thoroughly, at a quiet time without interruptions. Let its information sink in before you decide if it's worth subjecting your eyes to all these risks. After the orientation talk, some clinics want to do your pre-surgery exam immediately and will pressure you into it, saying it's free if you do it right now, but $100 if you wait, go home, and think about it first. They do not want you to think about it; they do not want you to google laser surgery and find websites such as mine or those listed on my site's laser surgery page.[5] If your eye clinic uses high pressure sales tactics like this, run the other way! Those people are only interested in lining their pockets; they do not have your best eye health at heart.

Dr. Bates of course did not write about laser surgeries – those came after his lifetime – yet it's common nowadays for me to have students who've had laser surgery and have either not benefited as much as they hoped, or have regressed since having the surgery.

If you have already had refractive surgery and are now suffering with negative side effects, you are likely wondering if the Bates Method can still be of help to you. I include the following email on this topic because it raises a typical question that appears fairly often in my inbox:

> Hello Esther,
> I have a question regarding the Bates Method after LASIK. I had LASIK surgery almost 5 years ago and now have many side effects including halos, poor night vision and a general feeling of poor vision. If I knew about natural eye improvement years ago, I would not have done LASIK. I'm wondering, is there any hope for me to improve my vision at this point?
> Sam

My answer to Sam is yes, the Bates Method can still be helpful to you. I say this with confidence because I've helped others in similar or worse situations since their laser surgery. A couple of examples:

- In 2012, I worked with Leo from Finland who had the early LASIK treatment in 1989 which had gone horribly wrong. They had cut too deep and too far, his vision was worse than before, and his eyes had since been tremendously tired and extremely painful every day. In his own words: "*That surgery botched up my eyes.*" His eyes were red, dry and tired; his eyelids were swollen, and he saw halos around lights. The first thing he had to do each day after work was lie down and cover his eyes for half an hour or longer to let the pain subside.

  After one day of following my instructions in using the Bates Method, he was much relieved; his eyes felt comfortable for the first time and his vision had already improved considerably. On the second day I met with Leo and his wife, he was sitting on the couch, looking out the window and marveling at how clear everything looked, and how relaxed and good his eyes felt for the first time in over 20 years.

- Judy from Berkeley took my email course three months after her LASIK surgery because her vision had remained blurry. She loved what she learned and wrote:

  I got the fastest result: In three weeks my staring, blurriness and dryness were gone. This course has given me 20/20 vision both at a distance and near. I'm not staring anymore. Also my eyes are not tired out any more in the late afternoon. Also, I am comfortable with both brightness and darkness. At last, my eyes have more tears because they're shifting. The course was fabulous! Thank you, Esther.

I much prefer to help people before they undergo LASIK or similar refractive surgeries, yet I know they often need my help even more afterwards. I do my best to help them minimize those nasty side effects. The Bates Method can help your eyes heal from these surgeries better than anything else can. There are no guarantees and I cannot promise miracles, yet much is possible, so stay positive.

Although laser surgeries have apparently improved since the first operations, and the risks are now reduced, such refractive surgeries still do not address the underlying cause of poor vision, which may lead to further problems after the procedure is done.

Other options offered by eye doctors

Phakic intraocular lenses (PIOLs) are thin lenses surgically implanted into the eye to help reduce the need for glasses or contact lenses. They are sometimes used for people with moderate to severe myopia or people with thin corneas who are not suitable candidates for laser surgery. The PIOL can be placed either in front of or behind the iris; the eye's natural lens is left in place. The PIOL is meant to be permanent, but the surgery comes with risky side effects and no guarantee of success.[6]

A non-surgical option is Ortho-Keratology, which involves wearing hard contact lenses while you sleep, which, through pressure, reshape the cornea enough to give clear vision during the day without needing to wear glasses or contacts. A few people I've worked with who used the Bates Method alongside or after Ortho-Keratology reported uncomfortable side effects from the hard lenses. Always remember that the side effects of natural vision improvement are likely to be far more pleasant!

Low-dose atropine eye drops are becoming a popular remedy for slowing myopia progression in schoolchildren. During eye exams, atropine eye drops, at their regular 1% dose, are used to temporarily paralyze the eye muscles, causing pupil dilation and inhibiting accommodation (the ability to focus up close). In low doses of 0.01%, a daily drop of atropine appears to slow down (but not halt) the progression of myopia in children. So far there are no studies that prove atropine treatment is effective long-term, and drawbacks can include blurred near vision as well as discomfort and light sensitivity from prolonged pupil dilation.

In recent years, research on the use of multifocal contact lenses (in this case: lenses that have a lower power in the periphery than in the center), show that such lenses tend to reduce the progression of myopia in children.[7] It is thought that this design slows "eye growth" because the peripheral retina receives inward stimulation through a blurrier image that's focused in front of it when looking into the distance. Slowing down the progression of myopia (aka Myopia Control) may sound positive, yet it means that vision continues to get worse, not better, when using these lenses. It's far from being a great long-term solution, as children still end up in glasses or contacts for the rest of their lives and may sign up for risky eye surgeries as adults.

> **Today glasses are prescribed for young and old generally without any previous effort to remedy the defects which are supposed to make them necessary, while at the same time it is common knowledge that glasses do not in themselves do our eyes any intrinsic good.**
> Robert Brooks Simpkins, *New Light on the Eyes*[8]

Summary
The old view tells you that vision can only get worse, never better. Glasses, contact lenses, surgery and drugs are the main tools of the current "eye care" industry and lens prescriptions are based on tests that induce temporary eyestrain. The choices provided are all crutches; there are no actual cures. Eye doctors typically conform to the established doctrine and often turn a blind eye to any reports of successes achieved by students of vision improvement methods.

A new point of view
Thankfully, some eye doctors think "out of the box" and realize there are better solutions than what they've been taught during their years of studying optometry or ophthalmology. Dr. Bates was the most prominent eye surgeon to question the status quo. Let's now look at his point of view.

3.   Insights into the Root Cause of Blur

The genes did it – true or false?

Bring your warm underwear and travel with me for a quick visit to Utqiaġvik, also known as Barrow, Alaska. In this northern-most settlement of the United States, 320 miles north of the Arctic Circle, the sun doesn't rise at all for two months in winter and shines continuously for eighty days in summer. The local Inuit used to live a hunter/gatherer lifestyle, until some industries came to town in the 1940s. This created jobs and thus a population growth that led to expanding their tiny school. By the 1960s, grandparents in town had not had any schooling, parents had at most six years of voluntary schooling, and their children were the first generation to go through compulsory education.

When two investigators noted an unusually high rate of myopia among Inuit children in Barrow while their elders showed virtually none, a study was done in 1969.[1] This study found that among the older age group of the first generation, age fifty-six and above, none were myopic. Between ages forty-one and fifty-five, only two were myopic, one of which had just -0.25 diopter, the mildest level of myopia. Those two meant that of all 131 adults in the 41+ age group, only 1.5% had any myopia. When the parent group was extended to include all those aged thirty and above, out of 191 adults only sixteen (or 8.4%) showed any myopia. However, their 227 offspring included 133 myopes – an astounding total of 58.6%. So, while grandparents had no myopia at all and the parents a very low level, the children had an exceptionally high prevalence of myopia, far exceeding the usual average in any American or European population at that time. The researchers concluded: "If neither of the grandparents nor the parents have myopia while the offspring have a significant amount of myopia, a genetic explanation is hardly tenable."

So they looked for other possible factors, such as diet (mainly unchanged for the mothers and children); indoor lighting (mostly still kerosene, gas and oil lamps, as electricity had arrived only seven years prior to the study, not all houses had it, and those that did had only one 40 Watt lamp per room); transportation (a change from dog sled and kayaks to mechanical sleds, trucks and boats); and schooling (the major environmental change for those born since 1940, causing many hours of reading in low light conditions).

Because siblings showed a high correlation (if one child in a family was myopic, chances were significantly higher that siblings would be myopic too) the researchers suggested that if the parents value education as a means of improving their situation and stress it, the children in that family will be pressured to perform adequately in school and to do their homework and read extensively. If, on the other hand, the parents are not basically oriented toward education, the children will tend to meet the requirements of school attendance but will not actually spend a great deal of time reading or doing homework.

Two similar studies have since shed an interesting new light on the possible causes of myopia. In the Orinda Longitudinal Study of Myopia, which followed 514 children from 1989 to 2001, time spent reading was dismissed as a significant connection to myopia.[2] However, both the Orinda study and the Sydney Myopia Study from 2003 to 2005 (which included more than 4000 children aged 6 and 12)[3] showed that the amount of time children spend outdoors proved to be a major factor in the development of myopia. Chapter 15 goes deeper into the important aspect of outdoor time.

As Barrow gets very little sunlight from October to March and indoor school hours occupy what little natural light the children might have enjoyed, it now is no surprise that their rate of myopia sky-rocketed when school attendance was made mandatory. What the study among these Inuit mainly proves is that myopia is not something you inherit from your parents. Yet this myth persists! I still hear people quote it so often that obviously the facts are not being taught much, if at all. So it is worth repeating:

> "If neither of the grandparents nor the parents have myopia while the offspring have a significant amount of myopia, **a genetic explanation is hardly tenable**."

If it isn't genetics, why does the eye "grow" too long?

According to Dr. Bates, the eyeball does not "grow" into any wrong shape, yet it can get pressured into elongation by its muscles. The eyeball is basically a small sack of liquid with an intraocular pressure that keeps the round shape. It resembles a rubber ball in some ways: squeeze a small rubber ball with your fingers and it will change shape. Let go of the pressure, and it instantly returns to a perfectly round little ball. Same with your eyeball: squeeze it with your eye muscles, and those muscles are very capable of changing the shape of the eyeball. Let go of the muscle tension and the eyeball instantly returns to perfectly round, due to its intraocular pressure. You don't have to squeeze the globe much to produce a myopic eye: an increase in axial length of just 1 millimeter can create 2 to 3 diopters of myopia! If you could lay a relaxed eye (with an average 24 mm axial length) and a 2.50-diopter myopic eye (with a 25 mm axial length) side by side, you'd barely (if at all) notice the difference in shape; so don't think the average myopic eye literally looks like a football.

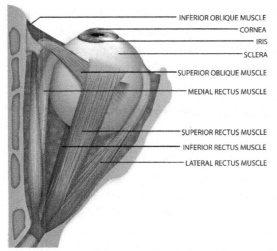

INFERIOR OBLIQUE MUSCLE
CORNEA
IRIS
SCLERA
SUPERIOR OBLIQUE MUSCLE
MEDIAL RECTUS MUSCLE
SUPERIOR RECTUS MUSCLE
INFERIOR RECTUS MUSCLE
LATERAL RECTUS MUSCLE

When you look at the various muscles attached to the outside of your eye, you can begin to picture how many different ways muscle tension can affect the shape of this one-inch globe. Dynamically-changing muscle tensions allow for eye rotations and focusing, while chronic muscle tensions create functional problems such as nearsightedness, farsightedness, astigmatism or strabismus. It simply depends on which muscles are chronically tense.

Top-down view of the eye and its extraocular muscles

When there is tension, you experience blurry vision. When your vision blurs, what is your typical reaction? Most people begin to squint, or they may stare at an object hoping that looking longer will bring it into clarity. You can see the strain in their face, wrinkles in their forehead, sharp lines above the nose, eyes that look small instead of relaxed and open.

But these are the wrong things to do when you experience blurry vision. Eye doctors say that using glasses at that point will reduce eyestrain. It is true that glasses tend to reduce this extra strain of frowning, squinting or staring, but they do not release the original strain on the eye muscles. In fact, glasses and lenses reinforce that strain, and add to it over time!

Eyestrain the major culprit
Dr. Bates realized that vision improves when glasses are not worn for some time, and thoroughly investigated everything that contributed to better vision in his patients. He found that eyestrain turned out to be the major culprit, and anything that released eyestrain contributed to better vision.

> **Eyestrain is always manifest when imperfect sight is present. The normal eye does not ordinarily have eyestrain. When it is acquired, the sight always becomes imperfect. When the sight is imperfect the eyes are under a strain. They are staring; making an effort to see. This condition is not cured by glasses.**
> William H. Bates, M.D.[4]

People with good eyesight do not strain to see; they gaze effortlessly out into the world and enjoy clarity. When strain becomes part of how you see, blurry vision comes right along with it. That blurry vision then feeds into the strain, as you try to clear it up, creating a vicious circle with more strain and worsening vision over time. You may wonder if you can ever break free from it. And there are many ways to strain your eyes, as every type of visual challenge has its own particular strain associated with it.

Eyestrain takes its toll on you, not only in blurry vision, but often in the form of headaches, tiredness, irritability, impaired mental focus, reduced depth perception, dull color perception, neck issues, poor posture, low self-confidence, a feeling that you are somehow less worthy or less smart than others because you don't see as well – and it does not improve your good looks either! To top it off, eyestrain can lead to eye diseases and blindness.

Physical strains

You may wonder what all falls under the heading of "eyestrain." Well, here's my handy reference list – patterns you want to recognize and avoid from now on. Let's start with the most obvious, the typical physical strains:

Staring – Staring is the big one. When I ask people to name a strained vision habit, staring is often the first one they mention. Staring has various components. It can be a combination of one or more tendencies, such as: little or nearly no blinking, a lack of eye motion, a lack of interest in what is seen, and "parking" the eyes while the mind goes off on its own. Your eyes and mind are basically out of sync when you stare; one has no clue what the other is doing.

Staring was my old "favorite." I used to be really good at parking my eyes somewhere in my blur zone and then letting my mind go a mile a minute somewhere else. My eyes would be frozen in place, I had only a minimal awareness of where I was, I would barely blink – and I could stay this way for five or ten minutes, while not even noticing it! Needless to say, I had to become aware of this tendency to stare, and changing this habit was my biggest step toward clear vision.

Squinting – This is very popular as well. It involves pressing your eyelids together and peering through your eye lashes. The resulting "pinhole effect" can really help clear your vision temporarily, but the strain it adds to your eyes is tremendous!

Posture adjustments – It is common, especially for nearsighted people, to crane the neck forward to get an inch or two closer for better clarity. Turning or tilting the head are common patterns too.

Habitually closing one eye – Less common but a favorite for those with different acuity in each eye. Closing the "bad" eye reduces its interference but only contributes further to the problem.

Eccentric fixation – Dr. Bates used this medical term often and considered it to be part of all errors of refraction. Eccentric fixation is attempting to see clearly where the eyes are not pointing, or to see a relatively large area clearly all at once. When you attempt to see clearly with peripheral vision, or disregard the detail provided by your central vision, you go against the anatomical design of your eyes and produce a strain. If eccentric fixation has become chronic, you may not notice the strain anymore, but your eyes may tire quickly and look strained.

Tunnel vision – Tunnel vision is an exclusion of peripheral vision so you can "concentrate" on one detail. It tends to go along with tense eyelids: you squint to "help" reduce your visual field.

Keeping tired eyes open – Not closing the eyes when tired and pushing past tiredness and sleep to the point of needing the proverbial "match sticks" to keep the eyes open. How helpful do you think this really is?

Doing eye exercises – Okay, this is my "pet peeve": Making the eyes move where they are not interested in going naturally is a strain. And moving the eyes without the head following along is contrary to how your eyes are designed to be used, so forget it; eye exercises done with strain will not help you see better!

Using glasses or lenses – Any glasses or lenses in front of your eyes create eyestrain. Not just prescription glasses or contact lenses, but also sunglasses, colored lenses, magnifiers, binoculars, microscopes and telescopes.

Mental strains

Mental strain often precedes any of the above examples of physical strain. Here are a few examples:

Wrong thoughts – Dr. Bates was well aware that "wrong thoughts" lead to blurry vision. Examples of wrong thoughts are: "My eyes are weak." "It takes effort to see clearly." "I am blind without my glasses." "I will never see clearly at a distance." "I have to try hard to improve my vision." Or you may worry about things beyond your control. Such thoughts are not helpful; they will cause worse sight in that moment, and the strain may linger well beyond the thought.

Lack of visual confidence – When you've had blurry vision for a long time, you can easily lose hope of clarity ever returning. You develop an expectancy of blur, which leads to a habit of no longer even looking for details because you are sure you won't see them anyway, so why bother?

Pressure to perform or live up to expectations of others – Letting other people's perspectives alter your own point of view can shape your life in many ways, and not always for the better. A perceived lack of freedom can impact how you use your eyes.

Environmental strains

Environmental strains are factors that are not always under your control but can impact your eyesight. Some examples:

A life mainly lived indoors – The higher the amount of time spent indoors where sunlight barely penetrates, the less likely it becomes that your sight remains good for life. Spending many hours exposed to artificial lights and/or looking at light-emitting screens is not conducive to healthy vision. If you live in a city shrouded in smog, or work in windowless rooms, this problem is exacerbated.

Lack of good vision role models – Growing up with parents and siblings who have visual challenges can leave you with few good examples to follow. Copying habits of eyestrain becomes more likely when you don't know how people with good sight use their eyes.

Night lights – Regularly working night shifts and sleeping during daylight hours, or sleeping while exposed to artificial light can also impact your vision.

Diet – What you eat and drink, as well as what you leave out of your diet, may affect your eyes.

Awareness of eyestrain

One big problem is that often you are not aware that you are straining to see. It happens subconsciously. You may not even believe that you strain at all! On the other end of the spectrum, you may be convinced that it takes effort to see better. Or you may believe it is normal for the eyes to get tired, sore, irritated, bloodshot, burning, itchy, twitchy, dry or watery, and that sleep takes care of it all and relaxes the eyes so you can assault them all over again tomorrow. Yet many of us tend to take our eyestrain with us into sleep, unless it is specifically released before going to bed.

Either way, whether you know you are straining or you believe you don't strain at all, if your vision is blurry you have probably been under the influence of one or more of the above visual strains.

Straining to see better

A whole lot of effort can be produced in the attempt to see better. This effort is counter-productive, and it is my job to prove that to you. Or, in fact, to make you prove it to yourself... Only when you are thoroughly convinced of the futility of using strained vision habits are you likely to be willing to let go of these crutches. You will become more and more at ease with periods of blurry vision once you learn to recognize its cause.

Any effort, any "trying to see," or any attempt to "force" an improvement in visual acuity will not only fail in the long run but will tend to produce worse vision instead of clarity. Even though many students intellectually understand that effort does not serve them, in practice I find they return to the tendency of straining to see far too easily. I will therefore begin with letting you test these strained vision habits, so you can put to rest the idea that they are actually useful...

4.   What Eyestrain Does to Your Sight

It is time to prove the futility of eyestrain to yourself, because personal experience is the best teacher and will convince you more than any theories ever will.

Note: Do the following demonstrations without glasses or contact lenses. You will need the medium letter chart (see page 279) and perhaps a mirror, as not everyone can sense their own eyestrain even though it is often clearly visible on their face.

 A. Staring demo

Hold the medium chart at the distance where your vision is clearest, then choose any one letter on the bottom line. Now slowly increase the distance at which you hold the chart until you notice that this letter has become a little blurry. Keep the chart at that distance. Okay, now stare at the letter you picked. By staring, I mean you hold your eyes still, fix your gaze on that one letter and avoid blinking. Hold still for ten seconds or longer, if you can.

How did that feel? How much better or worse did you see the letter?

The usual response is that the eyes start burning, they hurt, are uncomfortable, or want to look away. Most people notice the clarity of the letter diminishing, sometimes blurring dramatically. That is good! I hope you had that experience too. It will help get the message across that staring makes your vision worse.

Close your eyes briefly and blink to let them recover, then do the following test:

 B. Squinting demo

I am going to challenge you to break one of God's most feared commandments... Just this once!

> **The 11th Commandment: Thou Shalt Not Squint.**
> Mel Brooks[1]

Let's check what the dreaded squinting effort brings you…
Use the same chart, at the same distance where letters appear slightly blurry; look at the same line and just pick another letter for variety.

This time squint at this letter and do your very best to make it become clearer. Try as hard as you can to make the slight blur go away. If it seems to not be working, try a little harder…

If it seems to be working well, KEEP SQUINTING! Keep tensing those eyelids for a whole minute if you can and notice what happens then.

Did you succeed?

Perhaps you did see the letter more clearly for a while, as some people do. But, did the letter stay clear when you kept squinting? And how did your eyes feel after that effort? Is squinting an easy way of seeing? Can you sustain it for any length of time? I seriously doubt it. Typically, the letter will go in and out of focus and your eyes become more and more tired.

If you think squinting worked well for you, tell me something: Is this how you want to use your eyes for the rest of your life??? Check your squinting face in the mirror and answer that last question again...

> **You may temporarily improve the sight by effort,**
> **but you cannot improve it to normal, and**
> **if the effort is allowed to become continuous,**
> **the sight will steadily deteriorate.**
> William H. Bates, M.D.[2]

Squinting your eyelids or straining your face muscles to attempt to balance out the strain on your eye muscles is not a long-term solution, even if such double strain does provide temporarily clearer vision. When you squint, your eyelids create a narrow slit in front of the pupils, causing a pinhole effect that tends to provide a sharper image. Also, the squinting can affect the shape of the cornea and the eyeball due to the pressure created by the muscles in the eyelids. However, in this case, two negatives (two different forms of strain) do not make a positive! Seeing with artificial clarity gained by squinting is not a natural way of seeing, and it cannot be sustained for long.

C. Eccentric fixation demo

Attempting to see a large area clearly all at once, or wanting to see well where your eyes are not pointing, goes against the anatomical design of your eyes. It is called: "eccentric" fixation. It is a form of diffusion, or what I call "greedy vision." (Chapter 8 will explain this further).

Look at the top letter **B** on the chart and notice how easily and clearly you see it. Then pick a spot 3 feet or more away from the chart, look there, let your head follow your eyes, and notice how the **B** looks in your peripheral vision. Does the **B** look less clear than it did when you looked directly at it? Does it seem impossible to keep its original clarity? Yes? Good!

Now pick a spot nearer the chart and repeat this test. Let your eyes and head gradually approach the **B** on the chart and find out how near to the **B** you must look in order to see it with perfect clarity. You will likely end up looking directly at the **B** for the best clarity, and you may even notice that you can look at one part of the **B** and see that detail better than the rest of the **B**.

Let's go a step smaller with this demo. Keep the chart at a distance where you can see the bottom line clearly and pick a letter on that line. While you look at this letter, try to see the letter next to it with the same clarity as the one you are looking at. Don't shift your eyes to that other letter; keep your attention on the first one you picked, notice its details, and keep blinking.

My question is: Can you see both letters with equal clarity at the same time?

Most people will find eccentric fixation very hard or impossible to achieve, and the attempt itself makes the letter they were looking at blurrier. If you think you saw both letters with equal clarity at the same time, perhaps you saw them with equal blur instead.

Now, before going on to the next test, allow things you are not directly looking at to have less clarity. Then close your eyes and rest them for a few moments, or for as long as feels good.

 D. Tunnel vision demo

When you ignore your peripheral vision to "concentrate" on one detail, you fall into the habit of tunnel vision. Reading a book has often brought me to this point; a good book can easily absorb all my attention, and I forget that the outside world still exists. Call my name and I won't even hear you – I'm in another dimension! The book becomes all there is, and my peripheral vision goes to sleep. If I continue to read in this tunnel vision mode, my poor eyes strain more and more. On the other hand, when I stay aware of my peripheral field, I can read longer with less strain.

Test this: Same chart, same best-vision distance, same bottom line; pick a different letter for variety. Look at this letter and at the same time let 100% of your attention be on this one letter, so much so that the rest of the chart disappears from your awareness. All that exists for you right now is this one letter, in all its glory, with all its tiny details. It may take a minute to achieve such tunnel vision, but have a go at it.

Not so easy either, right?
Did your eyes like this tunnel vision or did it feel like a strain; like trying to do the impossible? Did the letter get clearer or blurrier?

Your answers will probably speak for themselves. Tunnel vision is not a relaxed way of seeing, nor does it bring clarity for any length of time.

 E. Mental strain demo

Dr. Bates claimed that eyestrain was a result of mental strain. One of his patients found that he was able to relax and see better on some days than on others. He realized that the days he couldn't manage to relax were the days he had received bills in the mail that caused him stress.

Look at the chart again and remember something that causes stress in your life.
Or tell yourself that effort is definitely the answer to all troubles in life; you must suffer to succeed!
What does this do to the clarity of the letters?
Does the chart reflect how mental strain negatively affects your vision?

Now let go of all stressful thoughts and think of something pleasant that makes you smile!
Can you pretend that you are an Air Force top gun pilot with the best vision in the world?
Does that make the letters clear up a bit again?

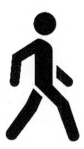 Please take a little break now. If you don't use glasses or contact lenses, skip F on the next page after the break. If you normally do wear glasses or contacts, come back in ten minutes for one more of these strain testers. While you take your break, please do use your regular glasses or lenses (I won't ever ask that again!). But before you put your glasses on or contacts in, have another look at the same line you just viewed on the letter chart at the distance just within your blur zone and remember what these letters look like at this distance.

Okay, welcome back. Please keep your glasses on. What follows is one last test, and then I promise that I will not ask you to do these tests ever again!

 F. Using glasses or contact lenses demo

With your glasses still on (or contact lenses still in), look at the letter chart at the same distance where you had it before you took this break – a little into your blur zone. Notice how the bottom line of the chart looks right now. Due to using the glasses/lenses it may look a little or a lot clearer, or it may even appear much the same.

Now take your glasses off (or contacts out) and look at the same line at the same distance. It looks blurrier, probably, but how much blurrier?
Does it seem worse or better than how it looked before you put your glasses on?
Usually it will be somewhat worse now than it was before you put on your glasses, although the difference may not always be very noticeable.

You have likely proven to yourself that the use of lenses tends to create worse vision without them, not better. Each time you use your lenses, your vision without them needs time to recover. You will find that the longer you leave your glasses off, the better your vision without them becomes.

Glasses always lower the vision at your optimum distance, and you can easily prove this to yourself too. With glasses off, hold the medium letter chart in the area of your best vision and notice how easy it is to read the letters. Now keep the chart at this same distance, put your glasses on and notice if the letters appear better or worse. Probably worse; your glasses lower your vision at your optimum distance.

 More strain tests to do?

Do you have any other "solutions" to see better? If so, let's test them too. For example; what happens to slightly blurry letters when you crane your neck, or when you close one eye for a minute or so?

You will likely find that any and all effort you make to improve your vision actually backfires on you and creates worse vision instead. That is GOOD TO KNOW!!! You *need* to know this! Without this personal experience of what happens when you try hard to see, you are unlikely to give up such bad habits. But now, having witnessed these negative effects yourself, are you ready and willing to let go of your visual efforts?

 Make your vision worse

Perhaps you still have a lingering doubt. That's okay. Let's take this one step further. I want you to make your vision worse.

ly: I *want* you to try and make your vision *worse*. Don't be
ion more. I want you to allow blur to be present, and to play
an, because you will learn from this.

distance where letters appear slightly blurry, and see what all you
kes it impossible to read that blurry last line. How can you make
things! Put in any and all effort.
orse vision? How much effort do you have to put in?
do, but it is *very* educational!

al to learn how to make your vision worse, because when you
sion worse, you've learned something valuable about how to
Now you can consciously stop doing what you unconsciously did
e. If you stare a lot without being aware of it, and you discover
n you purposely stare, it will help you break the unconscious
e that eccentric fixation is a strain that lowers your vision, then
void doing it unconsciously, and thus develop central fixation
I we'll go deeper into these things.

on worse is an important step on anyone's path to clarity!
need to repeat these strain demos, and you will always remember
its that made your vision blurry.

The John Denver Syndrome

Out of all the various reasons people become nearsighted, this one is slightly unusual, but
happens more often than you might expect – the desire to wear unnecessary glasses, either
to "look intelligent," "be part of a cool trend," or "look like a bespectacled idol."
Dr. Marc Grossman calls this "the John Denver Syndrome." Marc could not find anything
wrong with the eyes of a young girl who claimed to not see well, but from her parents he
learned that her best friend had recently started wearing glasses. So he gave the girl
"plano" glasses (no prescription, just clear glass), and she claimed those were perfect.
Luckily, she soon got fed up with the glasses and stopped using them.

Richard, a man in Ojai, California, told me that, as a boy, he felt he was not accepted in his
family. His young mind figured out the reason: both his parents and his brother wore
glasses – obviously, they were jealous of his good eyesight! The solution was easy...
After a few days of watching TV at a close range with as much eyestrain as he could
muster, he told his mother that his eyes hurt after watching TV. She took him to an eye
doctor after school the next day. Two weeks later, his glasses arrived, and he proudly wore
them to dinner that night. "Guess what changed?" Richard asked me. I knew the answer:

Nothing at all; he still did not feel accepted, yet his eyesight steadily got worse over the years.

Odaro, a woman in Nigeria, told me much the same story. At age ten she admired people with glasses, and she wanted glasses too, but knew her parents would only let her have a pair if there truly was a problem with her vision. So she convinced them her sight was blurry, and at the eye doctor's she pretended she could not read some of the lines on the chart. Success! She got her much-wanted glasses. The following year she could no longer read the blackboard without them, and now, 16 years later, Odaro has 4.50 diopters of myopia and needs her glasses for everything, and has come to hate those burdensome crutches that hide her true self...

Stacy, a woman from Chicago in her late 20s, started using colored contact lenses in her late teens, part of a modern "cool" trend. Hers were not prescription lenses; they didn't fit quite right and caused her to squint to see distance. After wearing them some months, she went to an eye doctor and was given her first pair of glasses for mild myopia. Ten years later, her prescription has crept up to -2.00 diopters with slight astigmatism. Not so cool…

Dr. Bates warned us that glasses only make vision worse, and this applies equally to healthy eyes that don't really need them!!!

Happy side-effects of releasing eyestrain
Now you are ready to release the eyestrain you have. Along with releasing this eyestrain, you will release blurry vision, but I invite you to view that as just a happy side effect, similar to the likely reduction of headaches, the disappearance of floaters, reduced light sensitivity and less neck tension. Other happy side effects are better depth perception, more vivid color perception, increased eye health, higher self-confidence and improved memory. Would you like some of these happy side effects? Then learn to release your eyestrain. The following pages show you how to do just that.

> **It is the things that we stop doing that promote perfect sight.**
> **We do not need to practice something new nor learn by mental**
> **training how to do something that we have never done before.**
> **When a patient is convinced of these facts [he realizes that] using**
> **his eyes correctly is so much easier and brings renewed vision.**
> William H. Bates, M.D.[3]

Part II

–

Release Eyestrain through Passive Relaxation

5. What's Good About Blur?

You have now proven to yourself that strained ways of seeing only make your sight worse. Whenever you respond to blurry vision with an increase in squinting or staring, or make any effort to reduce it, you take another step on the path to worse vision. If you would rather be making strides on the path to better vision, you will need to respond to blurry vision in a different way. This book shows you how to respond correctly to blurriness and provides effective options with which to replace the typical squint, stare, strain, craned neck, etc., that you may have applied until now.

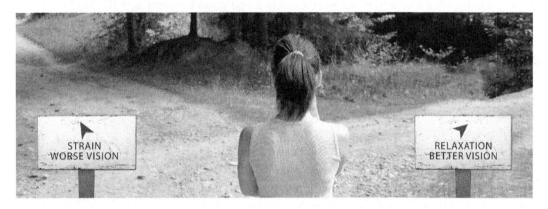

To begin with, the best thing to do is to accept your current blurry vision and stop fighting it in any way. Your blurry vision is a message: a gentle reminder that your eye muscles are currently under strain and that you need to release that strain. Once your muscles relax, you will have clarity. Until then, the blur will stay with you as this gentle reminder.

When you see blur as your friendly reminder and teacher, your level of strain will likely drop immediately. Mentally accepting your blurry vision, no longer treating it as an enemy or an illness, releases a lot of the strain. I know this is counterintuitive. You probably hate your blurry vision, which is why you picked up this book. But hating blurry vision doesn't help you overcome it. There is no need to be afraid of blurry vision, so give it permission to be there. Accepting the blur does not mean you accept going blind; it just means you stop fighting it, and thereby you paradoxically increase your chance of "winning this battle." Imagine shaking hands with "Mr. Blur" and accepting him as your friend. Once you get comfortable in his presence, he will leave of his own accord, and then his sister "Ms. Clarity" can take her place as your new companion! By the way, feel free to change blur's gender if it is easier to accept blurry vision's presence if you think of her as a woman…

It is actually good to simply forget about your eyes, if you can. Let them be; pay no attention to them. Instead, imagine that you see from the back of your head rather than with your eyes. Notice if anything feels different when you imagine seeing from the back of your head, as if your eyes are simply openings through which light comes in.

Vision fluctuates

In Chapter 2, I briefly alluded to the fact that vision is not static. You may have noticed that your vision fluctuates. Many people see better in natural light or when they are well rested. It is normal for vision to fluctuate a level or two (see the chart below). Even the eyesight of people with perfect vision fluctuates. Children often have great vision: 20/15 or 20/10, which may drop to 20/20 when they are tired. If a person's overall vision tends to be great, then the fluctuation between excellent and good vision is usually barely noticed. It's when overall vision drops to a "good" level that fluctuation becomes noticeable. At that point, cloudy days, evenings, or stressful moments may drop acuity down into the level of slight blur.

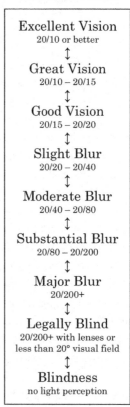

Levels of Vision

Excellent Vision
20/10 or better
↕
Great Vision
20/10 – 20/15
↕
Good Vision
20/15 – 20/20
↕
Slight Blur
20/20 – 20/40
↕
Moderate Blur
20/40 – 20/80
↕
Substantial Blur
20/80 – 20/200
↕
Major Blur
20/200+
↕
Legally Blind
20/200+ with lenses or
less than 20° visual field
↕
Blindness
no light perception

Without knowing or understanding the cause of your blur, you then tend to start trying harder to see clearly, and unfortunately that causes the blur to get worse. When the blur doesn't go away by itself, you are likely to visit an eye doctor. The doctor tests your visual acuity by having you sit behind a phoropter. You may have had an experience similar to this: the neck is held tight to keep the eyes in the correct position, the light is dim, the letters are viewed through a mirror above eye level, and the questions are fired at you rapidly: "Which is better, A or B?"

Does this sound stressful to you? Does it bring back memories of tense moments, of not wanting to "fail" this important test or not wanting to risk getting the "wrong" glasses?

Having just done the "strained vision habits" tests, do you think your eyes are likely to perform better or worse during such an examination?

Under such stressful conditions, visual acuity is usually at its lowest level in a person's current range, and the eye doctor is likely to prescribe compensating lenses. When you return a week later to pick up your brand-new glasses, you put them on and are likely to exclaim: "Whoa! These are **strong**!" What does the eye doctor usually say at that point? Right: "Wear them all day, <u>you'll get used to them.</u>" Yes, you will. If you wear these glasses a lot, your eyes will have to adapt and learn to keep the strain that you had when you were tested. So now that level of visual acuity becomes your mid-range, and your vision starts fluctuating around this new, lower level.

Glasses may provide clear vision, but they do not address the cause of the blur. By wearing such lenses, you actually send a false message to the brain. With the artificial clarity created by the lenses, the brain now receives the message that everything is A-Okay, there is no need to change; no need to release any strain. In fact, keeping the strain now seems better, because you experience clear vision with this strain.

When you take these glasses off, your level of blur is more than it was before you started wearing them. So you'll start straining even more without the glasses. Or you'll wear your glasses all the time, which reinforces the strain and makes it chronic. The strain basically gets locked into the eye muscles. The next time some stress enters your life, you will probably do what you did before: you strain a bit more to see, because you have not learned how to not do so. This means more blurry vision, and another visit to the eye doctor.

Do you recognize the start of a vicious cycle here? Unaware of the need to relax into clear vision, more strain is followed by more blur, followed by more strain, followed by more blur, followed by another visit to the eye doctor, followed by stronger glasses, followed by thanking and paying the eye doctor(!), followed by more strain, followed by more blur, followed by another eye doctor visit… etc.

Invite blur back into your life
If your current glasses or contact lenses give you perfect clarity, there is no blur to remind you to relax, nor do your eyes have any room for improvement. Such lenses will keep your vision at its current level. Eyes are very good at adapting to the lenses they are given (see the story of Luke in Chapter 22), and if you give them lower diopter lenses, they will begin to adapt to those, especially if at the same time you stop fighting the blur and begin to release eyestrain. So, in your journey to seeing clearly without glasses, a major part of the solution is to either not wear glasses at all, or to wear lenses with a lower prescription. A lower prescription allows room for improvement; it is a prescription that your eyes can "grow" into.

As you learn to see with ease and your eye muscles begin to release tension, these lenses reward you with better vision instead of worse, which helps the process of relaxation. You will soon see with as much clarity through such lower diopter lenses as you do with your current full prescription lenses. At that point, it will be time for the next lower prescription, and then you repeat the process, step by step, back down through the diopters, until lenses are no longer needed.

Note: See Appendix E for an explanation of prescription numbers and the abbreviations used on a prescription, which itself is often abbreviated to Rx.

Caution about under-correction without relaxation

Although medical research shows that under-correction of myopia is associated with a higher progression of myopia,[1] such studies do not include teaching people how to release their eyestrain. If you wear under-corrected lenses but do not know what causes blurry vision or how to deal with it, you will most likely strain your eyes even more and cause worse vision, rather than relax out of the strain and see better. Future studies on the use of reduced prescriptions should include appropriate education about eyestrain and how to release it.

Keep the blur to a manageable level

Having invited you to accept the blur into your life, I also realize that the amount people can function with varies. How much blur is acceptable? The answer is different for everyone. One person with 3 diopters of myopia can completely accept such blurry vision, does not miss glasses at all and loves the freedom this provides. Another person with the same level of myopia feels completely lost without glasses and can only manage to deal with a small amount of blurriness. The first one may choose to return to clarity without ever again using glasses, while the other will likely lower the power of their glasses by the smallest steps possible, a quarter diopter at a time, to keep their blurry vision in manageable proportions. You will need to find out how much blur you can comfortably tolerate.

Mirko, a student in Switzerland who started with a -3.00 prescription, found that lowering his Rx only one quarter diopter at a time was the easiest way to make progress. With such small steps, progress was noticed quickly, which encouraged him. He used contact lenses and when he felt ready for the next step down, he would go without lenses for two days and then start using his lower Rx the following morning. This worked very well for him. He wrote:

> I find it useful for a rational person like me to go down by small steps, because that allows me to see immediately if one day I see better or worse than the previous one, and thus makes me think about which habits and activities make my vision better and which ones make it worse. If I wear too low a prescription, I always see badly, and I cannot really notice a difference from one day to the other. I know mine is "the long way," compared to people who get down to zero within a few weeks, but it's teaching me a lot, so it's fine for me.

How much lower should the prescription be?

Full prescription glasses often provide 20/15 acuity and give your eyes no room to release tension. If you cannot go without glasses, use a lower power to bring some blur back. Usually anything from 0.25 to 1.00 diopter lower is easy to deal with, while some people can tolerate more blurriness and step down more than one diopter. Everyone is different, and it is up to you to choose glasses or contacts that are comfortable for you. Choose lenses that provide enough blurry vision to allow your eyes some room for improvement, yet that don't overwhelm you with blur. A guideline that is often used is to aim for 20/40 visual acuity with the strongest reduced prescription. 20/40 Visual acuity means that you can read the letters on the 40 line on the letter chart while wearing these glasses and while standing 20 feet from the chart. An acuity of 20/40 tends to translate into a 1.00 diopter reduction in power for most people. You may love the "perfect clarity" that full prescription glasses give you, but you are going to love the perfect *natural* clarity that your own eyes can give you much more when you get to that point!

In the U.S., most states require a minimum of 20/40 visual acuity for non-commercial driving. Various visual field requirements also apply. You can find your local laws listed on the internet. Please do stay within your local legal limits and wear the appropriate reduced prescription glasses when you drive, so you can be safe on the road. For other times of the day you may not need 20/40 "clarity" and you may want an even lower prescription – or to not use lenses at all. For example, a man who has been using -3.50 lenses, might start using -2.50 for driving and for work, while using -2.00 or -1.75 for other tasks, and going for walks without glasses. Having a few pairs of glasses of different lower prescriptions will give you the choice to wear what feels best for you at the time.

If your profession requires 20/20 vision, as is the case for commercial pilots, then your room for improvement in lenses is very small. Yet you still have a narrow margin to work with on your path to clarity: You can improve to 20/15 visual acuity with those lenses and then lower the diopter by a quarter to stay within the 20/20 safety limit while you work. Use those 20/20 glasses only for work, and have an extra pair of glasses with a lower diopter for other times.

Getting reduced prescription glasses or lenses from an eye doctor

Visit a helpful eye doctor (Yes, they do exist… see below) and ask for a prescription that gives you 20/40 visual acuity. Ask if you can try various lower diopters in a pair of trial glasses, then walk around the store for a few minutes wearing those trial glasses. If possible, try various options of either lower sphere and/or lower cylinder and find what level of blur you feel most at ease with.

Suggestions to keep in mind when you visit your eye doctor to get new lenses:

- Leave out astigmatism cylinders of 1.50 diopter or less. Amelia Salvador, M.D., recommends completely leaving out a cylinder up to 2.00 diopters. If your astigmatism cylinder is more than 2.00 diopters, aim to halve it. If possible, check how that looks and feels with a pair of trial lenses.

- Avoid bifocal/progressive lenses. These add to neck tension and therefore to blur. (See Chapter 12.)

- Avoid photochromic lenses and UV coatings. (See Chapter 15.)

- Anti-scratch and anti-glare coatings are useful.

Finding a helpful eye doctor

Some students report that it is not easy to find an eye doctor who is supportive of their choice to improve vision naturally. It may even be a challenge to find one who is willing to write a reduced prescription for you. Do keep in mind that the eye doctor is there to serve you, and that you are entitled to choose a pair of glasses that you are comfortable with, or that are within the legally accepted range of visual acuity if you use them for driving. If your eye doctor is uncooperative, you have the option of simply taking your business elsewhere. Behavioral optometrists (also known as functional optometrists) are usually more open to the notion of vision improvement and are more likely to be helpful in this respect. You will find a list of behavioral optometrists on my website.[2]

Tip: It is best to schedule your eye doctor visit at your best vision time of the day. Avoid going right after a long stint working at the computer. You're likely to get much better results first thing in the morning or after several hours walking outside in nature.

Personalized yet affordable glasses

Regularly buying new glasses can get expensive, even prohibitively so. There is absolutely no need for glasses to be so expensive. If a smart phone with all its advanced technology can cost only $100, why would glasses cost any more? At an online store they don't cost such a fortune; typically you'll pay $30 to $50 instead of $700 or more. I've listed some websites[3] that sell glasses at very affordable prices – a fraction of the cost of what an eye doctor charges, and at any prescription you want. I have no affiliation with these sites and cannot personally vouch for their work. I do know that most ship world-wide and some of my students have reported that they are happy with the services offered and the glasses received.

When buying glasses online (see Appendix E for a guide), look for sites that allow you to enter the pupil height, not just pupil distance. This is one detail often overlooked by the webstores that can make a difference in how well the glasses fit your sight. An eye doctor will make sure he gets that right, but it does not justify his much greater expense. Either way, you will likely use these lower diopter glasses for only a few weeks or months before needing the next lower step, so price is a big factor. You also don't need to worry much about how these glasses look because you won't be using them for very long! Some of these companies will even replace the lenses in your own frame if you send them in.

Determine your own prescription numbers

If you do not know your prescription and don't have a helpful eye doctor available, you can determine your own approximate prescription by measuring your far point for each eye (see Appendix B), or you can use something like EyeQue,[4] which is a small, affordable device that works with a smart phone to measure your refractive error. As such technology keeps advancing, I expect that the extreme prices that eye doctors charge for a pair of glasses will soon become a thing of the past. Once you have your diopter numbers for each eye you can step down 0.25 to 1.00 diopter when you are ready for new glasses and save money when you order them online.

Glasses or contact lenses?

I'm often asked: "Which is better, glasses or contact lenses?" In general, despite all their issues, I think glasses are better, simply because it is so much easier to take them off during the day, thereby allowing your eyes more freedom from compensating lenses. However, contact lenses can still be used while improving vision. You can either use lenses of slightly lower diopters or reduce the diopters more and combine them with a pair of low diopter glasses. For the latter, let's use a fictitious person as an example, I'll call her Ella.

Ella is very nearsighted; she has been using -10.50 contact lenses for the last two years. She is highly motivated to improve her vision, but she does not like the idea of wearing strong glasses, even if only temporarily. So she decides to order contacts that are -8.00 diopters, which is 2.50 diopters lower than her current prescription. She buys a 6-week supply of those. She also buys one pair of glasses of -1.50 diopters. When she wears the contacts and the glasses together, they add up to -9.50, which is one diopter below her 20/20 prescription of -10.50, so this gives her approximately 20/40 vision.

For most of the day Ella uses only the contact lenses. For driving, and other times when she needs to see more clearly, she also wears the glasses. She takes the glasses off again whenever possible and she practices relaxed vision habits a lot.

As soon as she notices that she can see clearly (20/20) when she wears both the glasses and contacts together, she orders a lower set of contacts. -7.00 contacts will be the logical next step in Ella's case. As her vision improves, she steadily lowers the power of her contacts, until she needs only glasses occasionally – and eventually she will throw those out too.

To buy contact lenses in the U.S. requires a valid prescription from an eye doctor. In other countries, such as Canada, the U.K., and most of Europe, no prescription is required, so you can buy any diopter contact lenses on the internet and have them mailed to you. When ordering, use the same brand, base curve (BC) and diameter (DIA) of your current lenses and only adjust the diopters (or power) for each eye as desired.

Pinhole glasses

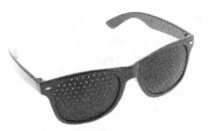

Some people with blurred vision can see surprisingly clearly through pinhole glasses.[5] These aren't actually glasses; they are made of black plastic with small holes in them. Although these pinhole glasses do not teach you how to use your eyes in a better way, they can be helpful as a transition tool. The advantage of pinhole glasses is that they can be used for any prescription, thereby possibly saving you the cost of buying several pairs of lower prescription lenses. The disadvantage is that they cannot be used for driving, as they restrict the visual field too much. Also, they do not work for everyone, so it is advisable to try a pair before you buy them.

What pinholes do is bypass the refraction problem by restricting light to central rays only. These central light rays do not get refracted (bent) and therefore provide a clear image to the retina (unlike light rays coming in at an angle, which depend on correct refraction to reach the retina in focus). As refraction is largely bypassed, it no longer matters what your prescription is; the images will come through with relative clarity, if the holes are small enough.

Pinhole glasses can become crutches too, so they should be used as little as possible. When used too much they cause increased light sensitivity.

The next step

When you invite some blur into your life, either through avoiding the use of lenses or through using lower diopter lenses, the logical next step is to release the underlying causes of this blur so you can start to move toward clarity.

6.   You May Close Your Eyes

Now that you've given your eyes some room for improvement by allowing blur to be present, let's look at how you can begin to truly release tension from your eye muscles. There are two ways to relax: passive relaxation and dynamic relaxation. This chapter is all about passive relaxation: the type of relaxation where you have your eyes closed, your body is comfortable, and relaxation becomes relatively easy to attain. Once you achieve passive relaxation, the dynamic form will be easier to realize, so let's look at passive relaxation first.

Sleep

Sleep is one way of achieving passive relaxation, but, as you are not conscious of what you do during sleep, and it is possible to continue eyestrain during sleep, sleep is not necessarily the best way to achieve relaxation, contrary to what you might expect.

A local woman who heard about my work asked me why she typically wakes up with better eyesight in the morning, but it doesn't last through the day. She is one of the lucky ones who truly relax during sleep, as evidenced by her lower eyestrain in the morning and accompanying better vision. Once she learns how to keep her eyes relaxed when open, her vision will improve each day. However, not everyone relaxes their eye muscles during sleep; it is fairly common to take the strain of the day into sleep with you and either not release it at all or even strain worse during the night, causing the same or worse vision when you wake up. I will talk about how to prevent eyestrain during sleep in Chapter 12.

Dark room

In Dr. Bates' time it was common to have people stay in a dark room, or with bandages over the eyes, for extended periods (weeks or months) to try to alleviate vision issues, as it was thought this would rest the eyes from what was considered the "injurious" influence of bright light. Bates found the opposite was true: that it was not light but darkness that is dangerous to the eyes. He said that such prolonged exclusion from light always lowers vision and may produce serious inflammatory conditions.[1] Florence Nightingale would have agreed. She believed that what hurt her patients most was a closed room and a dark room, and thus considered fresh air and sunlight to be essential.[2]

Although sleep and prolonged stays in a dark room are not the most effective ways of relaxing the eyes, sleep can be a great way to extend a visual relaxation session that is done just before falling asleep. Sitting in a dark room for a brief period can also be a calming experience.

Hot/cold compresses

Some people find it soothing to alternate hot and cold compresses on the eyes and thus achieve passive relaxation. This is not part of the traditional Bates Method, so if you find this too time-consuming or cumbersome, feel free to skip it; you won't need it to get to clarity.

To get ready: Fill one bowl with cold water and add some ice-cubes, if possible. Fill another bowl with hot water, but not scalding hot. Use two washcloths, one for each bowl. Have a dry towel within easy reach for when you are done. Dip one cloth in the hot water, squeeze out the excess, and gently press this cloth against your closed eyes for half a minute. Then switch to the other cloth, dip it in the ice water, squeeze out the excess, and hold that against your closed eyes for the next thirty seconds. Alternate between the two for as long as you like. This will likely release tension and increases circulation around your eyes. Don't worry about the length of time you use each cloth; let temperature and comfort levels guide your rhythm. In the morning, end with the cold cloth to stimulate circulation and get ready for the day. At night, end with the hot cloth to help you relax for sleep.

 You may close your eyes

Yes, you hereby have my permission to close your eyes, any time you want to and for as long as you want to. Simply closing your eyes is a form of passive relaxation that can be incredibly effective, especially when you then think about things that make you smile! Anyone can easily close their eyes for brief periods throughout the day. Whether for a few seconds or longer, closing the eyelids allows you to become aware of strain around the eyes, plus you may notice strain in facial muscles and postural strain, thereby giving you the opportunity to release that tension before opening your eyes again.

If you can't think of anything that makes you smile, pretend that you have perfect sight already. People with perfect sight are not aware of their eyes, just like people with perfect hearing are not aware of their ears. Or pretend that you have no eyes. When you pretend you have no eyes and imagine your eye sockets are empty, any eyestrain that crept in suddenly becomes superfluous. Clearly, if there are no eyes, then you have absolutely no reason to strain… Thus, in pretending to not have eyes, it becomes easy to let go of strain. Wait to open your eyes until you sense zero eyestrain, and at that point it will actually feel like you have no eyes! I really like to "empty my eye sockets" when I close my eyes, meditate or go to sleep. Test it out or create your own favorite thought that has a similar effect on your eyestrain (for suggestions see Chapter 11).

Giving your eyes many little mini-rests like this can be very useful on your path to clarity!

Gently rotate your closed eyes

You can make good use of your increased awareness of eyestrain when eyes are closed by using this time to find out if any of your four recti muscles are strained. Proceed gently as you play with this activity, because doing it with any effort will not yield the results you want.

A good way to start is to imagine a small coin magically floating inside your head behind your closed eyes (or floating at a comfortable distance in front of your closed eyes if you find that easier). Notice the outer edge of this imagined coin. Let your attention and eyes follow that outer edge, thereby slowly making a small circular motion, going around a few times in each direction; clockwise and counterclockwise. This should be easy to do. Now replace the small coin with a larger coin and repeat the process. Imagine being interested in the edge of this coin, so your eyes move smoothly around it, following your interest. Is it still easy? Then replace the coin with a tennis ball, with soft fuzzy edges. Again, notice its edge and let your attention (and eyes) gently go around this ball, a few times in each direction. If this is easy too, replace the tennis ball with a soccer ball and do the same. Replace the soccer ball with a hula-hoop that is so big that following its edge will create a large circular motion for your eyes.

Whatever your largest diameter circle is, does moving around this circle happen smoothly? If so, all four recti muscles are doing fine right now and you can stop. If there are any areas where it seems your eyes want to "skip" a section or move nearer to the center because the outer edge feels too hard to stay with, then notice where in the circle this typically happens. Is it while looking up in a 12 o'clock direction? Or is it to one side, either three or nine o'clock? Or down, or at an angle? Is it the same direction for both eyes?

If, for example, the 12 o'clock upward angle seems harder to do, then you likely have some tension on the inferior rectus muscle, the bottom one, which gets in the way of the eye's ability to freely move upwards. It is not a case of a "weak" superior rectus muscle (the upper one that pulls the eye upward) because even a relatively weak muscle is strong enough to pull up that small eyeball in its "greased" socket. But it can't do so if the opposite muscle doesn't cooperate and tries to pull at the same time! These recti muscles work as two teams. When the upper muscle tenses to rotate the eye upward, the lower muscle must release, else the eye will stay centered or will not go up with ease. The same applies to the left-right recti team. To look to the right, the right rectus tenses while the left releases, and vice versa. Between these four muscles, your eyes can move in all directions, but they must cooperate with one another to do so smoothly, and eyestrain on any of them will make this game of motion unnecessarily hard.

So, if you found any one direction hard to move to, I want you to focus your attention on the opposite muscle. If looking up is a challenge, focus on releasing the lower muscle in each eye. If looking to the right is challenging, focus on the left muscle of each eye, and if up to the left is your worst direction, then both the lower and right muscles need some releasing. How do you release them? By picturing them releasing as you make the motion that was challenging. Go gently, and definitely do NOT pull hard with the upper muscle if 12 o'clock is a challenge. Trust that the upper muscle can do this, no problem, as soon as you release that lower muscle. So "talk" to that lower muscle; tell it all is well, and that it can release now. Imagine this muscle becoming longer, and that in some way it actually "pushes" the eye upwards. If you can do this – if you can release the muscle(s) opposite the side that your eye doesn't like to move toward – you'll find movement in that direction becomes a whole lot easier. This is a quick and easy way to find and release rectus muscle tension that you can use anytime.

Palming

Most people find it easy to relax with their eyes closed. But since some light comes through closed eyelids, a still greater degree of relaxation can be obtained by excluding light. This is done by gently covering the closed eyes with the palms of the hands, which is called "palming." You cup your hands slightly when you palm the eyes so there is no pressure on your eyelids, and as much as possible you exclude all light.

The advantages of palming over merely closing the eyes are:

- With all or most light excluded, the darkness brings a deeper relaxation. Palming gives your eyes a power-nap.

- The flow of warmth and healing energy from the palms will aid in relaxation.

- The cupped hands touch many of the acupressure points around the eyes.

- The brain gets the message that this truly is a time for total rest, and that there really is no need to try to see, because even if you were to open your eyes, you still won't see anything other than darkness.

- Palming occupies your hands, so you aren't likely to do anything else; you truly rest.

- If you like to open your eyes while palming, you are unlikely to strain because you only see black. Palming can therefore be a practice of staying relaxed with open eyes.

- Once you become aware of how relaxed eyes feel while palming, you may find it easier to get back to that relaxed feeling at other times.

Palming positions

Palming is best done seated or lying down. If you sit at a table, support your elbows with books or pillows for optimal comfort, at a height that allows your spine to be relaxed and long. You can also support your arms with a firm cushion on your lap or use a palming support such as the one shown to the right.[3] Avoid hunching over with a rounded back; bend from the hips instead, if necessary. Place your feet flat on the floor.

For palming while lying on my back, I use a pillow on my chest to rest my arms against. I also like to slip my arms through a belt which prevents my elbows from dropping sideways while I relax. If you have a slant mattress[4] or slant board which allows your head to be lower than your feet, you may find that perfect for palming.

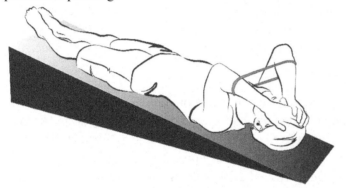

For your first palming session, take at least a few minutes to arrange good elbow support and to find your most comfortable position, whether sitting or lying down. Palming is most effective when you are truly comfortable, not fidgeting to alleviate postural tensions.

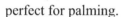 **Guided palming meditation**

To avoid common pitfalls while palming that interfere with relaxation and thus reduce the benefit you can get from it, I highly recommend that you listen to and follow my palming meditation (available from my website[3]) for your first few palming sessions. Once you are familiar with the routine, you can listen to what you enjoy most, whether silence, instrumental music or a guided meditation.

Seeing black while palming

What do you see when you close and cover your eyes? Some people see something like the aurora borealis, a show of gently moving colored lights. Some see flashes of lights streaking by, while others simply see mostly gray or a black field dotted with bits of color or light. What you see gives you some indication of the level of muscle tension around your eyes. The more lights you see, the higher your tension level. The darker and blacker, the more relaxed your eyes are. Once your eyes are totally at rest, you will see a perfectly dark black field. Ideally, you palm until you see black, but be careful – you cannot *try* to see black! The degree of black is just a barometer; black appears by itself when you reach a high level of relaxation, it cannot be forced in any way.

If palming is more like watching fireworks for you, the best thing to do is not stress about that or try to ignore the colors and lights. Instead, allow your mind to wander to those colors and see if you can remember any one color in vivid detail for a moment; then pick another color and do the same. If this gets tedious, imagine a bright white circle about half an inch in diameter, and imagine it as white as possible. Notice the color of the background. Usually it will be a shade of black. Let the blackness be there. If this isn't working, simply move on to the next suggestion.

Another way to relax deeper into black is by looking at a dark black object at a distance where you see it best. You can use black letters on a chart, black shoes, black clothing, a black hat, a black cat, a black car, a period in a line of text, a can of black paint, a black plush stuffed animal, etc.

Notice that the black seems blackest right where you are looking. Then close your eyes and remember the object's black details. Alternately open and close your eyes, and keep remembering the black until the memory is as clear as the actual object. Even in your memory, you can only see one part of the object best at a time, and if it appears to be moving, it may be even easier to imagine (Chapter 10 explains why motion helps). With that perfect memory of the black object, cover your eyes with your palms and notice that now the whole background is perfectly black. If it is not, or doesn't become so after a few seconds, open the eyes and look at the black object again. If you have several black objects, allow your eyes to shift from one to another, or close your eyes and do this in your imagination.

The degree of blackness you see can be used as a guide for the length of time you should be palming. David Kiesling, a keen student of the Bates Method, gives a fun guideline for how long to palm: "If palming looks like Las Vegas by night, you are not done yet!"[5]

Avoid staring while palming
Staring is a strain when eyes are open, and you also don't want to encourage a staring habit with eyes closed. Where do your eyes typically want to go during palming? Some people park them as if gazing at a near point, some gaze away at an angle, others gaze into the distance and some find their eyes like to move around.

Five tips to overcome a tendency to park your eyes while palming:

- Give your eyes permission to move without making them move on purpose. Pretend they are floating on a small lake with a gentle breeze creating wavelets for them to bob around on.

- Think about things in motion, such as watching birds fly in the sky, flowers sway in the wind, or imagine yourself in motion, such as dancing, bicycling, or pretending you are a bird soaring above the trees.

- Remember details of something that you are very familiar with that makes you smile (see Foundation Memory, page 95).

- The sensation of blinking can continue, even with eyes closed; it feels like a ripple going through your closed eyelids. Try it: let a blink traverse your eyelids and allow it repeat if it wants to. This too can help keep your eyes in motion.

- While palming, there is nothing for the eyes to see or do; they can't fall out through your closed eyelids, so there is no need for you to hold on to them in any way. Keep in mind that your goal is to simply let them be free for a while.

 One long palming session

I encourage all my students to do at least one long palming session. By long, I mean an hour or more, and preferably several hours. A long session will help you reach that deep relaxation, the point where you don't even feel your eyes anymore; they are so relaxed they seem to no longer exist. When you get to that point at least once, you will be able to use the memory of that deep relaxation, and your familiarity with how your eyes are supposed to feel, to help you reach a similar level of deep relaxation in brief palming sessions too.

Even properly supported, your arms can get tired or tingly after some time, and it is fine to then let one hand cover both eyes while you shake out the other arm. Another option during longer sessions is to temporarily use a "Mindfold"[6] to keep your eyes covered and in darkness without pressure on your eyelids while your arms and hands get a break.

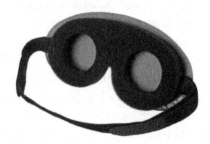

Tips for a long palming session

Here are a few tips for that one long palming session that I encourage you to do soon. My longest palming session was six hours, which I did after a period of intense stress associated with the passing of my 21-year-old niece who had leukemia. I had become so tense during the eight months of her illness that I had trouble reading anything. So, after I returned home from her funeral, I knew I needed some time for myself. I shut the door, prepared some easy-to-eat food, a large bottle of water, a box of tissues (for the tears I knew would come), switched off my phone, switched on my favorite music, grabbed my Mindfold, palming support and a pile of pillows, and I sat down to palm and finally relax and release those months of tension.

Although Dr. Bates recommends thinking of pleasant things while palming, I spent the first three hours processing the emotions I had gone through. I cried it all out until I reached the point of "empty" and started to truly relax. It took another three hours from there to reach that delightful stage of feeling super-relaxed, happy again, and knowing I had let go of all tension. I often switched positions in those six hours, as my hands do get quite tingly at times when palming. I also took a few bathroom breaks and didn't worry about these short interruptions – I simply got right back into it. When I finally opened my eyes, my vision had improved tremendously, and reading was no longer a problem from then on.

I do recommend that you pick instrumental music rather than listen to lyrics that may trigger memories of a broken heart... Also, avoid books on tape, lectures, or anything that requires paying a lot of attention to the spoken words. This is not your opportunity to catch up on work! It is an invitation to let go of the outer world; you want to go deep within.

Dr. Bates related the story of a man who palmed for twenty hours.[7] This man was nearly seventy years old and he had worn glasses for forty years for myopia, astigmatism, and later also for presbyopia. He had more recently developed cataracts too. His sight was so bad that he could not even see clearly with glasses anymore. He came to Dr. Bates as a last resort, as other eye doctors had been unable to help him. Dr. Bates did what he did with most of his patients: he told him to palm for about half an hour in his office. This helped somewhat, and the man asked if he could do more of it, or if there was a recommended limit. Bates told him he could palm his eyes as much as he liked; that he could not "overdo" relaxation. So the man went home and set his alarm for 4 a.m. the following morning, got up and palmed until midnight, then went to sleep. The next day he went to see Dr. Bates again, to report that he was seeing much better and wanted the doctor to test his acuity. Bates had him read the chart at 20 feet and was astonished that he read the bottom line, and the same with small print up close; his vision had completely reversed itself and, two years later, was still excellent. If that's what a long palming session can do for a nearly seventy-year-old man with major vision issues, think what it might do for you!

Regular palming sessions
Once you have done a long session, you can use it to help your eyes relax faster and deeper during short sessions. Bates recommended palming several times a day, especially first thing in the morning and last thing at night. When you palm before going to sleep you take that relaxation with you into your sleep and practically extend your palming session by about eight hours! You can palm for any length of time. Whether you do just a few

seconds when you are strapped for time, or several minutes or longer when your eyes feel particularly tense, each session will benefit you and increase your chances of reaching clarity sooner. If any one day you don't seem to have time for palming, you may find that remembering how wonderful your eyes feel while palming can be quite relaxing too.

Unable to palm?

If for any reason you cannot palm – for example, if your elbows get sore very quickly and that makes palming uncomfortable – then simply close your eyes and use your imagination instead. Pretend you are palming and imagine the warmth of your hands on your face. This can be very soothing and will likely help release tension. Although palming is greatly effective for most people, a physical inability to palm doesn't mean you can't reach clear vision!

Alternatively, perhaps a dear friend is willing to lend two hands for a few minutes, so you can experience the feeling of palming. He or she can stand behind the chair you sit on and gently rest both palms on your eyes while resting their forearms on your shoulders. Similarly, as a parent you can help your young child to palm by having the child sit in your lap, facing away from you, so you can gently cover their eyes with your palms. Tell them a sweet story to distract attention from their eyes.

 Transition to eyes open

Of course, at some point you will want to end palming and return to using your eyes. But if you end your palming session by going straight back into your old habits of straining to see, or by immediately peering at a letter chart to check if you made any progress, you will greatly reduce the benefit you just received from the palming rest. That's where flashing comes in…

Flashing

There is a "bridge" between closed-eye palming and eyes-open regular seeing that, when used for a few seconds or a minute, will help you keep the passive relaxation level you reached and allow that relaxed state to flow over and extend into the remainder of your day. This bridge into dynamic relaxation is a simple trick Dr. Bates often used called "flashing." Flashing is basically the opposite of blinking. Whereas in blinking your eyes are generally open and they simply close for a split second every few seconds, in flashing your eyes are generally closed and you allow them to open for a split second every few seconds. The eyes-closed interval can be longer than a few seconds too, especially when you first practice this.

The important key to remember when you practice flashing is that it should be done without any strain. The eyelids aren't "forced" open and then tightly shut; no, they are simply *allowed* to open. You open them all the way, but ever so briefly – and then you swiftly close them with ease, not effort. Try this right now: Close your eyes for a count of ten and relax any tension you may notice; then open them for a split second and quickly close without tension, keeping the eyes closed for another count of ten.

Go ahead, do that right now, and repeat as desired.

How was that? Was it easy? Did your mind receive an image from the brief flash of what was in front of you? If so, is it true that you did not have to "do" anything for that image to come into your mind? At least nothing more than just opening your eyelids – you did not need, or even have time, to try hard to get this image. It instantly appeared, right?

Do a few more flashes like that – eyes fully open for just a split second – and notice how each flash is like taking a quick photograph of what is in front of you. Feel free to turn your head in a different direction each time so you get different photographs. Don't attempt to hold on to the image from a flash, it comes and goes quickly; let it go. Flashing is simply a practice of receiving light. This should not create any tension whatsoever, but if it does, make sure you close your eyes long enough to release the tension that has crept back in.

Each image you receive with a flash, when you do not have time to try to see, shows that vision is meant to be receptive. Each image proves that the only thing you need to do to see is to open your eyelids, so that light floods into your eyes and instantly creates a picture in your mind. There is no *trying* to get that image, nor any conscious effort to focus; the image is already there! This is really important: Vision is meant to be receptive like this! If you can remain in this receptive mode with your eyes and mind – if you only ever practice staying receptive to light all day long – you will release much tension and experience better vision.

Transition into dynamic relaxation

To transition from flashing to effortless seeing, gradually increase the time your eyes are open, and reduce the time your eyelids are closed between flashes. Increase eyes open time from that initial fraction of a second to half a second, to one second, and then to two or more seconds. Make sure you stay in your new relaxed and receptive mode! To do this, simply notice various things that interest you in the moments that your eyes are open, and release any tension when they are closed.

Now, to help that receptive better vision stay and to improve even faster, you need to move into dynamic relaxation, so it's now time to check in with your blinking.

Part III

—

Increase Clarity through Dynamic Relaxation

7.   To Blink or Not to Blink

In essence, dynamic relaxation is action without effort. It is seeing and moving with ease; no undue effort interferes with the natural flow. In this third part of the book, you are going to explore the various facets of dynamic relaxation, and, one by one, replace unnecessary strains with effortless physical and mental habits.

The importance of blinking

When you extend the time your eyes are open after flashing, from the split second of the flash itself to gradually increasing to two seconds and longer, it is essential that you begin to blink when your eyes are open more than a second. Blinking is the most important (and most underrated) tool your eyes have for staying clean, moist, healthy and relaxed. It is easy to underestimate the importance of blinking, so let me give you the reasons why blinking is crucial for your vision.

First, blinking keeps your eyes clean. The cornea has more nerve endings than any other part of your body; its ultra-sensitivity will instantly alert you to small particles landing on it. With an abundance of blinks, your eyelids wash those particles away, your eyes stay clean, and you avoid many irritating problems.

Secondly, blinking keeps your eyes moist. Dry eyes feel incredibly itchy; they can become painful and prone to infections. Dry eyes are typically not due to an eye-drop deficiency (which are so often issued for chronic dry eye problems, see page 55) but could easily be related to a blinking deficiency – and just blinking at a healthy rate may solve this problem! I'll tell you what a healthy blink rate is, but first I'll cover the other reasons why blinking is so essential.

A third reason you need to blink is that your corneas do not have a blood supply. If they did, you'd be viewing the world through a network of tiny red lines. Thankfully, the eye was designed to not need little capillaries in the cornea; it was designed to get its nutrients from the aqueous humor behind the cornea, and from tear fluid on the front. Each and every blink nourishes your cornea and helps keep it healthy, as well as clean and moist.

Furthermore, each blink also gives your eyes a mini-rest, contributes to eye motion and helps the eyes refocus. When you also add the usefulness of a rapid reflex-blink when something comes flying toward your face, does blinking begin to sound like a good idea to you? I trust it does!

The problem with staring and low blink rates

Strained eyes never blink as much as relaxed eyes do, and they tend to blink with effort. As soon as you learn to release the strain around your eyes, you will find blinking returns with ease. And, vice versa, if you learn to blink often again, your eyestrain will be reduced.

Although the blinking frequency of healthy eyes varies, each blink is always quick and effortless. People with imperfect vision tend to blink with an effort, and this effort is evident in the slow or jerky movement of the eyelids. Due to the blur, you may tend to stare and avoid blinking because you are trying so hard to see better, however, it is only when you allow your eyes to move and blink that your vision improves.

To reinforce the importance of blinking, I'll quote British actor Michael Caine, who wrote the following paragraph in his autobiography, *What's It All About?*:

> It was in the library that I found a book on how to act in films, which claimed that actors should never blink before the camera. I walked around for months with a blank, unblinking stare in order to prepare for my film career, scaring the shit out of any strangers with whom I happened to come into contact – but I managed eventually to go without blinking for first ten, then twenty minutes at a time, and was well on my way to Hollywood. I also managed to get an eye infection from the filthy air as the particles of soot built up in my eyes. One has to make sacrifices for one's art I am told, and that is an early example of one of mine.[1]

Now you know why Michael Caine has red-rimmed eyes that hide behind glasses… It is clear from his experience that avoidance of blinking can have very unpleasant consequences! As far as blinking goes, please don't follow Michael Caine's example.

Here is another case illustrating the same point, provided by Dr. Bates, who felt good vision was impossible without blinking:

> In the year 1884, I roomed with a young medical student who was suffering from subjective conjunctivitis, a very painful symptom of eyestrain. During the examination period he could not read more than five or ten minutes before his eyes became so sore and painful that he was unable to read at all. His physician prescribed a spray which had no apparent benefit.
>
> One evening while I was reading, he said to me: "Why do you blink so often?" "Because it is an easy way to rest my eyes," I answered.

He practiced blinking and obtained complete relief. "My eyes are cool and comfortable, my sight is perfect, and best of all, I can remember what I read more easily," he stated.

We investigated the facts. He demonstrated many times that when he read without blinking the symptoms of eyestrain soon appeared, and his vision became worse. Other students tried it as well, and we all were positive that staring or trying to see without blinking always caused eyestrain. When blinking was practiced relief was always obtained. There were no exceptions.[2]

The blinking myth

I am often told by students that lots of blinking is supposedly a sign of nervousness, or even lying. This is a common myth that is perpetuated by popular media[3] and has caused presidential candidates in the U.S. to be judged by their blink rates. The candidate who blinks the most is not to be trusted… This is complete nonsense, and research confirms it as nonsense, showing instead that a tense person typically blinks less.[4-7] Yet the myth persists, so I want to set the record straight and make sure you know the truth. The person who blinks the most is the one who is most relaxed; it is a person at ease. With this myth thrown out the window, are you ready to change to a healthy blinking habit?

Catch your staring habit

When I first learned about the importance of blinking, I had a well-established staring habit. I clearly needed to become aware of times that I stared. I recruited my then-boyfriend and asked him to say something, nudge me or wave a hand in front of my eyes to get my attention whenever I stared. He had to do this quite often before I was able to catch myself in that stare. Each time I noticed (or was made to notice) that I was staring, I would break the stare, squeeze my eyelids, shake my head, and blink my eyes rapidly for a while to catch up with all the blinks I had missed. Slowly but surely, I got out of my staring habit, and these days I find it hard to even demonstrate how I used to stare, as my eyes instantly protest and feel uncomfortable when I do! You too will need to become aware of any periods when you stare. Like me, you can ask a friend to point it out to you, because change can only happen once there is awareness of a problem.

Once you catch those stares, it is time to turn your staring sessions into blinking sessions. Of course it is not normal or natural to have to consciously think about blinking all day long. Reminding yourself to blink every second is clearly not a viable solution. Your goal each time you catch the stare, is to trigger your latent blinking habit. The following seven suggestions will help you do that. Test any or all of them and find which suits you best.

Continuous blinking

Dr. Bates said that a few minutes of continuous blinking will help break the staring habit, and it counteracts the strain created by that fixed stare.[8] Continuous blinking means blinking without pauses, resulting in two or three relaxed blinks per second. If you do this every time you catch yourself staring, you will catch up with all the blinks you missed out on, and you will soon return to a healthy blinking habit.

 Rapid blinking

My personal favorite. If a few minutes of continuous blinking seems long, you can reduce the time to 30 seconds but then increase the blink rate to the maximum you can attain without effort. For me, that is four blinks per second. Thirty seconds of rapid blinking can change a forced blinking habit into a more relaxed blinking habit, because the higher the speed, the less effort you can possibly put into each blink. You must find a way to *let blinking happen* in order to blink that fast.

After continuous or rapid blinking, simply forget about blinking. Look around without caring about blinking. You'll probably find that the blinks continue by themselves. Likely not quite as rapidly, but probably faster than you are used to! Also notice that these blinks are effortless. Every time you use either of these two techniques, it will likely take longer before you find yourself caught in another stare.

 Think about blinking

When you have used continuous or rapid blinking for a while whenever you've noticed a stare, you will likely reach a point where just the thought of blinking will trigger more blinks. No doing, just thinking. The thought will create the blink effortlessly! Think about blinking without blinking on purpose, and simply notice what happens.

 Copy a good example

It may help to watch someone with perfect eyesight and copy their blinking pattern for a while. Don't mention what you are doing, so they continue to blink naturally and without conscious thought! Follow their example, if you can.

 Flashing

Some students with tired eyes find it helpful to close their eyes for a minute or two and then allow the eyes to open only briefly, quickly closing them again. Similar to flashing after palming, the eyes are closed much longer than they are open. As their strain releases, they gradually reduce the eyes-closed time until eventually they are happily blinking. This seems to "reset" their natural easy blinking mechanism, and they can let go of the effort they were making.

A long palming session

Renee, a student in Maine, found that letters on the chart looked worse when she blinked, which frustrated her and reinforced her staring habit. The strain in her blinking reduced her vision every time, and nothing seemed to fix this. It wasn't until she did a long palming session that her blinking became more relaxed. She was inspired by the story I quoted from Dr. Bates' book, about the man who palmed his eyes for twenty hours (page 44). He cured himself of incredibly bad vision in just one day of palming. She decided to do the same, and also palmed for twenty hours. Afterwards, to her delight, she found she was finally able to blink effortlessly. Her vision cleared up, colors became brighter, and even her hearing improved.

 Squeeze blinks

Another nice thing to do for your eyes whenever they feel dry from staring is a squeeze blink, which involves tightly squeezing the eyelids together. If you like, you can also make a funny face and purposely tense various facial muscles. Then breathe out and let all strain go at once, releasing that tension from your face and eyelids. The squeeze blink will aid circulation, which brings more oxygen, moisture and nutrients to your eyes. It may help overcome an itchy eye too.

Note: Squeeze blinks are not recommended for people dealing with high intraocular pressure (such as glaucoma).

No Effort

Be mindful of the fact that it should never take an effort to blink. The key is to increase your awareness of times that you stare, and then break those stares with some easy blinking, using any of the above suggestions.

It's only the eyelids that blink!

When I watch my students, it is obvious that blinking comes easier to some than to others. The muscles of the forehead and the upper cheeks should not be involved at all in regular, continuous or rapid blinking! You can use a mirror or make a video of your face while blinking to ensure only your eyelids are in motion and that your eyebrows, forehead or cheek muscles are not "helping."

Blinking is never metronome-like

Natural or spontaneous blinking does not have metronome-regularity to it, so do not aim for a steady rhythm in your blinking. Give it its freedom to adjust to circumstances while you simply aim to increase your overall blink rate and get out of any staring habit. Blinking sometimes continues with eyes closed or asleep, which Dr. Bates said was "nature's method of resting the eyes during sleep."

How often should you blink?

There is no standard answer to this question, because blink rates vary depending on conditions; nor is blinking something you should do consciously, except when briefly using continuous or rapid blinking to break a staring habit.

> **When most I wink, then do mine eyes best see.**
> William Shakespeare

Yet there are clear differences between the number of times people with good eyesight blink and the number of times people with blurred sight blink. The main difference is that relaxed and healthy eyes blink far more often than strained eyes.

Blinking frequency of relaxed, healthy eyes

Healthy eyes tend to blink a lot, averaging a blink every two seconds. That's thirty blinks every minute. This is an average; there are times when healthy eyes blink more and times when they blink less, ranging from ten to fifty blinks per minute. In general, people with normal vision blink almost continuously, even if somewhat irregularly. Dr. Bates stated: "In all cases where the sight was normal, blinking occurred almost every second."[9]

Relaxed, healthy eyes blink more when it is harder to see

Dim light, bad print, light reflections, or simply too far a distance – these are conditions that can challenge your vision. In such situations, a person with good eyesight simply blinks more often. If the blink rate is not increased, visual acuity lowers due to strain. So pay attention to your blink rate when such conditions make it challenging for you to see. Ask yourself: Can I avoid making an effort to see? Can I inhibit the stare or squint, and instead blink more? My advice is: **Always blink instead of squint!**

Your eyes will naturally want to blink faster than usual when:
- Adjusting for changing light levels.
- Suddenly facing a bright light or bright reflection of light.
- In dry air or air-conditioned rooms, as well as in very hot and very cold air.
- There are relatively high levels of dust in the air.
- Looking into the distance.
- Looking at pale or bad print.
- Your body is dehydrated.
- Loud noise or conversations distract you.
- Initially adjusting to using contact lenses.

Blink rates may vary depending on the task; one study claimed that "conversational" blinking averaged 10-30 blinks per minute (bpm), silence brought 10-20 bpm, reading lowered the rate to 5-15 bpm, and the use of computer screens dropped the blink rate down as low as 3-14 bpm.[10] The study referenced here reported large individual differences but did not state whether the people involved had good vision or not. Considering they concluded that a "normal" blink rate was 14-20 bpm and more than 20 bpm was considered "frequent," I suspect they had a large percentage of people with eyestrain in their group.

Blink rate of infants
The blink rate in infants varies too and can be very low in their first four months, averaging no more than four blinks per minute, while it gradually builds up to fifteen to twenty blinks per minute in young adults.[11] The likely reason for the slow blink rate of many infants is that their tear film is thicker, which keeps their eyes moist longer and gives them time to establish a regular blink reflex.

Blink rate of contact lens users
Contact lens users commonly have dry eyes, particularly in the evening. In the early stages of contact lens wear, people typically blink more because the eyes are trying their best to remove the foreign object. Once this natural rejection response is dulled, the rapid blinking response gives up and the contact lens wearer often ends up blinking less than normal to avoid displacing the contact lens. This results in dry eyes, especially by the end of the day.

Chronic dry eyes
Judging by the amount of dry eye drops for sale in drug stores, there must be a dry eye epidemic going around. Many of these dry eyes would likely be helped greatly by regular blinking. In healthy eyes, the cornea is continually kept wet

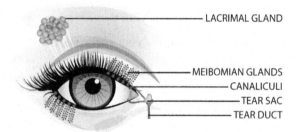

and nourished by a layer of tear fluid, which is topped by a layer of lipids secreted from the meibomian glands in the eyelids. This top lipid layer prevents rapid evaporation of the aqueous layer. Each blink spreads fluid from the lacrimal glands over the cornea, which, besides water and lipids, also contains mucin, sodium and proteins. To have enough tear fluid to keep the eyes moist, make sure you drink sufficient water and get enough essential fatty acids in your diet as well as minerals. Dehydrating drinks such as alcohol, caffeinated beverages and soft drinks may make dry eyes worse. Other culprits are medicines such as diuretics, decongestants, antihistamines, antidepressants, cholesterol-lowering drugs, beta-blockers and birth-control pills. Dust, pollen or the use of make-up can clog the meibomian glands that supply the lipid layer, so it is important to keep your eyelids clean.[12] Wearing contact lenses can also affect secretion from the meibomian glands, which is why some people have to revert to wearing glasses after many years of contact lens use.

Complete blinks versus partial blinks

Partial blinking, when the upper and lower eyelids do not touch each other, also contributes to dry eyes. For those who do not wear contact lenses, the impact of partial blinking is not as severe and typically their complete blinks outnumber any partial blinks. Contact lens wearers, however, are more likely to blink partially, rather than completely. When they become aware of this and consciously change to more complete blinks, their dry eye issues are likely to reduce in severity. Use the suggestions on pages 52 and 53 to improve your blinking.

> **Blinking irregularly but often is something that is done universally by people who have no trouble with their eyes.**
> Emily A. Bates[13]

Reminders

Blinking is good for your eyes because:

- Each blink cleanses your eyes; it washes away particles and reduces risk of infections.

- Each blink moistens your eyes; blinking avoids dry, itchy eyes.

- Each blink nourishes your corneas, which have no blood supply.

- Each blink gives your eyes a mini rest, preventing eye fatigue.

- Each blink contributes to natural eye motion, which is essential to focusing.

- A fast reflex-blink can keep insects or airborne objects from flying into your eyes.

- Rapid blinking keeps your eyes comfortable under adverse conditions.

Always blink instead of squint, and whenever you notice you're staring, do some rapid blinking to make up for it!

8. The Surprising Reality About Clarity

Now that you have relaxed your eyes with palming, practiced receptive seeing with flashing, and have become aware of the importance of healthy blinking, notice how much you see. How big is your field of vision? Unless there is damage to the retina, to the optic nerve or to the visual cortex, your visual field is large, spreading about 190 degrees side to side, and about 150 degrees top to bottom.

Observe this large field of vision: notice how many things you can be aware of all around you! There is much coming in. It is good to let in light from all angles, to not limit yourself to just a small part in the center where you happen to be concentrating. Rather than go into the strain of tunnel vision, it is better for your vision when you keep a relaxed awareness of the entire field. Stay open to receiving all of it, even though your attention is centrally focused.

Central fixation / Central clarity

Throughout his writings, Dr. Bates emphasized the importance of "central fixation." This is a medical term related to the eye using its central fovea to focus on details. Few people really understand what exactly Bates meant by central fixation, as he liked to use it as an umbrella for everything that his method stood for, as well as to point out how your eyes are anatomically designed to see best. Here is one definition he gave:

> **By "central fixation" is meant a passive, receptive, or relaxed condition of the eyes and brain. When the mind is sufficiently at rest the eye sees best the point fixed – in other words, the eye sees best what it is looking at.**
> William H. Bates, M.D.[1]

I consider central fixation to be a poor choice of two words to represent the natural state of relaxed human vision, which encompasses a large peripheral field and is designed to be in motion, not fixed. Technically, the term is correct: perfect clarity is only possible centrally with a brief fixation. A medical dictionary says that *fixation* or *visual fixation* is the maintaining of the visual gaze on a single location. But this sounds like a stare, which doesn't promote optimal eyesight. In fact, we do briefly fixate, else we would experience motion blur, but this fixation lasts only about 1/60th of a second. Someone with excellent eyesight doesn't perceive their natural rapid-fire fixations as a stare, and thus the term isn't helpful.

I prefer to use the term "central clarity." Optometrist Jacob Liberman uses the term "open focus" and describes it as the effortless way that your eyes are meant to see; the way to look at nothing and see everything. He adds that "it allows your eyes to be automatically drawn to that part of the visual field that is calling for attention in that moment."[2] Regardless of what term is used, the essential concept to understand is that your vision is meant to be effortless and receptive, and that it has a central point of best clarity within a large field of less clear vision.

> **Look at your eyes.**
> **They are small,**
> **but they see enormous things.**
> Rumi[3]

How the eyes focus ~ a little eye anatomy

The image below shows a schematic section of the human eye. When light enters the eyeball it is refracted (bent) by the cornea, it goes through the clear liquid called aqueous humor, passes through the pupil, is refracted some more when it travels through the lens, continues through the clear gel-like liquid called vitreous humor in the center of the eye, and then reaches the retina, where it activates your photoreceptor cells: the rods and cones.

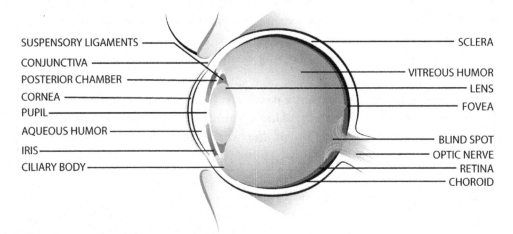

Meet the rods and cones in your retina

The rod and cone photoreceptors in your retina are triggered by incoming light and they transmit the impulses they receive via the optic nerve to the brain. Rods and cones have very different functions. The rods are very sensitive to low levels of light, thus providing your night vision. They are also good at picking up movement. However, these rods do not see very clearly; their acuity is around 20/100 at best, quite blurry in fact. The cones, in contrast, provide your sharpest vision; they have the capacity to see 20/10 or better. The cones also give you color vision, whereas the rods see the world in black and white and shades of gray. With such contrasting functions of rods and cones, you might think that they are mixed together and spread out equally over the back of the eyeball, but no, that is not the case.

The fovea centralis

Notice the little indentation in the center of the retina; this is called the Fovea Centralis, or fovea for short. The fovea is the size of a pinhead (about 1.5 mm in diameter) and this small area is packed tightly with... *cones*. It basically is "Cone City" with about 165,000 cones residing there per square millimeter. If you were to take a walk through the retina, beginning in the center of Cone City, you would be elbowing your way through these multitudes of tightly packed cones first, until you got to the perimeter (the edge of the fovea). Next, you'd find yourself in "Suburbia," the crowded macula (about 5 or 6 mm in diameter, depicted in the diagram below), which houses a high density of both rods and cones in a ring around the fovea. As you moved further away from the central fovea and out of the macula into the "countryside," the number of cones drops off dramatically and those you would still find are buried under the larger rods and other layers of the retina. That outer field is mainly populated by millions of rods; it is "Rod Country."

Your visual field in a diagram

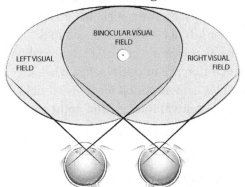

In this diagram, the center black dot represents the area of your best vision, provided by the fovea centralis (Cone City). This is your foveal vision, or central vision, and extends only 1 degree. The white circle represents the area of your macula (Suburbia). This is your macular vision. It is an area of good vision; you can see quite well here, but not with the same perfect clarity as foveal vision. Macular vision extends about 5 degrees.

The rest of the field represents your peripheral vision (Rod Country), which is everything else in your view. This outer area does not have sharp vision but is essential in creating the whole picture. You are good at detecting movement in this area, which calls your attention to things outside of your main (central) awareness.

The binocular field (seen by both eyes, shaded darker in this image) provides your depth perception and covers about 70 degrees horizontally.

"Two thumbs up" demo

Let's take a practical look at your field of vision. Hold your thumbs up in front of you, about 2 feet apart and at a distance where your sight is good. Look at your left thumb, being sure to also point your nose at the left thumb, not just your eyes. Allow your eyes to blink often. Notice the colors and details that you see all over that left thumb. Also notice that while you look at your left thumb, the right thumb is not seen clearly at all. In fact, out on the edge of your peripheral vision it will appear to be quite blurry. Wiggle the right thumb while continuing to look at the left thumb, and notice how easily your peripheral vision picks up the right thumb's movement. Now bring that right thumb closer to the left one and hold them about 12 inches apart.

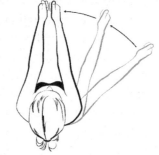

Notice that you continue to see the left thumb clearly and the right thumb is now seen somewhat better, but not yet as clearly as the left thumb. Correct? If so, continue to bring the right thumb closer, and check at 9, 6 and 3 inches away if you can see it as clearly as the left thumb that you keep looking at. Be sure to keep blinking! Finish by having both thumbs touch each other side by side. Keep looking at the left thumb (while blinking) and allow your eyes to notice details all over that left thumb. While you continue to pay attention to that left thumb (no peeking at the right thumb!), do you notice that it is still not possible to see the right thumb as clearly as the left one? If not, switch over and look directly at the right thumb. Does it look clearer when you look directly at it? It probably does, which proves my point. When you see a slight difference in clarity, even when the thumbs are touching side by side, congratulations! This demonstration turns visual field theory of your retina's design, into practical reality: **the central image – the point you look at – is seen most clearly, while the periphery is always seen less clearly**.

You can take this demonstration a step further and look at the fingerprint on any one of your fingers. Hold the finger close enough to your face that you can make out the lines with ease. Pick one line anywhere in your fingerprint and look at it, blinkingly. Notice the intricate detail of the curving lines so close together. Now, if you want to see the line next to this one as clearly as the line you are looking at, what do you have to do? Do you shift your attention to that adjoining line and thereby shift your eyes a tiny bit? Does the first line become a little less clear? If so, now you have a more accurate picture of how tiny your area of best vision is.

You can also do the two thumbs up demo by starting with one thumb held horizontally up above your head, and slowly bringing it down to the other thumb you are looking at. Notice how it becomes clearer as it comes closer to the thumb you are looking at. Or you can start with one thumb at arm's length, behind the one you are looking at, and notice a difference in clarity at a distance too. This shows that your area of clearest vision is not just two-dimensional; it is three-dimensional. If you imagine a tiny crystal ball and imagine that ball representing your area of best clarity, you are getting the picture. This "crystal ball of clarity" is miniscule (think the size of a pinhead), and the smaller it is, the clearer the details within that area will be.

Right now, while your eyes are still nearsighted, you may only be able to demonstrate the fact of central clarity to yourself at a close range. At a distance it may seem that both the periphery and the central point are equally blurry. This will change as your vision improves.

Eye-brain connection

About 60 to 100 million rods and 3 to 6 million cones[4,5] in each retina are all connected to the brain through roughly 1 million nerve fibers which are bundled into the optic nerves, one for each eye. Obviously, with the photoreceptor cells outnumbering nerve fibers at roughly 95 to 1, some road sharing must take place on the way to the brain. Yet sharing impacts your clarity; the more cells connected to one nerve fiber, the less accurately the brain can determine where exactly in your visual field a signal originated. To optimize clarity, each nerve fiber to the fovea connects to only a few cones, while rods in the periphery must share one nerve fiber to the brain with over a thousand neighboring peripheral cells. That results in poorer peripheral vision. Your eye-brain connection clearly favors central vision.

Peripheral blur leads back to central clarity

Before I improved my vision, I believed that, once my sight got better, it would get better everywhere; I expected my entire field of vision to become sharp. Some of my students similarly think that their peripheral vision must become clear, or else they've failed. But trying to see perfectly with peripheral vision is anatomically impossible, and attempting to do the impossible can only cause strain. Strain leads to worse vision, not better, so it is time to let go of this unrealistic expectation. When you are aware of the clarity of your central vision and the lack of clarity peripherally, you notice that you see best exactly where you are looking *and* you see all else less clearly. This happens without effort: it is simply awareness and allowing; it does not involve "doing." That is central fixation. Yes, it's as simple as that. You can't make central clarity happen by effort. You can only learn to simply allow it to be that way.

Six ways to improve central clarity by simply allowing it to be that way

 Peripheral vision awareness

A great way to effortlessly improve central clarity is by opening your awareness to your peripheral vision. When you see with this kind of total vision you take the effort out of trying to see any details. When you are aware of your peripheral vision, you can't *try* to see detail at the same time. So peripheral awareness causes you to let go of the strain to see detail, which, to your delight, results in details coming into better focus effortlessly.

Attention to details at a distance

When you are nearsighted and no longer expect to see details at a distance, you tend to stop looking for such details. This means you ignore the only area of your vision that can be clear, and you thereby diminish that central clarity even further. Turn this tendency around if you have developed it; start being curious about distant details again. Let your attention for details lead your eyes on a happy exploration of the world around you. You may not yet see distant details clearly, but you can imagine what those details may look like if they were clear.

Eye motion

Without eye motion, your central clarity is quickly lost, which the staring demo (page 20) proved to you. If you keep your focus on one small point for longer than a fraction of a second, that one central point will soon get blurry and it may even disappear. This also happens to people with excellent vision. For the central point to remain clear, your attention needs to continually and effortlessly shift. The next chapter explains shifting further.

> **In practicing central fixation, it is necessary for the patient to shift constantly and to blink frequently.**
> William H Bates, M.D.[6]

Imagine seeing a detail worse when looking away from it

For some people, vision improves simply by allowing the periphery to be less clear. You can use the letters on a chart to help you understand that you truly can only see well with your central vision. Pick a small letter on the chart at a distance where you see it clearly. Look a foot or more away from this letter and notice you can't see the letter as clearly anymore. Gradually reduce the distance from that letter and notice you still see that letter worse as you approach it, until you look directly at it and see it clearly again. Eventually you will find that you can look directly at the top of the small letter, which allows you to see that part clearly, while you notice that at the same time you see the bottom of it worse. Or, look at the bottom of the letter and notice that you see the top worse. Dr. Bates said: "The smaller the letter you use in this way, or the shorter the distance you look away from a letter in order to see the opposite part indistinctly, the greater the relaxation and the better your sight. … At first [perfect] vision may come only in flashes. The letter will come out distinctly for a moment and then disappear. But gradually, if the practice is continued, central fixation will become habitual."

 Practice central clarity with eyes closed
Look at the top of a large letter at a distance where you see it clearly. Then quickly look at the bottom of the letter. Alternate. When your eyes shift to the top, the letter should appear to move down. When your eyes move down, the letter likely appears to move up. (Chapter 10 explains this motion further.) Along with this movement, you may notice that you see one part of the letter best and all other parts less clearly or less distinctly. When you can imagine the letter moving, it becomes easier to see best where you are looking. You can then progress to smaller letters and repeat this process. However, if this becomes challenging, stop any effort, close your eyes and imagine how the small letter would look if you saw one part best. Mentally shift from one part of the letter to another while keeping your eyes closed. When you practice central clarity this way, you may find that when you open your eyes you can still imagine one part of the small letter best, even if only briefly.

 Prove central clarity by covering part of a letter
For this you want a blank 3x5 card with a corner cut out as shown.

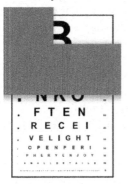 Place the medium chart (page 279) on a table in front of you and sit close enough to see it easily. Look at the large letter **B** and pay attention to the top of that **B**. Is it true that it is now easier to see or imagine the top of the letter best, and the bottom of it less clearly than to imagine both the top and bottom perfectly simultaneously? Now look directly at the upper right corner and imagine you see one quarter of the letter best. Then cover the remaining three-quarters of the letter with the blank card as shown in the image. Look at the exposed part of the letter and imagine you see half of it best.
Cover the part that is not seen distinctly, and demonstrate again that only half of the remaining visible part of the letter can be seen or imagined best, while the rest of it is not seen so clearly. Keep covering the part you see less distinctly, until an area as small as an ordinary period remains visible. Now remember this small black dot that remained as the part of the letter you were able to see best. Uncover the letter and imagine that perfectly black, small period forming part of any of the letters on the chart. When you imagine that you are simply looking for the clearest small dot in each letter, and you no longer expect to see entire letters clearly, it will help you read smaller letters on the chart.

> **The smaller the point of maximum vision, the better the sight,**
> **and the less the strain upon the eye.**
> William H. Bates, M.D.[7]

NOTE on wide angle vision or open focus

For anyone who is very much in the habit of using tunnel vision, switching to more emphasis on peripheral vision (or optometrist Jacob Liberman's term "open focus"[8] or Tracker School instructor Tom Brown, Jr.'s "wide angle vision"[9]), works well to bring you out of that narrow tunnel of strain and therefore "open" your peripheral field and allow for a more relaxed way of seeing. However, I've seen a few people take the emphasis on peripheral vision to an extreme, resulting in them walking around like sleep-walking zombies, literally disregarding all details as they attempt to stay purely in their peripheral vision awareness. If you allow peripheral awareness to get to the level of ignoring the detail provided by central vision, you have literally "missed the point" and are closer to staring and straining again. So, do spread your awareness, yet let interesting details gently guide your attention within this large field of vision.

Effortless central clarity

Here is a beautiful description of central clarity happening effortlessly to a woman who had been myopic and had an experience that created total relaxation for her.

> All things were the same in my little bedroom yet totally changed. Still sitting in wonder on the edge of my narrow bed, one of the first things I realized was that **the focus of my sight seemed to have changed; it had sharpened to an infinitely small point which moved ceaselessly in paths totally free of the old accustomed ones, as if flowing from a new source.**
>
> What on earth had happened? So released from all tension, so ecstatically light did I feel, I seemed to float down the hall to the bathroom to look at my face in the mottled mirror over the sink. The pupils of my eyes were dark, dilated and brimming with mirth. With a wondrous relief, I began to laugh as I'd never laughed before, from the soles of my feet upward.
> Flora Courtois[10] (emphasis added)

It is obvious that you must look directly at something to see it clearly. And now you know that you can only expect to see one small detail clearly at a time. But, if you stare, your only point of possible clarity quickly blurs! This means your attention can't stay in one place for very long, it needs to move... Let's talk about eye motion next.

9.   Set Your Eyes Free

Healthy eyes are not only relaxed, blinking, and open to a large visual field with central clarity, they also move. In fact, they are in constant motion. To begin with, they have what is called "saccadic motion" of 60 to 100 moves per second. This rapid motion is minuscule, not obvious when looking at the eyes. And yet, it's essential… as proven by A.L. Yarbus, a researcher who showed that without saccadic motion, eyesight blurs in five seconds and functional blindness follows in twenty seconds.[1] Obviously, since these rapid movements, or saccades, are supposed to happen at such high speeds, there is no way you can consciously move your eyes that fast – but you can certainly slow down this saccadic motion through eyestrain. In Chapter 15, I will show you how to stimulate saccadic motion. For now, I am going to focus on larger eye motions that are equally important for good eyesight.

In Chapter 4 you proved to yourself that staring makes your vision worse, so it follows that eyes in motion see better. However, *how* this motion is created makes all the difference in whether eyesight actually improves or not.

A very common misconception about the Bates Method is that it is based on eye exercises, such as purposely moving the eyes from side to side, up and down, diagonally, in circles, and alternately focusing near and far. The interesting thing is that Dr. Bates never did such eye exercises. Actually, he avoided the term in all his writings! He knew that eye motion created by such eye exercises went completely against the way nature intended the eyes to be moved. He therefore felt that eye exercises were unlikely to be helpful for vision improvement and could, in fact, slow down or hinder progress toward clarity.

In my mid-twenties, I tried eye exercises from a book about the Bates Method in an attempt to clear my mild myopia. The daily practice was boring and brought no results whatsoever, so, after a few weeks, I stopped doing them, concluding that the Bates Method was ineffective. I know I am not the only one who came to this wrong conclusion. The problem lies not in the Bates Method; it resulted from someone's wrong interpretation of the Bates Method long ago. Like that game of telephone I mentioned in the Introduction, the clear instructions Bates gave became more and more distorted as they were passed down from one teacher to the next; and now, a century later, what is typically taught as "the Bates Method" is nothing like the traditional method.

So, if you have been taught eye exercises and have been practicing moving your eyes consciously or with effort, I want you to let go of that concept, and explore eye motion the way nature intended; the way Dr. Bates taught it.

Test three ways of eye motion

Within your large field of vision, pick something to your left to look at, and then also pick an object to your right. Let's say you pick a chair to your left and a lamp to your right. First, keep your head still with nose pointing mid-way between these two objects, and move your eyes from the chair to the lamp and back. Do this a few times. This is the equivalent of forced eye motion typically done during eye exercises. How does it feel?

Now stop that, return your gaze to the center, and release your neck. Give your head permission to follow this time, yet do not purposely move your head. With eyes open and blinking, think about the chair or object to your left. What do your eyes want to do? The moment you think about the chair, your eyes naturally want to go there and look at the chair, right? Good, let your eyes go there. And what does your head want to do? It will likely want to follow your gaze. Let it follow. Now think about the lamp or the object on your right. Am I right that your eyes instantly want to jump over to the right to look at that lamp? And what does your head do? Did it follow along nicely? Go back and forth like this a few times, letting your thoughts direct your eye motion. Notice how it feels different in comparison to the first way of moving your eyes. Did you have to consciously move your eyes or your head? I expect not. Was this easier? Faster? Effortless?

Lastly, just to demonstrate a third option and a common misconception about the Bates Method, re-center your head between the two objects, and now move your head at the same time as your eyes. Let the head and eyes be in perfect sync as you look from the chair (or left object) to the lamp (or right object) and back a few times. How does that feel? Is it easy or is it more of an effort?

The natural order of motion

Sometimes the differences are subtle and you may not feel a big difference between these three ways of motion, but if you exaggerate the forced eye motions of the first example and the forced head motions of the third example, you will begin to get a clearer feeling and find that the only way that your eyes move rapidly in a relaxed way is when you let them follow your attention and let the head be free to follow as needed, as in the second example. *That is the natural order of motion.* Your attention shifts first, your eyes rapidly follow your attention, and your head follows your eyes, slightly lagging behind but happy to come along for the ride.

If the head does not come along, as described in the first way of eye motion above, the eyes soon feel uncomfortable looking at an angle. If the eyes are moved consciously like that, especially when done without an actual mental interest in where they are going, the movement becomes strained. If the eyes and head are kept in sync, as in the third way, a robot-like motion results where the eyes don't get any actual movement at all; they are stuck in center position which results in both neck and eyestrain.

Sketching

This third way is evident in "sketching," which I don't teach because it goes against the natural order of motion. Sketching was taught by the late Janet Goodrich, a Bates Method teacher from Australia. She used an imaginary nose-pencil or nose-feather and instructed her students to move the head and let the nose-pencil sketch the world around them. "Move your whole head as you sketch. [...] Your mental and visual attention is with the *end* of your pencil."[2] Following her instructions, wherever your nose points, that is where your eyes should point too, and when the eyes move, the head moves right along with it. Yes, it is correct that the head moves along with the eyes, but not rigidly! Janet did mention to sketch "loosely" but I have seen too many robot-like eyes come to me for help after failing to improve their vision with sketching and wondering why they don't yet see better. Margaret Corbett, a Bates Method teacher in Los Angeles, had a "nose-writing" practice[3] which also used an imaginary nose-pencil, but this was only done with closed eyes and didn't create such problems. If you have followed Janet's sketching advice and turned it into a robot-like form of synchronized head-eye motion, please throw out your nose-pencil or nose-feather, stop moving your head consciously, and instead let your head follow your eyes naturally. Your eyes will be grateful!

Edging

A similar misinterpretation of the Bates Method regarding eye motion is "edging," where students are instructed to follow the edges of a building, or the edge of a door frame, or window, or painting, or tree, etc. The aim is to get the student to move their eyes and to notice the most obvious outlines, but the mistake is that attention is skipped over in this approach. Are you *interested* in the edge of the building, the door, the window, painting or tree? Perhaps you are an architect and you do have an interest in the edges of buildings. If so, then edging a building is fine to do, because your interest leads your eye motion. But if your interest is not in that edge, it is a strain to limit your eyes to something that has no appeal while other items in your visual field are calling for actual attention!

Relaxed eye motion comes from attention

Let your eyes be free! Give them permission to follow your attention! I know, we have "societal rules" that say certain things must not be looked at, whether your interest goes there or not. For example, in person-to-person conversation, eye contact must be kept, to show the other person that you are paying attention to them. This culturally forced eye contact is also a strain, and I invite you to let go of it. You may enjoy finding details in this person's face. Notice their eyebrows, eyelashes, shape of the nose, hairline, freckles, and other distinguishing details. Your memory for faces may improve if you do this. Also, don't be shy to let your eyes move away from that face. One woman told me that she felt her husband never paid any attention to what she said, because he refused to keep eye contact with her. He claimed he did listen to her, but she expected eye contact to prove it. I asked her how her husband's eyesight was. Oh, it's excellent, she responded. I smiled and told her that his habit of not keeping eye contact is likely part of why he has such good eyesight, contrary to her eyes, which are trapped in that mental rule. What mental rules do you have that limit the freedom of your eyes?

So, have a look around. Use your large field of vision to find things of interest to you. Blinkingly, of course. Where is your attention drawn? What do you like to look at? Do you notice your gaze keeps shifting from one item to the next? Do you have to put conscious thought into moving your eyes or do they move by simply following whatever catches your attention?

Shifting

To summarize: Relaxed eye motion, or "shifting" as Bates called it, happens as a result of shifts in your attention. Whatever you are interested in, whatever you are curious about, that's where your eyes want to go. And the greater your interest, curiosity and attention for small details, the more motion your eyes get.

So how do you practice shifting? You don't. Eye motion or shifting should never be something you have to do consciously. Instead, you practice having attention for details. And while noticing details, I recommend you forget your eyes, forget your head, get out of their way and let them move naturally. If you are highly myopic, your practice for noticing details starts up close, while at a distance you may recognize a tree, a car, a house, a mountain, a cloud, without seeing much detail within those shapes yet. However, I encourage you to imagine the smaller details; pretend you *can* see some tiny parts of the bigger object you recognize. You may surprise yourself like one of my students in Los Angeles who, standing on his balcony, looked out across the street to brick houses on the other side, and was surprised that once he imagined seeing the mortar between the bricks, he could actually distinguish it.

 Experience natural eye motion

Have a look at the smallest letter chart (page 281). Hold it in your area of best vision, so even the small letters are clear for you. Notice how nice it is to look at something with such clarity. Also notice how easily and rapidly your eyes move from one letter to another. Because each letter is seen clearly, there is no reason to stop and stare at any one letter, and your eyes therefore happily move in a smooth and continuous way... Is that true? It is good to be aware of this way of motion. It is fast, easy and continuous! Remember how good it feels; remember how rapidly and easily the eyes move here at this close range where your vision is best. That is the type of shifting that you want at all distances, not only up close!

Now move this small chart a little further away from you, to where your blurry vision begins. Right there, on that edge between clarity and blurry vision, where your blur is minimal, can you stay relaxed and copy the easy shifting habits your eyes have when the letters are clear? Remember that these letters are not printed with blur – they are absolutely black and clear; you only need to bring them a tiny bit closer to prove that to yourself. So knowing that they are still black and perfectly sharp, can you scan for their details, notice their white background, and let your attention shift all over this chart with ease? What happens when you do that?

For some of my students, this is the easiest way to see instant improvement happening. Like Mario in Canada, who at -10 myopia finds practicing in his slight blur zone far more satisfying than any attempt to see at a distance. Within 4 inches from his eyes he has perfectly clear vision, but at 4¼ inches blurriness begins to show. Yet it's a slight blur, and when he uses a little relaxation (blinking easily and often, open periphery, interest in the details, and remembering or copying the easy feeling he has when looking at 4 inches) he finds this minor blur starts to clear. It comes and goes for a while, then settles into a steady clarity. This is exciting to him, as it's his first proof that his eyes do respond favorably to relaxation, and it allows him to move the card to 4½ inches and repeat the process.

When practicing with a chart like Mario did, you can also break any staring habit you have by simply moving the chart from side to side a bit. This chart motion should be small and gentle, not fast or jerky. With the chart in motion, your eyes have no option to stare, because now their target is in motion. Many students find that they instantly see better when the chart is in motion, which proves that they were still staring, trying to see clearer. Let go of this desire to see clearer! I know I repeat myself, but improving your eyesight through any kind of effort is counter-productive. Let it go, accept the blur, and simply notice any details in the chart. When you lose interest in the chart, look at something else!

When you practice with distant objects, you cannot make them move to break your stare, but you can gently move your whole body from side to side in a swaying motion, which will have the same effect.

The Easy Shift

Dr. Bates had a few patients who tended to always try too hard, causing a complete lack of vision improvement. If you also have a strong tendency to stare or to try too hard (including trying hard to not try), or if palming is not your favorite thing to do, then perhaps the "Easy Shift" will work for you. Dr. Bates would simply tell you to sit down in his office and instruct you to look from one side of the room to the other and back, without paying actual attention to what is seen, while remembering a room in your own home with your own pieces of furniture. This way your mind is on something familiar, you are not making any effort to actually see things in front of you, yet your eyes are kept in constant, easy motion. If you make any kind of effort, this will not work, but if you can find the ease in it and keep going until you feel relaxed and all trying has been abandoned, you may find this easy shift can help your vision considerably!

Using an Eyeport to practice effortless shifting

A modern tool to help learn effortless shifting is the Eyeport, created by Jacob Liberman, O.D. The current model is shown here. It has a series of small red and blue LED lights equally spaced on a white strip. The machine has three programs (varying in order of how the lights come on) and a variety of speed settings. It is 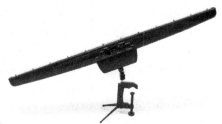 used with a pair of reversible red/blue glasses, causing one eye to see only the red lights, the other to see only the blue lights. The purpose is to simply sit and watch the lights come on, and as each light catches your attention, your eyes will quickly shift to it.

Dr. Liberman's instructions tell you to keep your head still and let your eyes move without the head following. I amend those instructions slightly because I do not want you to end up with a stiff neck or unnatural eye motion. It is better to let your neck be loose and let your head follow as desired, without purposely moving your head. When the Eyeport is used at a speed that you can keep up with – not too slow, not too fast – you will get into a nice rhythm of relaxed shifting and following the flashing lights. This is very beneficial for your eyes. The speed can be increased over time as your ability to shift rapidly and easily improves. At high speeds your head will not be able to keep up with your eyes, so do not attempt to keep the head in motion yet do keep your neck soft and relaxed. The Eyeport is also a great help in increasing depth perception, which I cover in Chapter 23.

Two important points to remember about eye motion:

- Eyestrain, staring and trying to see interfere with both saccadic eye motion and natural shifting motion, thereby reducing clarity.
- The natural order of relaxed eye motion is: Your attention shifts first, your eyes rapidly follow, and the head moves along smoothly as needed to keep the eyes from straining to see at an angle.

Eye move, you move, we all move

Once your eyes move effortlessly, you may notice more movement happening in your field of vision. The next chapter explores the bigger picture of visual motion… Come along for the ride!

10. Getting into the Swing of Things

When your eyes are in constant motion, the content of your entire visual field is also continually changing. This can create an "apparent motion," which means that stationary objects can appear to be moving, even though you know for sure they aren't. Take a wall, for example. Most people will agree with me that walls typically do not move, except perhaps during an earthquake. Walls are solid things, and quite reliable in their immobility. Motion simply is not something you are likely to associate with a wall. That, at least, was my solid conviction when Tom Quackenbush tried to teach me about walls that move. I thought he was crazy, and I thought this was the weirdest part of the Bates Method. My history with motion sickness as a child had made my logical mind as argumentative as could be regarding whether or not to perceive stationary objects – and certainly walls – as moving. I thought: "They don't. Period." I ignored this "motion-nonsense," until I was proven wrong, a few years later. Walls do move. Even without earthquakes…

A shift in reality?

Let me invite you to a little game. Yes, with a wall. Stand about 5 feet from a wall. You don't need to be able to see the wall clearly, so don't worry about any blurriness, but do pick a wall that has a few obvious features or decorations on it. If your wall has a window or door, that is fine too.

Face the wall and hold up one hand 2 inches in front of your eyes with the palm facing you and the fingers spread out and pointing up. (I know, that's really close to your face… You should just about be able to kiss your palm.) Hold your hand still. You can ignore your hand for a while but do keep it steady in place, right in front of your face.

Now look at the wall behind your hand. Blink easily and be aware of your peripheral vision. Shift your attention, eyes and head to an interesting item on the left side of the wall (ignore any blur) and then turn your attention, eyes and head to look at an object on the right side of the wall. As your nose moves past your hand, simply ignore the hand and look "through" the spread fingers at the wall behind the hand, not at the hand itself. Alternate looking to the left and right for a while.

What happens when you do this? Does your hand seem to move? Does it pass by in the opposite direction of your head motion? If so, excellent; you can move on to the next part.

If not, have another go at this: Play with shifting your attention from side to side at different speeds, and imagine that the hand moves by "letting it go" as you look away from it; that may help. Although the hand is not actually moving, it is correct to perceive it as moving. This is a "hand swing."

Next, facing the same wall, still keep your hand 2 inches in front of your eyes with fingers spread out and pointing up. Now bring your attention to the tip of your thumb. Ensure that your head follows your attention and eyes, so your nose points directly at the thumb. Now shift your attention to the tip of the pinky and let your nose also turn to the pinky. Go back and forth like that several times: Looking from your thumb to your pinky and back, letting your eyes and head gently follow your attention from side to side. Oh, and keep your peripheral vision open!

While you do this, what is moving now?
No, not the wall?!? Really?? Yep, the wall… Ha, I told you! ☺

First of all, if you did see either your hand or the wall in motion despite evidence to the contrary (you held your hand still and there was no earthquake), I congratulate you – because you reached this point of perceiving apparent motion a whole lot faster than I did.

If you didn't see it, don't worry about it. It took me two years to see it, and even longer before I actually enjoyed it and was fine with letting it happen. You will likely still get there faster than I did. It can be a little frustrating (as well as counterintuitive) to see solid objects move, so if the other practices in this chapter don't come easily to you either, feel free to focus more on the other techniques in this book and come back to this later.

Let's review what happened here. While I may have crushed your possibly long-held belief about whether walls move or not, the real issue is: What caused this apparent motion of a solid, stationary object, and why is it important for vision?

To answer this last question, and speaking from personal experience of the difference between viewing the world first without and later with motion, perceiving apparent motion in stationary objects is a more relaxed way of seeing. The difference between the two is subtle; yet suppressing motion is a strain on the eyes and mind, while allowing motion is relaxing. It didn't seem that way when I first tried it, but that was because I was putting far too much effort into trying to perceive motion and failed to understand how to simply let it happen.

As to the question of what causes apparent motion – the answer is found in the design of your eyes, specifically in the rod photoreceptors that populate your peripheral retina. Those rods are good at perceiving motion. Remember the two-thumbs-up demo where you held one thumb in the edge of your visual field, and it was barely recognizable as being a thumb? When you wiggled it, didn't it become more obvious that it was there? Your peripheral rods can't see your thumb clearly, but they do pick up on its motion! Because the rods are located in the retina's periphery, while absent in the fovea centralis, your awareness of apparent motion is also mainly peripheral. It will elude you if you try to see it centrally, while it becomes more obvious when you stay aware of your peripheral vision.

Swinging

In order to help his patients keep their eyes open to peripheral vision and in continuous motion without inducing any effort, Dr. Bates used a mental trick for them to become aware of apparent motion. He called the apparent motion "swinging" and invited people to imagine or become aware of a variety of swings. Beginning with a long swing that most people could see, he'd gradually let them work with smaller swings until they were able to distinguish what he termed "the Optical Swing."

The good thing is that it does not require perfect vision to be able to see these swings. Even people close to blindness can perceive apparent motion and will benefit from practicing that awareness.

> **The eye with normal vision never regards a point for more than a fraction of a second, but shifts rapidly from one part of its field to another, thus producing a slight apparent movement, or *swing,* of all objects regarded.**
> William H. Bates, M.D.[1]

Dr. Bates used the name "swing" for both the apparent motion observed and for the body's movement. However, this can create some confusion, as some students erroneously put emphasis on the body movement, yet completely miss relaxing into the perception of apparent motion, which is the actual goal.

Just remember: **A swing is not something you do; it is something you see.**

For clarity, I use the following definitions of shift, swing and sway:
  Shift = the natural motion of the eyes in response to the mind's shift in attention.
  Swing = the apparent motion of stationary objects in response to motion of the body, head, and eyes.
  Sway = the deliberate motion of the body to stimulate the appearance of the swing of stationary objects.

When the eyes shift, or the body sways, the world around you responds with swings. Because healthy eyes are always shifting, the world appears to be continually swinging.

Dr. Bates said: "The world moves. Let it move. All objects move, if you let them. Do not interfere with this movement or try to stop it."

When the world stops moving, you are staring! If you attempt to see the world as stationary, the eyes will become uncomfortable, strain sets in, and vision lowers.

When you learn to accept the perception of apparent motion, you reduce your tendency to stare. As your peripheral vision gets stimulated in this process, the strain of tunnel vision is overcome, and central clarity becomes effortless.

Tip: Do not try to see clearly while swinging! Clear sight is not the purpose of the big swings at all – that's an important fact to remember. Nor is clear sight possible when you experience motion blur. Clear sight comes when the eyes follow your attention in natural, easy motion. The purpose of the swings is to stimulate motion awareness and induce relaxation by encouraging the eyes to let go of tunnel vision and of straining to see.

There are several different swings offered on the following pages for suggested practice. You do not need to master one before you go to the next, but they do gradually get smaller, and starting with larger motion is usually easier. I'm presenting them in the order I have found most effective for my students.

Ready? Let's get into the swing of things!

1.a. The Long Swing

The long swing is probably the most well-known of the swings Dr. Bates taught. It consists of a 180° movement of the hips, upper body and head while letting the attention go out to the distance, yet without trying to see anything clearly. The side-to-side turning of your body results in a long 180° swing of all objects around you.

Pick a location with some prominent feature in front of you – whether a window, a painting, a tree, or building doesn't matter, as long as it's something obvious, stationary and not too far away. Stand with your feet hip-width apart, toes turning out a bit. Slowly turn your hips 90° to the right and let the left heel come up a few inches to make that motion easier. Check that your upper body, nose and eyes have also turned 90°; they should not turn beyond that. Then come back to center and do the same to the left. The turning movement comes entirely from the hips. Meanwhile, your torso, head and eyes simply move along, and the arms hang loosely. Keep your ears in line with your shoulders, and simply let your eyes flow through the room in a 180-degree arc, without making any effort to see anything clearly. Blink regularly while turning from side to side.

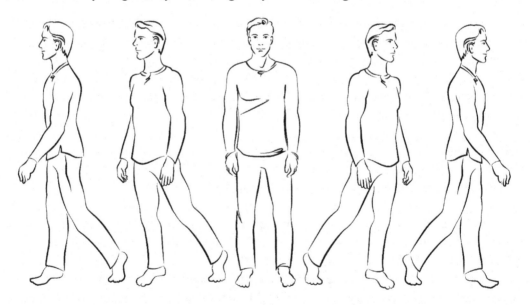

To begin with, pay attention mostly to the motion itself, not to what you see. Many people tend to torque the upper body beyond 90° either side and turn the head and eyes even further. If you notice yourself doing that, align your upper body with your hips again and avoid torqueing your spine. Go slow enough that you can comfortably keep up the same speed and motion with your eyes closed. Practicing the swing with closed eyes makes it easier to detect and notice muscle tension in your body and around your eyes. When you let go of this tension before you open your eyes, you will make faster progress.

With open eyes, notice that as you turn from side to side, your chosen obvious object appears to move in the direction opposite to your movement. As your body turns to the right, your object swings from your right peripheral field to the center and into your left peripheral field. And it probably isn't the only thing that appears to be moving. This is the long swing. Seeing such oppositional motion is the key; it means your peripheral vision is engaged and the eyes are relaxed, not attempting to clearly see objects that move by.

If you don't see any movement, you may be trying to "lock on" to objects as they move by. To overcome this, hold up your index finger about 10 to 12 inches in front of your eyes and slowly repeat the swing while looking at the finger. Keep blinking. The surroundings will speedily swing by your finger in the opposite direction. Now lower the finger slightly and look over the top of it into the distance behind the finger and keep turning from side to side. The pointing finger will help guide your eyes. Do you still perceive the swing? If so, then drop the finger out of the picture while continuing to turn from your hips. Imagine that the world around you is still moving. The long swing will seem less obvious without the finger to compare the motion to, but it should still be there to some extent.

When you are able to just *imagine* that things are moving, you take the effort out of trying to see motion, and the long swing will likely come to you more easily. It's important that you do not try to see objects clearly while they swing by. Your eyes should not get time to focus on anything; everything will be blurry because of your motion, and that is normal. Allow this motion blur to be there. The less you attempt to clear the blur, the easier it will be to notice the swing itself.

The main reason for practicing the perception of the long swing is to help your mind relax into seeing the illusion of movement and letting that swing of objects simply happen, without any "trying" to either see it or make it happen.

If your eyes are tense and you have the tendency to lock on to a few objects in your visual field, your eyes will not move smoothly; they will likely cover the entire 180° arc in three or four big jumps. But the more your eyes relax, the smaller and therefore more frequent these jumps become. With practice in letting objects go and move, the eyes will no longer jump so noticeably but move more smoothly with your body.

On a physical level, when done correctly, the long swing helps relax the extraocular muscles and promotes saccadic motion of the eyes. This can help improve both your central and peripheral vision. If the long swing feels relaxing to you, do it often! It's great to do for a minute or two just before going to sleep. If it doesn't come easy yet, try the two variations below, or skip to the sway.

Four tips for the long swing:

- When you first learn the long swing, practice it without a letter chart anywhere in your view. As you become able to see the objects swing, a chart can be added, but keep the level of your eyes either above or below the chart as you turn. Do not look directly at the chart or try to read the letters when practicing the long swing. When you avoid looking directly at the chart it will be easier to maintain its long swing. Later you can move the chart into your line of sight and you may notice that the letters gradually appear blacker as they swing by.

- If you do not easily see peripheral movement while looking at your finger (which may happen, don't worry), then get a laser pointer and do the "laser swing" (courtesy of George, a student in Mississippi who discovered this trick really helped him see movement). Yes, a laser can be useful in improving vision; just don't shine it in any eyes… Point the laser in the same direction as your body is turning, and let your attention follow the dot of color light it projects as it glides along objects in the room. Don't try to see the point clearly, just effortlessly flow along with it.

- When practicing the long swing without the aid of your finger or a laser beam, be careful not to "stare into space." Do let your attention go to whatever is on the horizon as it swings by, without attempting to lock on to anything. The long swing is a practice of continuously letting go, letting go, letting go…

- Before you finish, close your eyes and continue the long swing (see also the memory swing on the next page). With eyes closed you can imagine the movement continuing around you, and you can imagine it to be even smoother than you experienced it with eyes open. With eyes closed, it may also be easier to "tune in" to the feeling of the swing, and thereby increase the amount of relaxation.

Feel free to practice the long swing often, until motion awareness becomes easy. Do it for three to five minutes at a time, or up to 100 times (50 times to each side) if you find it relaxes you. Keep the body movement slow, smooth and easy, about two seconds for each side-to-side turn. Go slow enough so you don't lose your balance or get dizzy.

 1.b. Long Swing variation – the Gate Swing

Hold both hands out in front of you, about 10 to 12 inches apart, and look through this "gate" between them while you practice the long swing. The hands help guide your eyes and stop you from staring at objects that pass by. You may find it easier to keep your eyes moving along when they are limited to the area within the gate. It may also help keep the head from turning further than your body, so your upper body moves more easily as one.

1.c. Long Swing variation – the Head Sway

If body mobility is an issue, the long swing can be done with a slow easy motion of the head from side to side, looking first in line with one shoulder and then the other. Treat this head sway the same as the long swing: the aim is to relax into noticing apparent motion. Blink often and do not try to see anything clearly!

 2. Memory Swing

If you cannot imagine that objects swing when you have your eyes open, you may find it much easier to imagine a swing with the eyes closed. Doing so is good practice, especially if you find it more relaxing. Another advantage is that the memory swing can be done in a dark room or while lying in bed, thereby extending your vision improvement practice.

With your eyes closed, imagine that you are looking over your right shoulder, then your left, as far as you can possibly look. You may move your head along from side to side, but that's optional. Do this for a few minutes, then gradually decrease the distance between looking left and right by imagining looking a shorter distance to each side, until finally imagining that you are looking from one side to the other of a small letter.

If you let your fingers rest lightly on the closed eyelids, you will feel the movement of your eyes underneath the lids. This movement will be large as you imagine the extra-long swing of looking over the shoulder to the right and left, and small when you imagine looking to each side of a small letter.

Memory Swing with the Hand Swing. Using the hand swing from pages 71-72, alternate three closed-eye swings, thinking: "The fingers move to one ear, then to the other," with three open-eye swings, noticing the fingers swing by while you let your eyes blink often. Repeat this until it is easy.

You can mix the memory swing with all the other swings in this chapter too, alternating eyes-open and eyes-closed swinging. Here's how to do it: With eyes closed, simply *think* of looking in each direction. You may be able to imagine that you see the same objects swing that you saw with your eyes open. If you are not yet able to imagine seeing objects swing while your eyes are closed, just relax into the movement of the eyes themselves.

The memory swing can help you to accept movement at the mental level by simply imagining the apparent motion with closed eyes as you think about looking from one side to the other. When you can easily imagine such movement, it will become more comfortable to perceive it with your eyes open.

3. Perception of smaller movements

When apparent motion becomes easy to see with either the hand swing or the long swing, you can progress to smaller swings. Even if you don't yet see apparent motion, the following sway sometimes does the trick and can help you see it when the long swing does not.

 ### 3.a. The Sway

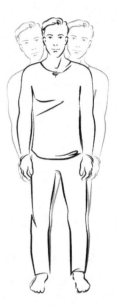

The easiest way to practice the sway is to stand somewhere with a view. Face a window or glass door if you are inside, while outside you want to stand fairly close to something like a tree or tall object in front of you. Stand with your feet shoulder-width apart, facing the view. Slowly sway your body a short distance from side to side by shifting your weight from one foot to the other. When you sway to the right, let your attention and eyes also go to the right. When you sway left, your attention and eyes go left too. Do no make any effort to see clearly in the distance; just let it all flow by easily.

While swaying from side to side, does it seem like things in your view are swinging? If not yet, be more aware of the door frame/window frame/tree/tall item in your peripheral vision. Compare its position to other things in your view while you sway.

Notice also how objects near you seem to move opposite to your motion while things in the far distance can appear to move with you. Dr. Bates called this the variable swing, meaning that whether an object swings with or against your motion is relative to its distance from you and also relative to other objects in your view.

Five tips for the sway:

- It's important to shift your *attention* from one side of the view to the other, instead of consciously shifting your eyes. (Let attention lead: think of looking right, then think of looking left; the eyes naturally follow.)

- While swaying, move your attention and eyes in the same direction as the movement of your body, as a crossing motion may cause strain and discomfort.

- Avoid tipping your upper body from side to side; simply shift your weight. The sway is mostly a leg and hip movement. The upper body moves with the hips.

- You can vary the speed of the sway. To begin with, feel free to practice the movement relatively fast and wide, yet for best vision you gradually reduce the sway to a slow, short and easy movement.

- Blink often and easily.

Important: Once you see the swing, gradually decrease the width of your sway, while noticing a corresponding decrease in the swing. Start by reducing the width of your sway by half, and if you still observe motion, cut it by half again. And again, and again, until you are barely moving at all. Yet that tiny side-to-side motion of your body likely still produces a tiny swing, true? If so, stand still and simply notice the most interesting items in your view. As your attention moves around, let your head and eyes follow along easily. Now, do you still see slight motion happening as you lazily scan around for interesting items to look at? If so, congratulations! This is the swing that always happens when your eyes shift naturally, yet you likely have not noticed it before. Allowing it into your awareness helps keep your peripheral vision engaged and your eyes relaxed. The effort of staring or trying to see should be gone.

> **No matter how long staring has been practiced, the sway at once lessens it.**
> William H. Bates, M.D.[2]

If the sway does not come easily to you, go back to the long swing, because the longer motion may make it easier to move the eyes in the same direction as the body moves.

4. Motion in any direction

So far you have practiced noticing side-to-side swings, yet all movement produces a resulting swing: up and down, obliquely, circular, near-to-far and randomly! So don't think the swing is a side-to-side motion only; it will happen in any direction.

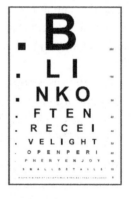

Bates used a variety of swings, including circular, elliptical, square and rectangular, because their continuous motion reduces any tendency to stop and stare which can happen at each end of a sway or long swing. When used with a letter chart you may find that a simple slow sway improves your clarity, while, if you also let your attention, head and eyes move slightly up the chart at one side then down the other side, you create a more continuous motion. When you do this, the chart makes a rectangular or elliptical swing and the letters may clear up even more because you reduced your opportunity to stare.

I suggest practicing with your eyes closed at first while imagining the chart responding with a swing; then practice with eyes open and play with gradually decreasing your motion. Notice how long you can imagine a corresponding swing.

Near-to-Far Sway

A useful variation on the sway is the near-to-far sway which can also be put to good use with a letter chart. Stand in front of the large chart with one foot further forward than the other and at a distance that when you sway forward, the chart is read easily, whereas when you sway backward it appears somewhat blurry.

Let your attention drift down to the lower lines as you sway forward and up to the bigger letters as you sway back. The chart may appear to move away and closer, as well as up and down in the opposite direction of your movement. With the near-to-far sway you also alternately stimulate and release the focusing muscles in a gentle way.

This near-to-far sway provides a general relaxation of your body through gentle motion, and your eyes will enjoy the perception of the swing. Notice how easy it is to see the chart when you sway forward and then imagine keeping that ease of seeing clearly as you sway back into your blur zone. Pretend that you bring the clarity back with you. If you do this sway for several minutes, you may find it reduces that blur.

5. Even smaller swings

The previous swing practices helped you get the illusion of apparent motion by moving your body or head, yet you ended the sway without body motion while still noticing a swing. And that's your goal. The purpose of the following practices is to gradually let go of the need to move the body to create the illusion of motion in stationary objects.

Eventually you want to become able to see motion simply by imagining it, without any conscious movement of your body, head, or eyes. It's through this *imagination* of swinging that you encourage awareness of your peripheral field along with giving your eyes permission to move continuously and smoothly. Imagination of swinging therefore helps to effortlessly regain the natural shifting motion of your eyes.

 5.a. The Short Swing or Optical Swing

The short swing, or optical swing, is the normal swing that you'll see when eyestrain is gone. It is the small, slow, smooth and continuous apparent motion of a stationary object in response to the natural, continuous shifting motion of your eyes. It appears by imagining its presence. Any lack of apparent motion is caused by staring or straining.

The width of the short swing is not more than the width of a letter and a letter swings from side to side and back, or up and down, in about one second. By Dr. Bates' definition, in the long swing objects appear to move anywhere from an inch to a foot or more, while in the short swing, objects appear to move an inch or less or about the width of a letter.

The most important thing is to maintain the short swing easily; no effort or strain should be involved, just imagination. Effort distorts or stops the swing. While the long swing is often easier, the short swing is more beneficial, as long as you see best where you are looking and see everything else less clearly.

Note: Seeing the short swing does not require any conscious physical movement of the head and eyes, yet neither does it exclude such movement. If it did, you'd only see the short swing when you hold the body perfectly still, whereas the aim is to maintain it easily – simply through your awareness of it.

When you look at the three dots below, shift your attention from the left dot to the right one and back, and imagine the dots to be gently swinging. Notice if the imagination of the swing helps you to shift your attention effortlessly.

. . .

Practice this for a minute or two, and, as always: blink and breathe rather than stare or hold your breath!

 5.b. The Letter Swing

Now look at the O below and let your attention shift from the dot on the left of the O to the dot on the right, and back. You can practice this with eyes closed too: Notice that every time you think of the left dot, the O appears to move to the right; and when you think of the right dot, the O appears to move to the left.

▪O▪

Can you do the same with this small O?

▪o▪

When this swing becomes easy to imagine, practice on the O below without the dots. Shift your attention from a black spot on the left side of the O to a black spot on its right side, noticing that the opposite side of the letter is seen less clearly than the side you are thinking of. As you do this, imagine the O swinging too.

O

Vary this by picking a spot at the top of the O and then at its bottom. Shift between these two spots, remembering each one alternately as the blackest part of the letter. Feel free to start with eyes closed. Notice that every time you think of the top spot, the letter appears to move down, and every time you think of the bottom one, the letter appears to move up.

If the O does not swing in the opposite direction of the movement of your attention, try to imagine the O stationary. See if you can hold it perfectly still for five seconds or more. If you succeed in doing this, it will likely be through staring and straining and the O will blur or disappear. As soon as you release the strain, you will probably find that the O does appear to move, and it becomes impossible to imagine it stationary. This experience can be a great help in imagining the swing!

Practice the letter swing with the large chart at a distance where the 10-line E is only slightly blurry. Or, if you prefer, practice it first with the E on the 50, 40 or 30 line, and then progress to a smaller E on the 20, 15 or 10 line.

Note: It really doesn't take much straining to stop the letter swing and blur the whole chart. If the short swing stops, play with increasing the swing or the swaying of the body from side to side, until you can imagine the chart moving again.

> **Perfect sight is not possible unless one imagines a letter to be moving, and an effort to imagine a letter stationary always fails**.
> William H. Bates, M.D.[3]

6. Continuous motion awareness
Now that you have experienced various degrees of motion awareness, the next step is to allow everything and anything to move, and to be able to perceive this motion at any time you choose to be aware of it or to imagine it.

6.a. Universal Swing
Going from the awareness of a short optical swing of one object to an awareness that everything else moves along with that object is the universal swing. You'll become able to imagine anything seen, remembered, or imagined to be moving with a slow, short, easy swing. This universal swing is usually easier to imagine with eyes closed than with eyes open.

Learning the Universal Swing
Sit 5 to 10 feet from the large letter chart. Hold the index finger of one hand about 6 inches in front and to one side of your face. Look toward the chart and move your head a short distance from side to side, without looking at the finger, and without trying to read the letters on the chart. Does it seem the finger is moving? Now close your eyes (you can put your hand down) and remember the side-to-side swing of the finger. Imagine that your hand, which is attached to the finger, also moves at the same speed and to the same extent. Realize that when your hand moves, the wrist, the arm, the elbow and your whole body, all

move with the finger. Now try to imagine the elbow as stationary while the finger is moving. It will be hard or impossible to do this.

When the finger moves, you can imagine that not only your body, but also the chair you sit on, the floor on which the chair stands, the walls of the room, the letter chart, the whole building with its foundation, are all moving with the finger. The ground, on which the building stands is also swinging. When the ground swings, other buildings connected with it swing. You can imagine your whole town is swinging, as well as this continent and all other continents on the earth. In short, you can imagine not only that the whole world is moving, but also the universe, including the sun, the moon and the stars. This is the universal swing.

One unusual characteristic of the universal swing, when it is imagined with the eyes closed, is that it is possible to imagine objects to be moving in the same direction as the head and eyes are moving. With eyes open this is only possible if a nearer object moves opposite to the movement of the head and eyes.

Remember that the universal swing is not limited to movement from left to right! Your eyes can move in any direction, so the universal swing can move in any direction too.

Practice observing the world move at least twice daily. Better yet, practice it all day long. When practicing imagination of the universal swing with a letter chart, let the movement of the letters and the chart be slow, short (about 1/4 of an inch), and easy.

When you get it and become comfortable with allowing this universal swing to be present, it will appear like the whole world is drifting like a ship on an ocean, gently moving on the waves. This is how it seems to me: with each breath, each slight head movement, each eye shift, everything responds with gentle motion. It's very soothing.

The world moves ~ let it move

Basically, all objects move if you let them. Your vision is best when you do not interfere with this movement or try to stop it. Trying to stop the movement is an effort which impairs the efficiency of both the eye and the mind. If you imagine a letter to be stationary, you'll fail! Try it, and you'll prove to yourself that the letter (and the whole world) really *is* moving.

6.b. Thumb Swing

Dr. Bates learned a useful aid to swinging from a couple of patients in 1921 who reported that with the help of the thumb they were able to maintain the swing easier and that this "thumb swing" improved their vision. It is easy to learn.

Rest one hand against an immovable surface. Lightly hold the ball of the thumb against the ball of the index finger, as if you are holding a small piece of paper. Look away from your hand or close your eyes. Now move the tip of the thumb in a circle of about 1/4 of an inch in diameter over the index finger. When the thumb moves in one direction, the index finger should appear to move in the opposite direction, although in reality it is stationary.

When the thumb is moving continuously, you can imagine that the whole body is moving with the thumb. This sense of soothing motion prevents any staring or straining. Once you get the feeling of the thumb swing, your hand no longer needs to rest against an immovable surface to use this swing. Test it out in front of the letter chart. Look at the chart first, then add the thumb swing and notice if the chart looks different, or if your eyes feel different.

It is easier to control the movement of the thumb than the movement of the eyes. So the thumb swing helps take attention away from the eyes, allowing them to relax more. Like the memory swing, the thumb swing can be used in conjunction with the other swings.

7. The Optimum Swing

The optimum swing is whatever swing works best for you under the circumstances. That's the one to practice!

When vision is good, the optimum swing is the optical swing, because it is always present. When you reach that level of good vision, everything you look at can easily be imagined to have a slow, short, easy swing. However, for those who are nearsighted, the optical swing will likely be easy to imagine only at a close range, not yet at a distance. At a distance, a different, bigger swing may be the optimum; it's whatever swing helps you imagine motion the easiest. Often this larger swing is not spontaneous, but has to be produced by a conscious movement of the body. It is usually wider and faster than the optical swing, yet this practice of a larger swing at a distance will help you to eventually be able to imagine the optical swing at a distance too.

Summary

Don't let these swings overwhelm you; you do not need to master them all! Your job is to find one or two that you like and that work well for you, so you can use those whenever your eyes feel strained or when you catch yourself staring.

Remember, the right way to shift is by moving your attention, rather than thinking that you should move your eyes. Let your attention move smoothly and effortlessly from one point to the next. Forget about your eyes; they move as a result of your attention moving. The eyes follow the mind's lead, and the world responds with motion.

Thinking of the swing as something you do is a misunderstanding of the Bates Method. The illusion of oppositional movement *is* the swing, not what you do to produce it. If your head or eyes turn left, everything appears to swing to the right. Look up, and everything appears to swing down. The point is to simply notice the swing and to let it happen all the time.

So, all you really need to practice is to imagine that the world is moving, all day long.

Once you notice a swing through making a long shift, you can then gradually reduce the distance until you can shift from the top to the bottom of the smallest letter on the letter chart, or any other small object, and still imagine it swinging. As your vision improves the letters will appear to swing gently any time you choose to notice it. Swinging may not seem simple at first, but a little practice will trigger the first perception, and with some dedication it soon becomes easy, thereby taking its rightful place as your normal way of seeing.

Nearly all ophthalmologists put glasses on people because that is all they know. I can recall the time when that was all I knew. If a patient left the office without a prescription for glasses it was not my fault. Now when persons with imperfect sight, wearing glasses, become able to practice central fixation and the optical swing in the right way, their vision becomes normal without glasses.
William H. Bates, M.D.[4]

---

11. Think Right for Your Sight

Here you are: friends with your blur, blinking happily, open to receiving light from a large field of vision, noticing best clarity where details catch your interest, and shifting effortlessly to other attention-grabbing details while you imagine the world swinging gently. These are essential elements of vision improvement that may already provide you with better sight. For some students, especially children who have not yet used glasses, these basics can be enough to reach clarity. For most people, however, habits of strain are deeper ingrained and need a little further digging to be uncovered and released. So, let's now delve into the mental side of vision before adding further physical aspects, because your mind can deliver an enormous boost to your progress.

The mental side of seeing is an essential and large part of the Bates Method. It is also the least understood. Bates was deeply into using memory and imagination for better vision and he had a wide array of techniques that use the brain to improve sight.

Bates experienced the benefit of mental relaxation himself

From the very start of his practice as an ophthalmologist in 1885, Dr. Bates studied cases of eyesight that improved without glasses. He drew his conclusions, started testing his theories on more patients, and slowly but surely developed his relaxation techniques for the eyes. As he became more confident in his ability to cure first myopia, and later hyperopia and astigmatism, he began writing more articles about his discoveries, and by 1912 he had become well-known for curing people's defective eyesight without the use of glasses. However, he had not yet had success with presbyopic patients. He did not expect his relaxation methods to be effective for that type of farsightedness, and, at age 51, he was quite presbyopic himself, for which he used reading glasses. That year, a friend of his sarcastically remarked: "You claim to cure people without glasses, so why don't you cure yourself?" Dr. Bates took those words to heart and set out to find a way to cure his own eyes.

For months he tried everything he could think of, but he made no progress at all. He asked various colleagues for help, only to be told that he himself was the only authority on the subject. He then enlisted the help of a minister, taught this man how to use a retinoscope, and asked him to examine his eyes to determine when, if at all, his eyes were focusing correctly up close. While Dr. Bates tried various techniques to focus on something within 14 inches, the minister reported that Bates' eyes were not responding as they should, and that they remained focused for distance.

Then, "One day…" wrote Dr. Bates…

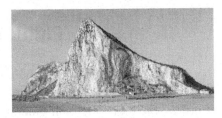

… while looking at a picture of the Rock of Gibraltar which hung on the wall, I noted some black spots on its face. I imagined that these spots were the openings of caves, and that there were people in these caves moving about. When I did this my eyes were focused for the reading distance. Then I looked at the same picture at the reading distance, still imagining that the spots were caves with people in them. The retinoscope showed that I had accommodated, and I was able to read the lettering beside the picture.[1]

Dr. Bates and his minister friend discussed this in order to figure out what had created the difference:

I tried again to remember the black caves while looking at the newspaper and my memory failed, I could not read the newspaper at all. He asked, "Do you remember the black caves?" I answered, "No, I don't seem to be able to remember the black caves." "Well," he said, "close your eyes and remember the black caves," and when I opened my eyes I was able to read – for a few moments. When I tried to remember the black caves again, I failed.

The harder I tried, the less I succeeded, and we were puzzled. We discussed the matter and talked of a number of things, and all of a sudden, without an effort on my part, I remembered the black caves and, sure enough, it helped me to read. We talked some more. Why did I fail to remember the black caves when I tried so hard? Why did I remember the black caves when I did not try or while I was thinking of other things? Here was a problem. We were both very much interested and finally it dawned on me that I could only remember these black caves when I did not strain or make an effort.

I had discovered a truth: *a perfect memory is obtained without effort and in no other way.* Also, *when the memory or imagination are perfect, sight is perfect.*[2]

By using his memory and imagination in an effortless way, Dr. Bates had temporarily corrected his presbyopic eyesight. After this discovery he made slow but steady progress with his near vision. He reported that it took six months before he could read a newspaper with any kind of comfort, and a year before he had cured himself completely and could focus easily on small print from as close as 4 inches to 18 inches.

Because of his experience in improving his own eyesight, Dr. Bates concluded that when the eyes are out of focus, the mind is also out of focus. He therefore began to teach his patients to use their memory and imagination for mental clarity and better vision. This turned out to be very effective. Releasing mental strain helps release eyestrain.

Exploring mental strain

Clearly, when eyestrain is "stubborn" and does not yield readily to any of the physical relaxation techniques, it is time to dig a little deeper and explore the underlying mental strain.

> **Mental strain of any kind always produces a conscious or unconscious eyestrain and if the strain takes the form of an effort to see, an error of refraction is always produced.**
> William H. Bates, M.D.[3]

Dr. Bates stated that we see largely with the mind, and only partly with the eyes. Margaret Corbett claimed that vision is 90% mental and only 10% physical.[4] Whatever the percentages may be, it is obvious that your mind interprets the stimuli received from the photoreceptors in the retinas and can "color" the images that it creates. The mind can enhance the image and make it more vivid, yet it can also add imperfections and dull or distort the image. When the mind is under strain, it will probably interfere with your clarity.

Examples of mental strain

My own blur started around age eighteen. It was the year that I learned to drive a car, which was scary at first; especially driving at night, as I feared I could be "blinded" by oncoming headlights. Coincidentally, it was also the one year of college that I failed and had to take over again, which was embarrassing. On top of that, and perhaps most influential, it was a year with great challenges in my personal life as I attempted to somehow reconcile my love relationship with the opposing desire of my parents for me not to date this man. For some months, I lied to my parents in an attempt to conceal that I was going against their wishes. With the benefit of hindsight, it now is no surprise that I tried to limit my view of reality that year. There was much that I did not really want to deal with and plenty of stress that I began to hold in my eyes because I preferred to not see these challenges as clearly as I should.

For a woman in Belgium, blurry vision started with the marital problems of her parents which included explosions of violence from a drunken father. A similar issue affected a woman in Ohio whose vision problem began when she was a little girl. Her father drank excessively, had a terrible temper, was abusive to her mother, and could scream and swear all night long. She says, "I know this started my eye problems as I did not want to 'see' his madness."

A young doctor in Arizona recalled that his first major change in vision was the summer after a visit to Palestine to see his grandparents and other relatives. He was 16 at the time and he "saw too much" during this two-month trip. The tragic and appalling situation he witnessed affected him deeply, and his vision noticeably changed in the months following that trip.

School stress

For many of my students, school years were stressful and likely played a part in causing their initial blur. For example, I asked a man in Minnesota what went on in his life right before his vision became blurry. His answer: "I was a teen in high school. What more can I say?! The whole experience was stressful."

Most people have to think about this question for a minute, but one woman in New York had an instant answer. She immediately knew it was her third-grade teacher that caused her to go into blur. She had adored her second-grade teacher, Miss Brown, who was "absolutely wonderful." However, in third grade she got "Mrs. Spaghetti," who she did not get along with at all. Spaghetti was not her teacher's real name, but it sounded like that, and thus became the nickname. She hated Mrs. Spaghetti so much that she decided to "blur her out." Mrs. Spaghetti of course noticed her inability to read the blackboard and sent a note to her parents for her eyes to be tested. This resulted in glasses for myopia. As soon as she started using these glasses in school, Mrs. Spaghetti appeared crystal clear again, which was not the solution this young girl wanted. So, she managed to blur her teacher out again. She needed three progressively stronger prescriptions that year! After third grade, her vision stabilized.

Here are some general examples of mental strain that you may put yourself through:

- Any kind of worrying, whether about vision, health, relationships, finances, responsibilities, or work
- Any fears you have about such issues
- Any dislike you have of what you see, feel or hear
- Anything you do beyond the point of tiredness
- Any boredom
- An expectation of imperfect vision
- Any negative expectations
- A disconnect between what you see and where your attention is
- Anything you do that you would much rather not do
- And even telling any lies

All these create some level of mental strain, which may affect your vision to some extent.

Stress links to start of blur

Not everyone recalls when their blur started, and not everyone went through a stressful period around that time; some simply spent too many hours on a computer, or indoors in general, and they simply lacked sunlight. However, many people do have a clear link between their blur and a particularly stressful period. Stressful school years and "hiding" in books seem to be common themes, as are relationship issues. Reading for extended periods commonly gets the blame for causing nearsightedness, yet why can some people read extensively without becoming myopic? And who even looks at the reason for wanting to spend so much time reading?

My colleague Bobby Lichtman delved deeply into this topic and wrote an interesting article about it.[5] From questioning many students, he concluded that blur often begins with fear of not being able to cope. Fear leads to a temporary fight or flight response, he reasoned, which, besides effects such as increased heart rate and respiration, causes pupil dilation and a focal shift to distance vision. When this happens in a classroom setting for a child who feels that they must pay attention, must try harder and who needs to read despite the fear they feel, they will double their efforts to focus close up despite the larger pupils and distance vision focus caused by the stress. To overcome the blur they experience while attempting to read under such circumstances, the extra-ocular muscles learn to grab the eyes and create near focus with extra strain. This additional muscle tension feeds into anxiety, and anxiety feeds into even greater muscle tension. If the child isn't taught how to release the strain, this myopic strain becomes chronic and glasses are likely to be recommended, which exacerbates the chronic nature of the strain.

You can explore your personal reasons for, and contributors to, your blurry vision on page 110, which may clarify a few things about the origin of your eyestrain.

Your response to stress

Many people experience stress in their daily lives, yet not all get blurry vision. Some get ulcers instead, or other dis-eases. Interestingly, others seem to not be affected by stress at all. I think the key may be found in how we deal with daily stresses. For example, one child at school might respond to a fear by looking out the window and letting the fear pass before focusing close up again, thus avoiding the eyestrain that leads another child to myopia. Depending on differing values, expectations and beliefs, what is experienced as a "stressful storm" by one person can be "a breeze" to the next. What is your typical reaction to a situation in your life that you perceive as stressful? Does it become a mental strain? Do you choose to focus on this "imperfection," or are you generally able to see the bright side?

Your goal: release mental strain

This chapter provides a variety of ways to release mental strain. Dr. Bates excelled in ways to reconnect your mind to your eyes without causing strain on either. You will learn how to use your memory and imagination for better sight. You will explore the part played by your subconscious mind – how it holds you back and how it can be of help instead. Because these three elements of the mental side of vision (memory, imagination and the subconscious mind) are interconnected, overlap is inevitable. Your goal is to have all three work together toward effortless clear vision, which, by the time you finish this chapter, will be easier than you may expect!

 What if it was easy?

I am not a psychologist, but I have learned to ask one simple question that I find very useful any time I notice my own mental strain increasing. I ask myself:

What would this be like if it was *easy*??

This simple question, as I let myself consider its answer, greatly reduces the effort I'm making, and allows me to take a different approach to whatever I was trying so hard to do. I usually don't even need a concrete answer to this question, because just the general feeling of ease it generates is enough to avoid further straining. The answer is likely to follow soon enough, especially when I don't force it.

> **If only we could give up, let go, let the thing be done for us,**
> **of how much strain would we rid ourselves!**
> **What a difference between trying to do a thing and doing it;**
> **between trying to see and seeing!**
> L. M. Stanton, M.D.[6]

A wrong thought

Bates felt a "wrong thought"[7] lay at the foundation of many vision challenges, and he wrote that those who would argue and question his approach were his hardest cases to cure. So, let's begin by laying some wrong thoughts to rest.

The wrong thought I hear most often is: "My eyes are weak." If you believe your eye muscles are weak, you may be inclined to also believe you need to do eye exercises to strengthen them. But as you have learned by now, it is not muscle weakness that prevents proper focus; it is chronic muscle tension that stops the eyes from working correctly. Doing eye "push-ups" is unlikely to solve that problem; the strain simply needs to be released.

Here are two similar wrong thoughts that are also quite common: "It takes effort to see clearly" and "If I try harder, I will see better." If this is your belief, it is important to know that people with good vision never try hard to see better. This is not because they always see perfectly well; an object can be too far away, too small, or too dimly lit to be seen clearly. In that case they simply relax, blink, and either choose to ignore it as not important, or, if curious about it, they imagine what the details might be. That's how they keep their good vision. In contrast, someone with blurry vision confronted with something outside their visual range tends to instantly strain, which leads to worse vision. Trying harder never helps you see better. I trust you have thrown out this wrong thought by now and replaced it with the knowledge that says, "I see better when I relax."

Another pervasive wrong thought that exists, even among many vision teachers, is that "it is hard to improve vision." Thinking it is hard creates a tendency toward strain. I invite you to think that it is easy to improve your vision. It typically takes much less time to return to clarity than it did to get to your current level of blurry vision. My sixteen years of myopic blur disappeared, for the most part, in two weeks, and completely in two months. As blur is mainly due to strain, and clarity comes from relaxation, how can clarity possibly be hard? To the contrary, it is relaxing! So, even if it does take some time, thinking of it as hard to achieve only slows down your progress, while if you keep in mind that relaxation is easier than straining you are likely to reach your goal sooner.

Bates recognized that the subconscious thoughts and beliefs that underlie your mental strain are a hindrance. He once told of a man who had so many negative beliefs that it took a very long time for him to return to clear vision.[8]

> One of the most striking cases of the relation of mind to vision that ever came to my attention was that of a physician whose mental troubles, at one time so serious that they suggested to him the idea that he might be going insane, were completely relieved when his sight became normal.

> [...] His memory was very poor. He could not remember the color of the eyes of any member of his family, although he had seen them all daily for years. Neither could he recall the color of his house, the number of rooms on the different floors, or other details. The faces and names of patients and friends he recalled with difficulty, or not at all.

> His treatment proved to be very difficult, chiefly because he had an infinite number of erroneous ideas about physiological optics in general and his own case in particular, and insisted that all these should be discussed; while these discussions were going on he received no benefit. Every day for hours at a time over a long period he talked and

argued. Never have I met a person whose logic was so wonderful, so apparently unanswerable, and yet so utterly wrong.

[…] He finally became able to read 20/10 or more, and although more than fifty-five years of age, he also read diamond type* at from 6 to 24 inches. His night blindness was relieved, his attacks of day blindness ceased, and he told me the color of the eyes of his wife and children. One day he said to me: "Doctor, I thank you for what you have done for my sight; but no words can express the gratitude I feel for what you have done for my mind. *(* Diamond type is a small font. See pages 182-183.)*

Perhaps Bates found that he wasted much time when arguing with people's subconscious beliefs. Instead, he showed them truth. His method was simple yet ingenious. He found that once a person can imagine something perfectly, such as the blackness of a small period, they can often see clearly in reality, because in order to imagine something perfectly they must release their mental strain.

Of course, this mental strain might return, but having achieved mental relaxation once, the brain can figure out how to achieve it again and eventually learn to make it last, thereby affecting the mental strain and underlying subconscious beliefs in a subtle way.

> **Myopia is not a permanent condition of the eyeball.**
> **It can be demonstrated that when the mind is at rest,**
> **and there is no mental strain when the patient**
> **remembers or imagines a letter, a color, or some other**
> **object perfectly, the myopia disappears.**
> William H. Bates, M.D.[9]

Dr. Bates' research shows that when vision is perfect and the mind relaxed, it is very easy to have a perfectly clear mental picture of something. Conversely, if a person can imagine a perfect mental picture, their strain will be gone in that moment, and vision will clear. Repeated practice then makes the clarity last.

Your next step, then, is to work with your memory and imagination, and discover how they can be used to improve vision.

Sensory memory
Scientists tend to divide memory into long term, short term, working, and sensory memory. For vision improvement we will focus on sensory memory, which includes visual memory. Sensory memory also includes auditory memory and memory for smell, taste, touch and movement. For example, you can hear a catchy tune play in your head or recall the delightful aroma of a beautiful rose, the delicious flavor of your favorite food, the texture

of your coat's fabric, or the steps of a popular dance. Each of these types of sensory memory, when recalled easily and in perfect detail, as if real in this moment, will relax your mind and can thus help you regain perfect vision.

This means that if you have a hard time with visual memory, perhaps due to blurry vision, and you find it difficult to create a perfect mental picture of anything, you can substitute an auditory or other sensory memory for similarly relaxing results on the eye muscles.

Be aware that your memory cannot be forced any more than your vision can be forced. You have probably experienced the name that was "on the tip of your tongue," but which would not come to mind until you stopped trying so hard to remember it. The harder you try to remember or the harder you try to see, the less you are able to do so. You remember best without effort, just as you see best without effort.

Foundation memory

When your mind is relaxed, mental pictures will appear easily, instantly, and with perfect clarity whenever you choose to think of something familiar. It's really useful to have a favorite memory – one that you can recall so easily that it will help you relax the moment you think of it. Dr. Bates called this a "foundation test."[10] I call it a foundation memory.

The things you are more likely to remember are those that are interesting and meaningful to you. Anything that is exciting or familiar is easier to recall than something that bores or frustrates you. For a sailing-loving, computer-hating friend of mine, I can safely bet that the carefully polished tiller on his beloved sailboat will likely pop into his mind much clearer and quicker than the keyboard for his computer ever would.

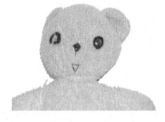

An easy memory for me is of a little white teddy bear that I've had my whole life. One of its button eyes has long since fallen out, and in its place a piece of black felt was stitched on with green thread. I may be the only person in the world who thinks this is adorable! Whenever I think of this little teddy bear, a smile comes to my face and I can easily picture its details in my mind – especially that black felt eye.

When you close your eyes and think of something you love, what is the first thing that effortlessly comes to mind? It may be the eyes of a loved one, the smile of a baby, an adorable pet, a favorite item of clothing, a piece of jewelry, a detail of your car, a colorful flower, or any hobby-related object. Children may think of their most loved toy, a favorite doll, a teddy bear, a cartoon character, or perhaps the black ears of Mickey Mouse!

Your foundation memory can also be a melody or a song, the sound of waves rolling onto a beach, or even a feeling of sheer joy that you fondly recall. It can simply be a color, like the bright white of fresh snow that you used to play in as a child; or it can be a shape – even just a small dot will do.

Your foundation memory can also be an abstract thought that makes you happy. Did you see the movie "Hook" in which Robin Williams played Peter Pan? To rescue his children, the adult Peter Pan needs to regain the ability to fly like he did in his youth. He keeps failing, while Tinkerbell, his little fairy companion, keeps reminding him of the solution, telling Peter, "*It only takes one happy thought to fly!*" When Peter finally remembers the immense love he felt at the birth of his son, his ability to fly returns, and all ends well.

You too need just one happy thought. It may or may not help you fly, but it will help you see! What is your most powerful happy thought? What makes your heart sing? What makes you laugh out loud? I will tell you a happy thought that I have used – a thought that still tickles my funny bone each time I recall it. Some time ago, a friend described to me his "home in heaven," providing elaborate details of a dream he had about this place. Only one detail stuck irrevocably in my mind, a detail that had surprised him. Even though he hadn't been there in many years, he noticed *there was no dust on anything.* Imagine that: no dust in heaven! What joy! I totally love this! Whether it is true or not is irrelevant, as the thought of it fills me with delight, and that's good enough for me. After years of trying to keep up with the dust brought into my home each day by six dogs freely running in and out, a dust-free space sure sounds heavenly to me. You may not be too concerned about heavenly dust, so tell me: What is your one happy thought to help you fly?

Whatever your foundation memory is, you'll know that it is the right one for you when a perfectly clear image or other sensory memory of it appears instantly and easily in your mind as soon as you think of it. That is the one to use. If it is a picture, it will appear with perfect clarity, with the exact color and size as the actual image, and it will be gently swinging.

If your foundation memory is something small, you may be able to physically carry it with you and look at it whenever you want to relax. The main objective, however, is to easily "carry it" in your mind, where you can put it to good use on your path to relaxed clarity at any time.

Paul, a man of sixty-three who started needing reading glasses at age fifty, used a "curvaceous glass teapot" for his "focus object," as he liked to call it. He loved how keeping his favorite teapot in mind changed his outlook on everything; it very effectively kept him out of his habit of straining to see. This gave him a much more relaxed outlook, which clearly showed in his face.

> **A familiar object, or one with pleasant associations, is often easier to remember than one which has no particular interest. One patient was cured by the memory of a yellow buttercup, and another was able to remember the opal of her ring when she could not remember a period. Whatever the patient finds easiest to remember is the best to remember, because the memory can never be perfect unless it is easy.**
> William H. Bates, M.D.[11]

 When to use your foundation memory

Start by using it during palming, when you are not tempted to try to see anything. Just enjoy the details of this easy memory and let it help you relax more deeply.

Whenever you notice eyestrain and can't seem to relax out of it, whether with eyes open or closed, bring your foundation memory to mind. Your eyes and mind will relax due to the ease and clarity with which it is remembered. Simply recall this very familiar item, take a few moments to relax with it, and then bring your attention back to what you were doing. If simultaneously you can keep your foundation memory swinging in the back of your mind, you may find that your actual vision improves!

Feel free to switch to a different foundation memory anytime you like; as long as your current choice is easy for you to remember perfectly and instantly, it will serve its purpose.

 The period

As smaller is better when it comes to seeing effortlessly, Dr. Bates recommended that you develop the memory for a dot the size of a period. He wrote:

> Of all the methods employed in obtaining normal vision, the memory and the imagination of the small black, white or any color period is among the best.[12]

Dr. Bates preferred a black dot himself, as he felt black would look equally black regardless of the intensity or source of light. But if you find black to be a depressing color, paint the dot your favorite color. Once you can imagine a small dot with the same ease as your foundation memory, you can use either one to relax with.

At first a small dot may be challenging to remember, even though you have likely seen millions of them: at the end of each sentence; atop every i and j; two in each colon and one in each semi-colon. Yet you may find it easier to first remember a somewhat larger area, such as a letter on the chart, and then imagine one part of that letter blacker than the rest. Continue to smaller letters until you get to the size of a period. You will then likely find that it is easier to remember a small area than a large one, and that the black is more intense in a small area. However, if you end up staring at this small dot, you will want to turn it into a colon or a group of dots so you can shift your attention from one dot to another and imagine them swinging.

Mario, my Canadian student with high myopia, thought that to imagine a period was the hardest thing to do, until I told him to imagine a sheet of white paper. I asked him to imagine a black pen in his hand and told him to make a small dot on the imagined paper. I asked him to make several more dots; he made hundreds. Then he imagined looking from one to another, hopping around from dot to dot in his mind. Now it was easy to do. After this, the text he had been reading looked a lot clearer.

Dr. Bates wrote the following about the memory of a period:
> When the memory of the period becomes habitual, it is not only not a burden, but is a great help to other mental processes. The mind when it remembers one thing better than all other things possesses central fixation, and its efficiency is thereby increased, just as the efficiency of the eye is increased by central fixation. In other words, the mind attains its greatest efficiency when it is at rest, and it is never at rest unless one thing is remembered better than all other things. When the mind is in such a condition that a period is remembered perfectly the memory for other things is improved.
>
> A high school girl reports that when she was unable to remember the answer to a question in an examination she remembered the period, and the answer came to her. When I cannot remember the name of a patient I remember a period, and behold, I have it! A musician, who had perfect sight and could remember a period perfectly had a perfect memory for music; but a musician with imperfect sight who could not remember a period could play nothing without his notes, only gaining that power when his sight and visual memory had become normal.[13]

Memory and property – there is common ground
I've heard there are three things that matter in property: *location, location, and location*. Guess what: location is also an important consideration in memory and imagination, so ask yourself: Where do you place your image?

When I first learned about using the mind for vision improvement, I had a habit of trying to place mental images in front of my closed eyes. I could not really do it well at all; it was frustrating, and I didn't find it helpful in clearing my sight. So, I set it aside and continued with other elements of vision improvement instead. Much later I came back to that topic and had another go at it. I closed my eyes and attempted to visualize a black dot. I still projected it in front of my eyes, and I still didn't succeed. However, this time, having already improved my vision to 20/15 by other parts of the Bates Method, I recognized how my eyes were straining as I *tried* to visualize the image in front of my eyes. With the recognition of the strain, I was able to let it go. The very moment I let go of the strain, the image of the black dot appeared, almost like magic! Yet it was interesting to me that it did not appear right in front of my eyes where I had tried so hard to place it. Instead, it appeared inside my head, behind the area commonly known as the "third eye." Also, the darn thing would *not* stand still… When I tried to make it stand still, I immediately noticed the strain return in my eyes. Now when I imagine something with my eyes closed, like a red elephant for example, I check for any feeling of strain in my eyes and let that go first. Then I smile, because I already see the red elephant triumphantly trumpeting in my imagination.

Avoid my mistakes and use the following tips to help you succeed with the period faster than I did!

 Tips for remembering a period

- Begin this practice during a time of relaxation, such as palming.
- Pick whichever color is easiest for you to remember. The size or shape that you remember this color in does not matter, but smaller is usually easier. Palm your eyes and imagine a ball of this color floating on the waves at a beach. Imagine it slowly being carried out into the ocean. Watch it becoming smaller and smaller until it seems to be just a small dot.
- Do not project the period out in front of you floating in mid-air. It doesn't exist there, so trying to place it there is a strain. Let it appear in your mind, behind your eyes.
- Use central clarity; imagine seeing one part of the dot best. No matter how small the period is, you cannot see or imagine all of it perfectly at the same time.
- Shift your attention continually to any part of this dot, also away from it and back, and imagine it swinging.
- To help see the period swing, turn it into a colon, and notice one dot best at a time. To imagine the colon requires constant shifting from the upper to the lower dot and back.
- Avoid any effort. You cannot remember the period perfectly by any kind of effort. The more you concentrate, stare and try hard to imagine a small period, the less likely you are to succeed.
- Always carry the memory of the small period with you and use it whenever your vision becomes blurry.
- With eyes open, imagine a black dot in a corner of a black letter on the letter chart and notice it is even blacker than the rest of the letter. This isn't the same as projecting the dot out in front of you – this is seeing with central clarity. It applies to colors too. When you look at a colored object, yellow for example, imagine a small yellow dot on its surface. Avoid imagining a black dot on a yellow surface (or any other color) however, as this can create a strain.

A tiny ant (your new imaginary friend)

If you think a small dot is boring, employ the services of a tiny ant instead!

 (This is the big sister of the one on the right.)   *i*

> I love to help you see details easily!

To help you use your central clarity in a fun and effortless way while looking at objects that you do not yet see clearly, imagine that there is a small ant walking on the object you want to see. This ant is tiny, and it has chameleon skills: it has the exact same color as the surface you are looking at. Imagine seeing this chameleon ant walking here, there and everywhere. This little ant is your friend: similar to the imagination of a small period, the ant helps you focus on small details and shift continually without strain.

You can use this imaginary friend at any distance. Notice it walking over the letters on the letter chart, at which time it is a deep black color, or see it happily skipping on top of letters on distant road signs. Imagine it walking over letters on this page; see it sitting on a bright cloud; imagine it everywhere, smiling back at you with blinking eyes. Notice how you zoom in on smaller details as you imagine the ant walking across the object, and how it makes focusing effortless. If you happen to have a phobia about ants, you can of course use the small period instead. Experiment, and have fun. If it seems hard to imagine an ant where there isn't one for real, then skip this, and look for the actual details!

Memory of clear vision

I asked Marian, a woman with 6 diopters of myopia and polyopia (seeing multiple images around a single image) to imagine what a letter on the chart would look like if she had clear vision. She told me she had no memory of clear vision without glasses. Her first memory of clear vision was when she received her first pair of glasses at age eight, and she described her surprise back then at seeing individual leaves on a tree instead of a green blur. She also remembered an odd moment that day when the optometrist placed a frame on her nose and she experienced seeing better already. She then realized that frame was empty – it had no lenses in it yet. At the time, she was too embarrassed to mention her experience of better vision through empty frames, but 40 years later, she still remembered it clearly.

I made use of her memory of clear vision while she palmed her eyes. I asked her to remember seeing the leaves on that tree clearly like that day long ago, while also imagining that she was wearing those first glasses. This was easy for her. Then I asked her to imagine those glasses being just empty frames, and to continue imagining that she could see the tree clearly. She was able to do that. From there it was a small step to imagine seeing the tree clearly without the empty frames. She could do that too. At that point I asked her to open her eyes, and she was delighted to see the chart distinctly better. The key to this first improvement lay in using her existing memory of clear vision to reduce her eyestrain.

Do you have a memory of clear vision without glasses? If so, use it like Marian did and use it often, so the resulting extra clarity can become permanent. If you don't have a memory of clear vision, you can build it with practice and you can use your current near vision clarity as a starting point.

The face sketch, or: "May I use you for target practice, please?"

Ask a loved one if you may please use them for "target practice." It may be wise to explain that you want to practice memorization by visualizing their face with your eyes closed. The familiarity of this face and the fact that you love this person will make it easy and fun. Sit at a distance from each other where you can clearly see their facial features. Glance at this dear person in a relaxed way, blinking often.

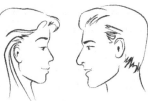

Notice that you cannot possibly see the whole face clearly all at once. When you look at the left eye, the right eye is seen with less clarity. When you look at the pupil of one eye, the iris is not seen as clearly. Look around the iris and notice all its details. Go around other facial features, seeing one best at a time. Then do the same with your eyes closed and notice that here, too, only one detail can be imagined clearly at a time.

You may be surprised at how many details you need to re-check before you can see their face more clearly in your mind. If you remember details in rapid succession, you may create an impression of seeing the whole face clearly, but the reality remains that you only see one detail clearly at a time. Open your eyes and check for more details that you may have missed. Can you see the individual hairs of the eyebrows? Close your eyes and go over all the facial details you can remember now. If any details are still missing, use your imagination to improve on this picture! Have fun with this; a smiling face will be your treasured memory.

Mental pictures of letters

You may have memorized the letters on the chart by now, but do you actually have clear mental pictures of these letters? When remembering a letter, it is not necessary to recall the entire letter. The memory of its color or of one small part of the letter is enough. The brighter white you imagine its background to be, the easier it will be for any part of the black letter to stand out. The smaller the part of a black letter that you remember, and the blacker you imagine it to be, the easier it is to picture in your mind. The less you stare at it physically and mentally, the more you let it swing gently, the longer the memory of the letter lasts.

Flashing to improve mental pictures

Dr. Bates often used the flashing technique with letter charts, and you may find it helpful too. Use two identical charts for this practice. Hold one in your hand, close enough to your eyes that you can easily read the smallest letters. Hang the other on a wall and position yourself so the wall chart is at a distance where it is seen with slight blur. This may be only one inch from the chart in your hand, or several feet from it.

Look at one of the smallest letters on the chart in your hand. Then close your eyes for anything from a second to half a minute or longer, and remember the letter as well as you saw it, one part best at a time. Now, with eyes still closed, imagine identical clarity of the same letter on the far chart. When you can imagine that you see this letter just as easily and clearly on the wall chart, open your eyes, remember the clear letter, and briefly glance at it on the wall chart. Quickly close your eyes again within a second, regardless of how well or how blurred you saw the letter. The key is to avoid staring or straining.

Alternate until the imagination of a letter on the wall chart becomes equal to the vision of the same letter on the hand chart. When you reach that point, your vision of the letter on the wall chart will clear too. You can then slightly increase your distance from the wall chart and repeat the process. If at any distance you fail to imagine a letter clearly on the wall chart, move closer – close enough to imagine it successfully without effort.

Flashing is a great help in improving mental pictures. With the eyes open, one may see a letter quite perfectly, and have a mental picture of that letter with the eyes closed for a fraction of a second. By repeatedly flashing the letter in this way, the mental picture becomes more frequent and lasts longer. When the sight becomes more continuously good, the memory is also benefited, and with the improvement in the memory, the mental pictures become more perfect.
William H. Bates, M.D.[14]

Add a gentle sway to this practice to help you see the chart and letters swing smoothly. Blink often. Ignore any blur you may still see and keep remembering details of the clear letter in your mind. If the swings don't come easily to you yet, imagine their presence while your eyes are closed. That may be easier and can help you imagine this motion with eyes open too.

The above practice employs the flashing technique to transfer your clear vision close up to a longer distance. You can also use this technique to transfer the ease with which you see a large letter and letting it help you relax with the same letter in a smaller font size. Or you can use it to alternate between bright and dim light, to help increase your ability to see in less favorable light conditions. You can even use it to transfer better visual acuity from one eye to the other (see Chapter 23).

Extend the flash

As your ability to stay relaxed with your eyes open improves, the mental picture you have of a letter will become clearer. You can then choose to advance your practice by gradually increasing your distance, reducing letter size or altering light conditions, or you can advance by extending the time you keep your eyes open.

To extend the eye-open time, go from the flash that lasts for a fraction of a second, to keeping your eyes open for a full second, and then closing them. Always relax any tension that you notice as you close your eyes to rest them after this second. When you open your eyes, notice how many more details you can see during a full second of looking at the chart.

Now extend the time your eyes are open to two seconds, then close them for as long as necessary to feel relaxed before you open them again for another two seconds. How many details can you notice during these two seconds? Let your attention be on noticing details, not on judging clarity! This relaxed mental attitude of simply noticing lots of details will help your eyes shift naturally and effortlessly while they are open. With your eyes open two seconds or longer, do allow them to blink!

When you practice this, you are teaching your eyes and mind to stay relaxed while open. You are practicing inhibition of your habitual strain pattern. The better you get at avoiding the strain and the longer your eyes stay relaxed, the clearer your vision will be.

Remember Mr. Blur from Chapter 5? He is the messenger that gives you an indication of your level of strain, which is why he is your friend. It is best if you imagine that you can already see clearly, with total ease, even when the letter you want to read is too far, too small or in too dim of a light to distinguish. Use your memory of the clear letter to fill in details that you don't yet see. When done just with your mind, and not with your eyes or eyelids or any other way of straining and trying, you will truly relax into seeing. And that gives Mr. Blur a chance to leave, because you no longer need his message.

As you increase the challenge, you'll want to increase the relaxation

You can practice with larger objects at a greater distance, for example, a tree that you walk by every day. Glance at the tree and close your eyes. Can you recall its colors, its shape? Do you have a memory of what one of its leaves looks like? How would it feel if you touched that leaf? How would the leaf look if you held it in your hand? Imagine details, color and texture. Maybe even add the sense of smell, recalling the pleasurable fresh scent of the tree's blossoms in spring. Alternate closing your eyes, remembering the tree, and opening your eyes to briefly look at it again. Is the image of the tree getting clearer? If not, make it more realistic; pick a leaf to actually hold in your hand.

 Mental pictures

With the practices above, you are using your memory to create mental pictures, whether it is a visual foundation memory, a period, an ant, a familiar face or a letter on a chart. Mental pictures may be the best tool for improving both memory and vision effortlessly. You can use any image you like, but choose ones that come to your mind easily.

You may find that it helps to add a non-visual sense to your picture. Perhaps you can hold a familiar object in your hands and feel its texture and weight. Gaze at it; notice its details and feel its weight, shape and texture, then close your eyes and remember them, both visually and kinesthetically. Flash your eyes open and re-paint your mental picture when you close them again. With practice, this flashing and taking quick vision photographs will greatly improve your ability to remember details and create mental pictures.

If you are not yet successful at getting mental pictures, change the size of the object you are looking at, change your distance from it, or choose to remember just its color. Avoid the temptation to try to see the entire object in one go. For a better chance at success, notice one small detail. Central clarity applies with your eyes open as well as with them closed! You will likely not get a good image of, for example, an entire apple, but you may find it easy to remember the tip of its stem best while you imagine the rest of the apple with less clarity and then shift your attention to another spot. Add your memory of taste to the apple image!

> **I do not know of any method of obtaining relaxation or perfect sight which is as efficient and certain as the imagination of mental pictures. It should be emphasized that a good or perfect imagination of mental pictures has in all cases brought about a measure of improvement which is convincing that the imagination is capable of relieving organic changes in the eye more quickly, more thoroughly, more permanently, than any other method.**
> William H. Bates, M.D.[15]

 Imagine seeing clearly

It is one thing to remember or imagine clarity when the same letter on the same chart is available, both in your area of best vision as well as in your blur zone; but it's another thing to do so when you do not have the perfect copy available in your hand to compare to. In some instances it can help to use a digital camera to zoom in on what you want to see, but relying on such technology doesn't compare to relying on your own eyes and mind. Your foundation memory comes to the rescue here – your perfectly easy and instant memory of something very familiar to you. Think about that memory, perhaps with eyes closed at first, and then keep the details of this memory in mind while you take another look at whatever you want to see with more clarity. You are not trying to get extra clarity; you are only recalling your foundation memory, and then you'll simply see what happens.

If you have seen the object you are looking at before or you have seen something similar to it, you can use those memories to imagine what the details of this current object would look like at the distance that you are seeing it now, if you were seeing it clearly.

For example, you are walking down a street in your hometown and notice a stop sign at a distance where it is blurry. From the shape and color, you can tell it is a stop sign, but the word STOP is not easily seen. You probably have a memory of what a stop sign looks like – you've seen them many times before while driving or walking around town. So, without any effort to clear up the blur, imagine what the distant stop sign would look like if you did see it clearly right now.

What details would you see that you aren't yet seeing? How white would the letters be? Do you remember the curves of the **S**? The shape of the **T**? The rounded **O** with its red inner oval? Can you imagine seeing the straight left side of the **P** clearly? Do you remember the white line on the edge of the sign, making the eight edges stand out against the background? Can you imagine the white to be even whiter?

👁 Imagine details you don't yet see

When you imagine that you see clearly, always imagine details which you don't yet see but which you expect to be there (details of the object's texture, lines, shape, color) and add other senses as applicable (touch, smell, taste, sound). The smaller the details that you can imagine, the easier it becomes to see. Of course, it helps to imagine the object swinging too. Stay with familiar items when you practice this, because anything that you have not seen clearly before will only make this harder, causing tension that creates blurry vision.

Dr. Bates said that the eyes of someone with perfect vision are relaxed and moving all the time. He also stated that someone with imperfect vision can achieve the same relaxation for their eyes **by the imagination of perfect sight.**

> **The only time the eye is at rest is when one has or imagines perfect sight.**
> William H. Bates, M.D.[16]

Are you remembering or imagining?

For added clarity, the difference between memory and imagination is quite simple. If you have just looked at an object in front of you, and you close your eyes and see a picture in your mind of that object, exactly as you just saw it, you are using your memory to visualize it. If you then mentally change the color, shape or size of it, or paint red spots on it, or have it sing to you, you are using your imagination to create something you have not actually experienced. Your imagination is not limited by any restraints of reality, or by any blurry perceptions.

Imagination

Imagination is vital to clear eyesight because when you imagine you see with clarity, or imagine how you would feel if you already had perfect vision, you take all effort out of seeing.

> **Most people have an imagination that is good enough to cure them if they would only use it. What we see is only what we think we see or what we imagine we see. When we imagine correctly we see correctly; when we imagine imperfectly we see imperfectly.**
> William H. Bates, M.D.[17]

Shortly after meeting Marian, who saw multiple images, a friend gave me a book about Neuro-Linguistic Programming, called *Trance-formations*. It basically is a transcript of various hypnosis seminars given by the authors, Richard Bandler and John Grinder. In one of their seminars a man asked if he could use hypnosis for giving up his glasses and having normal vision. My interest deepened as I read the reply. Apparently one of the authors had used hypnosis to age-regress a man who was wearing glasses. As this man was regressed to a five-year-old boy, he found he could no longer see through the glasses he was wearing, so he took them off to see better. When he was brought out of hypnosis, he needed his glasses. Regressing him to five years old once more allowed this man to again see fine without his glasses. The author then gave him this suggestion: "Now your eyes are going to stay five years old, and the rest of you is going to grow up."

That was all it took for this man to see clearly without his glasses! Quite an amazing effect, even if it only lasted two months. That's when his old subconscious beliefs regained the upper hand and his vision blurred. This is a prime example of how the mind can influence vision. If you can change your mind, you can change your vision. Whenever you imagine that you see clearly, when you consistently imagine that you can see smaller details than you usually see, you are changing your mind.

Ellen Langer, Professor of Psychology at Harvard University, studied how mind-set affects vision by helping people imagine they have excellent vision. Her research shows that vision can improve instantly when you change your mind-set regarding visual performance.[18] She therefore concluded: "Believing is Seeing."

> **You can't depend on your eyes when your imagination is out of focus.**
> Mark Twain[19]

 Develop a curiosity for details

Nearsightedness can foster a habit of not looking for details at a distance anymore, as the expectation is to only see blur out there. Remember my student in Los Angeles who looked across the street from his balcony and was surprised that he could actually see the mortar in the brick wall of a house? He had been wearing glasses of -6 diopters and certainly did not expect to see the mortar. He would not normally have looked for such detail if I hadn't asked him to.

Your natural curiosity keeps you interested in life and all that is around you. When you lose it, life becomes dull, depression may set in, and your vision may deteriorate. Keeping or developing a curiosity for detail will help keep your mind and vision fresh and sharp.

Imagine that you are from Jupiter and you're visiting planet Earth for the very first time. Walking through the streets of your town, you take a great interest in all that's around you; you have an intense curiosity. You may be wondering what all the signs mean, why people go where they go, why they are dressed in different colors, why buildings have different sizes, why there is only one moon, etc. Your awareness is heightened, and as your interest in details of objects around you increases, your vision responds accordingly. It's a fun way of being in the present moment, asking yourself all sorts of questions to which you may normally not give a second thought.

Nearsighted beliefs?

In *The Power Behind Your Eyes,* optometrist Robert-Michael Kaplan writes that nearsightedness is a pulling in of one's perceptual reality. He says this begins with thoughts like "I don't know how to handle what's out there – my world is too confusing. I feel too much when I look beyond myself. I can't cope with what's out there. I feel safe when I focus mentally inward. I will feel less by thinking more. Give me a book to read. I'll master this computer program. I'll take courses at a university. I'll excel at school."

You may recognize your own thoughts in some of these statements. Such thoughts and beliefs may have been part of your life for many years, and it may be a challenge to let them go. You can become so used to them, like you become used to your glasses. Your beliefs become part of your identity, your sense of self. Consequently, you develop habits that support your beliefs. These habits serve a purpose. In her book, *The Down Comforter,* Juliene Berk writes:

> Habits have no innate ability to keep you in their thrall. The only reason they persist is that they are offering some satisfaction, serving some purpose, answering some need. You allow them to persist by not seeking any other, better form of satisfying the same needs. Every habit, good or bad, is acquired and learned in the same way – by finding that it is a means of satisfaction.[20]

Obviously not all habits are bad for you, and they certainly don't all require changing. They simply fulfill a need. So let's examine your "need" for blurry vision.

Blurry vision has its "benefits." It can…

- Reduce your irritation from things you prefer not to deal with, like a nasty 3rd-grade teacher.
- Be an excuse for reading less (hyperopia/presbyopia), or reading more (myopia).
- Help develop your other senses, such as hearing.
- Make the world "softer," which may be nicer than "harsh" reality.
- Reduce the amount of visual input, creating less overwhelm.
- Allow you to wear glasses that make you look smarter, or that look like your favorite artist's glasses (also known as the: "John Denver Syndrome," see p25).
- Provide a sense of "protection" – now your eyes feel "safe" behind glasses.

Your blur served a purpose at one time, and, possibly, on some level, it still does. Take a few minutes to examine the beliefs hidden beneath this list of "benefits" and similar thoughts that may apply to you. You may find that you jumped to a wrong conclusion, or made an assumption that did not reflect reality, and ended up blurring out more than you needed to.

Once you uncover the underlying belief, you may be able to come up with a better way to deal with the reason for the blur. It's definitely useful to explore this, because next time a similar situation appears in your life, you will have the option of taking a route that is different from "blurring it out." You can develop a new way of reacting that allows you to keep your clear vision.

It is time to delve even deeper into your blurry vision. To get you started, I'll give the example of a myopic woman named Jaya. When Jaya was a young teenager, her family moved from a small town to a big city 500 miles to the south. She was shy and felt quite different from her new classmates. Jaya thought nobody really liked her much, and she spent a great deal of her free time alone. She would rather read or write in her journal then risk being rejected by her peers.

By the time Jaya and I met she was in her thirties and using -3.25 glasses all day. Jaya liked the idea of improving her vision because she hated her glasses; they were uncomfortable, seemed heavy on her nose, restricted her peripheral vision, and she just did not like being dependent on them. Besides that, she already had plans for the money she would save from not needing to buy glasses again.

Jaya had tried contacts for a while but they irritated her eyes and made her tired. The idea of laser surgery scared her, and she preferred to not even think about doing that to her eyes. Basically, Jaya viewed her glasses as a royal nuisance, and an expensive nuisance at that. She longed to be free from them.

When she looked at possible reasons for her myopia, she thought that her family's move was the pivotal point; that's when her comfortable small-town life ended and the unknowns of the big city were thrust upon her. Her blurry vision allowed her to see less of the things she dreaded dealing with, whether those were her new classmates, or life in the new city itself. She could hide from the "inevitable" rejections by reading, rather than going out; and she could use the glasses as a "protection" between her and the rest of the world.

After looking at these things, she realized that a fear of the unknown and a fear of rejection had been hiding behind her glasses. But today she is no longer a shy teenager; she's a successful business manager, and she has better skills in her bag of "life tools." She can consciously employ these skills in any future situation that puts her in unknown territory. Due to her business training, it is no longer hard for her to simply ask others for help. She recognizes that her fear of rejection does continue to simmer underneath the surface of her life, but here too, new skills plus a strong spiritual foundation give her better options for dealing with this fear.

Jaya now promises to spend a few minutes each day visualizing herself dealing with a variety of people, while imagining that she is not worried about any rejection at all. She can see herself giving her best, then letting the other person choose to accept it or not. Either way, she visualizes herself as happy that she had the opportunity to meet them. And she knows that soon she will find herself able to put this into practice in real life.

What is your perception?
What if your perception of something being hard is just that – your perception? And what if you can change your perception by shifting your point of focus? And what if that turns

out to be easy? Would you do it? Or do you prefer to resist change, resist letting go of your perceptions, even when they don't or no longer serve you? Digging a little deeper than usual into your own patterns can be very useful when you want to achieve any kind of change, so let's now look at your own thoughts and beliefs regarding your vision.

First, write down five or more reasons why you want to change your blurry vision, and/or why you want to change your need for glasses.

-

-

-

-

-

Look over the reasons you came up with. See if you can consolidate them and find three main reasons.

-

-

Next, write down five or more advantages of, or reasons for creating, blurry vision and/or reasons for continuing to wear glasses or contact lenses. This serves to make these reasons conscious, so they no longer mess with your good intentions on a subconscious level.

-

-

-

-

-

Here too, distill them into three main reasons, if possible.

-

-

-

Now, guided by these lists, can you begin to tell what needs are being served by the blur? Write down those needs.

-

-

-

The logical next step is to think of better ways to serve these needs. You may be able to think of some instantly, or perhaps you'd like to sleep on it. When you have your answers, write those down too.

-

-

-

Now take a few minutes, palm your eyes, and imagine what you would do, how you would feel, if you were completely free from blurry vision. Imagine being free from any fears you may have found beneath the blur. See yourself using your new way of dealing with the old challenges and imagine being very comfortable doing so. Do this as often as you like, until you are comfortable in your new mental habits!

Perhaps you can now see the blur as your personal gateway into your own fears. It has brought you in, it can show you the way out. Rather than judging the blur as something bad that you need to get rid of, ask yourself questions about the blur and the needs it serves. When you find answers that make you feel more at peace, that help you see clearer on a mental or spiritual level, then you know that you are heading in a direction that takes you out of the blur and back towards clarity.

One of my students, Zdenko, in Italy, happily told me after he passed his driver's test without glasses, that for him the key was to become thankful for his blurry vision. If you ever meet Zdenko you will see his joy in life, his newfound confidence. and his relaxation regardless of outer circumstances. (Zdenko started at -1.75 with slight astigmatism; he took about one year with two weekend workshops to get to clarity).

When you want to learn how to be healthy, it is best to study health and healthy people, not disease and sick people. The same goes for your vision. Clarity cannot be attained by worrying about blur. It can be good to simply forget your visual blur and study how to reach clarity instead.

Bruce Lipton, a well-known cellular biologist and author of *The Biology of Belief*,[21] wrote that the old belief that health depends on your genes has become outdated because it is now understood that your environment – and especially what your thoughts and interpretation are about your environment – is what really controls the actions of your genes. He says:

> This new perspective of human biology does not view the body as just a mechanical device, but rather incorporates the role of a mind and spirit. This breakthrough in biology is fundamental in all healing for it recognizes that when we change our perception or beliefs we send totally different messages to our cells and reprogram their expression. The new biology reveals why people can have spontaneous remissions or recover from injuries deemed to be permanent disabilities.[22]

 Watch your language

What you say about your vision reveals a great deal about your thoughts and subconscious beliefs. Not only is your language influenced by your subconscious beliefs, your beliefs are also influenced by your language. It's a two-way street. I often hear people say things like: "I can't see anything without my glasses!" or "I'm *blind* without my contacts." They don't literally mean it, but what kind of message are they sending to their subconscious?! Precisely. Such messages reinforce their dependency on compensating lenses. If you say "I am nearsighted," then, subconsciously, you close the door to the option of no longer being nearsighted. On the contrary, "I am improving my vision" is a much more positive statement and swings the door wide open.

Someone who believes they can't manage without their glasses will be unlikely to take a single opportunity to look around without those lenses. Would they get up in the morning and take time to relax into the blur and discover what the world looks like through their "naked" eyes? No, they probably grab their glasses and ignore the message that their vision is trying to tell them. They may stuff down any emotions associated with the blurry vision and "put on a brave face," along with their glasses.

So, listening to what you typically tell yourself and others about your vision helps you become aware of your subconscious beliefs. When you become conscious of the stories you tell yourself, you can start to change these negative patterns into positive ones.

The next page has suggested sentences that may help build your happy vision language. Amend these words to your specific situation, and only choose sentences that you believe in, because lying to yourself – even with a positive affirmation or mantra – only adds to stress.

1.   As I become more aware of my eyestrain, I release it more each day.

2.   I choose to accept my vision the way it is in this moment.

3.   I accept what I see, and I see more clearly.

4.   Acceptance and love lead to clarity.

5.   The more ease and relaxation I allow myself, the more clearly I see.

6.   I notice all that I can see; I trust what I can see.

7.   I am improving my vision.

8.   Clearing my vision is easier than I thought.

9.   The muscles in and around my eyes move freely and easily.

10.   I love making progress in clearing my vision.

11.   I have faith and confidence in myself and in my eyes.

12.   I love myself; I love my beautiful eyes.

13.   My eyes love lots of easy blinking.

14.   As I shift my attention, my eyes easily follow.

15.   My breathing is becoming effortlessly deep.

16.   I can easily imagine seeing with great clarity at all distances.

17.   My posture cooperates in clearing my vision.

18.   My emotions cooperate in clearing my vision.

19.   My memory and imagination cooperate in clearing my vision.

20.   I think, expect, remember and imagine perfect vision.

21.   My eyes love sunshine.

22.   Clarity is my natural state.

23.   I know I can see clearly without glasses.

24.   My eyes are healthy.

25.   I have clear intentions; I have clear sight.

26.   The more I relax, the more I accomplish.

27.   There is enough time for me to clearly see anything I choose.

28.   I happily take the next step on my path toward clarity.

29.   I choose to see solutions. I see the way things CAN work.

30.   I choose to see all the beauty and love in me and around me.

31.   As my heart opens, my vision clears.

32.   I choose to use constructive language; I enjoy an optimistic outlook.

33.   _____

Pointers

- **Let it be easy.** Use the tips and techniques above and enjoy the process; don't worry about the end result. You'll get it when you let it go.

- **Begin your memory practices under your favorite conditions**, as this will help you reach your best results! Have your eyes either closed or open, depending on which works better for you. Use the distance of your best vision, an object size that is easy, and the level of light that you prefer. When you can create a perfect mental picture under your favorite conditions, you can use that picture to gradually increase your ability to keep a perfect memory under any condition.

- **Memory can only be perfect when you are relaxed.** Making an effort to create an image in your mind is similar to making an effort to see – it's a strain. Memory works passively, it comes as a result of relaxation. And equally, you may not consciously know how to relax, but if you have one perfect memory, that'll do it. That's your foundation memory. By continuing the memory of it, you're continuing the relaxation.

- **Remember that smaller is better** – that's the law of central clarity! Your imagination works better in small bites too, so don't attempt to clearly memorize Rembrandt van Rijn's huge *Night Watch* painting all at once. Even a simple chair is too much to tackle in one go. Memorize one detail best at a time, while letting the rest of the image be in your "peripheral memory."

- **Be careful to not stare in your imagination either**. Let your attention wander smoothly from point to point.

- **Even in your memory, imagine that stationary objects are in motion,** gently swinging. This supports the shifting motion of the eyes, which is more relaxing.

- **Follow your bliss**: your level of interest is a good indicator of your ability to remember.

- **Practice regularly**. Anything repeated regularly (preferably daily) will build and strengthen neural pathways in the brain, resulting in an increased ability to do more of the same. Use it or lose it! An active mind stays healthy longer.

- **You see what you believe...** Do you believe you can imagine clearly?

> **I advise you to think, expect, remember and imagine perfect vision and you shall have it at that very moment you need it.**
> William H. Bates, M.D.[23]

12. Looking at Posture, Sleep and Massage

Having thoroughly explored the mental side of vision, let's get back to additional physical aspects of dynamic relaxation that can influence your sight. Not many people realize that poor posture can have a big influence on vision. And vice versa, poor vision can easily influence your posture. Eye doctors fail to point out the connection despite research clearly pointing to a strong correlation between posture and astigmatism[1] and between head tilts or turns and double vision (diplopia.)[2] Giving you glasses that have a cylinder to compensate for astigmatism or a prism to compensate for double vision only reinforces the underlying postural issue. I believe that before cylinders or prisms are put into lenses, postural issues should be addressed, because a little somatic education can go a long way in resolving such issues without lenses.

For the extraocular muscles to be as relaxed and balanced as possible, good posture is essential. The outdoor lifestyle our bodies are designed for is far from reality for most of us. Too often we end up sitting indoors for many hours and don't get enough exercise to keep our body's musculature in balance. This leads to bad posture, which leads to knee problems, hip issues, back pain and neck tension. Any part of your body may attempt to compensate for trouble elsewhere in the body, and once neck tension has established itself, the head no longer follows the eyes smoothly and the eye muscles will attempt to compensate too. Such compensating eyestrain affects your visual clarity.

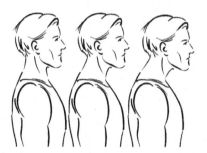 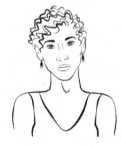

Most of us are not aware of our own bad posture habits. Bad posture is easy to spot in others, but awareness of your own posture is a very different matter. A few months before I learned how to improve my eyesight, a friend of mine took a photo of me driving a Jeep in Costa Rica. I distinctly remember the fun I had driving this beat-up Jeep that would even drive without its key in the ignition, and I remember that I more or less "posed" for that picture. When I saw the actual photo after it was developed (yes, pre-digital days), I was shocked to see myself terribly stooped behind the wheel! I threw that photo out, too embarrassed to show it to anyone, and checked my posture more consciously from then on, especially if I knew a photo was being taken.

👁 Awareness of your posture habits

Ask a close friend or check photos of yourself. Do you stoop forward or crane your neck to get closer to things you want to see? Do you have a habitual head tilt to one side, or a head turn that makes one ear more visible than the other? Does your chin look level or is it typically slightly up or down? Is it the same with or without glasses? Notice how bifocal glasses or progressive lenses affect your neck and posture. Do you tilt your head to look through the lower section of the lens in order to focus clearly close up? Become aware of these habitual posture adjustments!

Stand in front of a mirror, close your eyes, and find the posture that feels comfortable and "straight" to you. Then open your eyes and check, paying special attention to where your nose points. Does your posture look as straight as it feels?

The Alexander Technique

In my mid-twenties I was fortunate to live near Yael Israeli, a wonderful teacher of the Alexander Technique. This technique is named after F.M. Alexander, an actor who lost his voice and regained it after studying his body posture in a mirror and realizing that what he felt to be a straight posture certainly did not look straight. As he learned to adjust his posture and his sense of his body, his voice came back. I took a lesson from Yael once or twice a month during a few stressful years in my life. After each lesson I came home with a taller body, a more relaxed attitude, new insights, and a clearer mind. Yael helped me realize that there were better ways of moving my body that involved less muscle strain than I had been using. Basically, what she and other Alexander Technique teachers aim to achieve is better posture through dynamic relaxation.

The Alexander Technique is about undoing tension in the body that causes you to lose good posture. For example, you may have been told to "sit up straight," and you likely reacted to this request by using muscular effort to oppose any existing tension, resulting in a forced tall posture that you are unable to maintain for long. The approach of the Alexander Technique, to the contrary, would be to help you relax the muscles that pull the spine out of alignment. When that relaxation is achieved, a tall posture returns effortlessly. At first, you may need a teacher to help you find and release the strain, until muscle memory kicks in and allows you to do so by yourself. You can then habitually maintain a relaxed, tall posture.

👁 You can start to release tension by cultivating a habit of not forcing yourself into any posture, and instead close your eyes whenever you notice that you have slouched, tensed up or let your head tilt. With closed eyes it is easier to sense the tension that is pulling you out of alignment. Allow it to release – visualize those muscles relaxing and loosening up. Imagine that you *let* your head come up, that you *let* your neck lengthen, your chest lift, and your back widen. Notice how this changes your posture with ease. Take your time, as there often is more tension underneath the first layer you release.

British author, Olive L. Brown, wrote *Your Innate Power*, in which she combines the Bates Method with the Alexander Technique. She says: "FREE the head forward and up from the neck. Let it go up itself, do not deliberately put it there. It is not so much what you do as what you do not do that matters. In learning the new use you simply make a calm decision: 'No, I am not going to tighten. I am not going to pull that head back. I will not close in or sink into myself.' If you refuse deliberately to do any of these things the right thing does itself."[3]

When your posture needs work, I suggest you get some personal guidance from a somatic professional who can pinpoint and alleviate your most chronic postural issues. You can study and apply the work of F.M. Alexander, Milton Trager M.D., Esther Gokhale, Françoise Mézières, Moshe Feldenkrais, and others. Massage or osteopathic bodywork can also help vision considerably. Combine such somatic training with regular exercise to keep the postural improvements you make. A relaxed, tall body posture and a natural body alignment while in motion will help your vision improve more quickly.

Here are a few simple practices that may help release body tension for you and thereby reduce eyestrain.

Extend your eyes-closed mantra

If, for example, you notice an upper body slouch and a craned neck to compensate for the slouch, give yourself an extended mantra, similar to the "empty my eye sockets" suggestion I gave on page 38. Whenever you close your eyes, say to yourself: "Chest floats upward, shoulders drop down, neck releases, I have no eyes." This brief mental check of your most common strain patterns interrupts these patterns. I suggest you don't make conscious motions in response to such a mantra but simply allow the words to help you visualize the better posture and then "float" into it. The more often you interrupt your strain patterns, the sooner new relaxation patterns can establish themselves. So, close your eyes often and create your personal mantra to counterbalance each postural strain.

Neck stretches

A set of neck stretches can help release muscle tension when done gently and within your range of comfort:

- Left ear to left shoulder, then right ear to right shoulder (keep both shoulders down; just let your head drop sideways).
- Turn your head from left to right (chin to shoulder) and pull the opposite shoulder back to increase the stretch.

- Chin down to your chest, then gradually let your head tilt back as far as comfortable.
- Gentle head rotations. Do this a few times in both directions. While your head rotates, keep your eyes open (with blinking) and notice how your surroundings swing in the opposite direction!

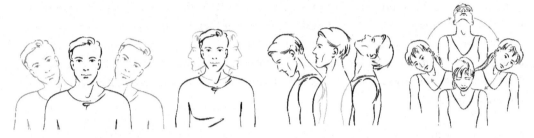

The Walking Swing

When some patients complained that their eyes felt strained after walking a short distance, Dr. Bates investigated the facts and taught them how to walk without straining their eyes. His advice was simple and effective – he encouraged them to imagine a swing.

You can practice the walking swing with the help of a straight line on the ground, such as a plank's edge in a wood floor, a grout line in a tile floor, or you can use an imaginary line that begins at your feet and stretches out in front of you.

Stand with the right foot to the right of the line and the left foot to the left of the line. Your chin is directly above the line. Now practice the relaxed way of walking and using the eyes. First take a few slow steps forward. When you lift your left foot to take a step, notice how your weight shifts to the right. Your body (including head and eyes) shifts slightly along with your weight to the right of the line. When the right foot steps forward your body moves back to the left. You may notice that your head and eyes cross the line with each step, which causes the line to swing in the direction opposite to the body's motion.

Outdoors, you can use a tall object to walk toward, such as a tree or lamp post. Do you notice the background behind the tree gently swings from side to side as you walk toward the tree? You may also notice a slight up and down motion with each step. When you walk at a regular pace, your own side-to-side motion becomes more subtle, and so does the swing, but it doesn't stop entirely.

Lastly, there is the more obvious far-to-near swing of all objects you pass by. The resulting motion in three directions is the walking swing. It happens with every step you take, yet how often do you notice?

The Running Swing

The walking swing can also be used while running. When Bates decided to take up long-distance running in his late 40s, he soon discovered from personal experience that any amount of strain during running created a major problem.

> About fifteen years ago I was ambitious to learn how to run long distances. At that time I was, it seemed to me, the poorest runner ever invented. I could not run a mile or even a quarter of a mile. To run a block brought on palpitation of the heart and the loss of breath and fatigue was sickening.[4]

A fitness trainer at his local gym told him that he did not breathe naturally but instead held his breath the whole distance. This knowledge was a great help to Bates, but he realized there was a more important key factor. He wrote: "The strain I was under when running interfered with my breathing and was a more important factor in the cause of 'fatigue' than the lack of air." So he decided to experiment further...

> In one race I ran about eight miles and I made all the effort possible, planning to keep running until I dropped. The experience was valuable. Before I fell, I lost all sense of effort, my sight failed, the ground appeared to be rising in front of me, I lost all perception of light, everything was midnight black. I had literally, actually, run myself into the ground. In a few minutes I was conscious. In spite of my protests they carried me away in an automobile.
>
> In another experiment I entered a race of twelve miles. Just as soon as my sight failed I stopped running and walked until my vision was again normal, when I would again run some more. By alternating the walking and running I was able to finish with a sprint. A policeman invited me to sit down. Before I knew it they had me in an ambulance, galloping to the hospital, with me protesting all the way. I have run in many races since, finished in good condition and have escaped the kind attentions of the police and the ambulance service.

Bates overcame his inability to run by learning not to strain his mind or his body while running. He used the swing to achieve this. According to a New York Times article in May 1918, Dr. Bates ran a marathon at the age of fifty-seven. He also encouraged others to run with relaxation, as evidenced by this letter from a young man who visited him in December 1919.[5]

> Besides improving my sight, the swing did many other things for me. I had never done any running before coming to New York, but I now began to experiment with that form of exercise, not expecting in the least to distinguish myself. In a week, however, I was able to run eleven miles, without fatigue or loss of breath, and without even

feeling sore or stiff afterward. This I attributed to the swing, which I kept up all the time I was running. When I did not do this, I quickly became tired.

Good posture prevents eyestrain during sleep

Posture is even important while you sleep. Dr. Bates discovered that most people strain their eyes much more in their sleep than they ever do when they are awake, and they aren't even aware of this. If you tend to wake up with worse vision, and feel tired first thing in the morning, you will want to prevent eyestrain during sleep. Here is Dr. Bates' advice:

> Posture during sleep has been studied. Lying on the face has generally been accompanied by an increase of eyestrain. Sleeping on the back with the arms and limbs extended with slight flexion is undoubtedly better than sleeping on the right or left side. A cramped posture is always wrong.

> The patient is not always conscious of his posture when asleep. In a number of cases observed by friends of the patient, one or both arms were held behind the head while asleep and this was strenuously denied by the patient when awake. The correction of this and other strained positions of the arms and limbs has been followed by decided benefit to the vision. Eyestrain during sleep produces or increases the symptoms of strain in various parts of the body.[6]

If you have worse vision in one eye, do you sleep mainly on that side? If the side of your face is pressed into the pillow for several hours, the resulting pressure on the eye can change the shape of the cornea and affect your vision in that eye for many hours. Ortho-keratology makes clever use of pressure on the cornea by specially made hard contact lenses that are worn overnight. The pressure of these lenses changes the shape of the cornea sufficiently that vision is good for the rest of the day. Of course, none of the original muscle tension has diminished, so clear vision doesn't last more than a day or two before the cornea reverts back to its previous shape and the hard contacts have to be used again. However, it does clearly show how pressure on the eyeball during sleep can influence your vision during the day, both for better or for worse.

Mirko from Switzerland noticed his astigmatism was worse in the morning and got better during the day. He realized that his mattress was somewhat worn out, causing him to wake up with a sore neck each morning. He decided to turn the mattress around. The next morning his vision was better, and over the next few days his sore neck disappeared – along with his astigmatism.

Going to sleep with your eyes in their most relaxed state allows you to effortlessly add eight hours of Bates Method practice per day! The cumulative effect of this extra relaxation time can make a huge difference to your vision over a period of a few weeks.

Additional tips to promote relaxing sleep

To help you fall asleep easier, switch off any full spectrum lamps an hour before bedtime, dim other lights if possible, and avoid using light-emitting screens during that hour. (See Chapter 15.) If any nagging or troublesome thoughts tend to keep you awake, keep a notebook and pen next to your bed and write those thoughts down. Journaling before bedtime has been extremely effective for me, as it allows me to let go of these thoughts. I know they will still be there in the morning if I want them back, and in the meantime, I can sleep without worrying that I'll forget something.

 Here are some excellent ways to prevent eyestrain during sleep.

- Observe the long swing or sway for a few minutes before going to bed.
- Read small print up close for a few minutes (without any effort!).
- Pretend to empty your eye sockets from all strain when you go to bed.
- Palm your eyes for a few minutes or longer, or until you fall asleep.
- Switch off or cover up all artificial lights in your bedroom.
- Sleep on your back with your arms at your side.

Pick one or combine all six! Then notice if you wake up with better vision than usual.

 Sleep in darkness

Researchers have found a strong correlation between the development of myopia in childhood and exposure to ambient light during sleep at night in the first two years after birth.[7] Babies who slept in darkness had a 9% prevalence of myopia in childhood, while more than triple that number – 31% – of babies exposed to just a small nightlight developed myopia, and as many as 48 out of every 100 babies who slept with room lights on in their first two years of life developed myopia in childhood. Sleeping in darkness is of great importance in those first few years, and it will benefit you too if you start adopting that habit now. If you don't do so already, turn off any bedroom lights, cover up digital displays such as from an alarm clock, and use curtains that minimize artificial light entering from streetlamps. The less artificial light in your bedroom, the better the rest you and your eyes will get. If you live in the country and don't have streetlights shining into your bedroom, you may not need curtains. Moonlight will not interfere with your rest like streetlights do; it isn't static, has a low intensity, and it resembles the full spectrum.

Exposure to sunlight helps regulate your wake-sleep cycle too, so both sun and darkness are important for a restful, regenerating sleep and better sight. A gentle awakening in the morning from the rising sun is also very beneficial; it helps decrease light sensitivity. If you can, keep a window open for a steady supply of fresh air.

If you still tend to wake up with worse vision, the following suggestions may be useful:

- As much as possible, sleep until you wake up naturally. If you must get up by a certain time, go to bed earlier so an alarm clock is not required. Regular use of an alarm clock basically guarantees that you are sleep-deficient, and you may need to sleep ten to twelve hours on some nights to catch up.

- When you wake up, keep your eyes closed and check for tension. If you notice any strain, let it go as much as you can. Gentle movement of your closed eyes may help achieve this – imagine watching birds soar in the sky.

- Keep your eyes closed until they naturally open by themselves. This may take some time, but it is very much worth waiting for, so reserve weekends or days when you can sleep in for this practice.

- To relax your eyes mentally before opening them, imagine that you have perfect vision. Notice if your eyes feel different when you imagine clear vision.

- Keep a favorite picture or object near your bed to look at when you open your eyes.

Sleeping outside in the daytime

If you find yourself tired during the day and in need of some sleep, it is actually nice to sleep outside, provided of course that you take precautions not to burn in summer, or get too cold in winter (set an alarm, sleep in the shade or cover up if necessary). I remember walking on a beach in the middle of a summer's day. An unusual tiredness I felt was causing my eyes to strain against the light, even though the sky was semi-overcast. I lay down on the beach to rest my eyes, and promptly fell asleep. I awoke an hour later with my eyes feeling incredibly rested, and the sunlight no longer bothered me at all. Dr. Bates wrote that sleeping in the sun is good for the eyes. He recommended that mothers do not cover their baby's eyes when they fall asleep outdoors in a stroller. Having experienced the difference it made to my tired eyes, I very much agree! It is only artificial light that I prefer to minimize or eliminate. (Also see Chapter 15.)

Massage and acupressure

Through the fascia, all muscles are interconnected, and therefore the eye muscles can be affected by tension in any part of the body. A full-body massage can be very beneficial, allowing you to reach a deep level of relaxation and a comfortable good posture, which will help your sight. A regular full-body massage isn't always an available option, but you can give your vision a boost by encouraging muscles around the eyes to release with a gentle self-massage, with or without the use of acupressure points.

Acupressure is based on acupuncture, but there are no needles involved. For acupressure you'll use the tips of your fingers to stimulate the points on the face that are related to vision. The pressure and movement from your fingers will bring circulation to these points and help release tension. I recommend doing acupressure and massage with your eyes closed. The exact location of the points is not so important; you will find the points that are in most need of massage by how sore they feel – those are the ones that need attention!

 Acupressure Points for Myopia

The image below shows the acupressure points which are related to myopia. It's good to regularly go over all these points and check them for any soreness. You can check them by putting light pressure on them with your fingertips or thumbs. If a point feels sore, don't press hard! Instead, give it a gentle massage with small circular motions or alternately press and release it with a soft touch. Choose according to which feels best to you. The length of time spent on each spot depends on the soreness. When the soreness has gone, move to the next spot.

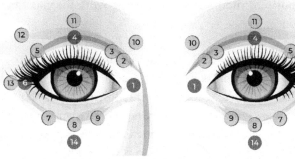

I typically start at point 1, at the corner of each eye next to the nose. Place the tip of your index fingers on each side of the nose and press them toward each other. Most people find these spots feel fine, but if you find either side is sore, linger there and massage it.

For point 2, use your thumbs, and press upwards on the underside of the bony ridge above the eye. Between points 2 and 4, approximately at point 3, still pressing upwards on the underside of the bone with your thumbs, you will feel a ridge in the bone. This point can be quite sore, so be gentle and take as much time as you need there. Then continue to press upwards against the bone while you move across to point 5 and toward 6. Feel free to check out the entire upper ridge, not just the spots shown in the image. Linger at any sore spot, while you can move on quickly from any spots that feel fine.

At point 6, switch back to using your fingertips. For points 7, 8 and 9 (and all along that lower bone) use gentle pressure downward on the top of the bone, taking care not to put any pressure on the eyeball itself.

When you have completed the rim circuit and find your fingers back at point 1, move up to point 10 on the inner edge of your eyebrows. From there, let your fingertips explore outwards over the entire length of your eyebrows (points 10, 11 and 12 and all points in between), looking for any sore spots to massage. From there, continue to your temples (point 13), and also check point 14 on the center of your cheeks.

According to Chinese Medicine, the four points shown in darker circles (1, 4, 6 and 14) may require stimulation to reduce myopia, rather than relaxation from gentle massage. To stimulate a point, rapidly shake it with your thumb or fingertip. Don't shake your head in the process; just shake the finger that's in contact with the point. Instead of shaking a point or alternating pressure on it, you can also hold a point steadily until you feel it softens up or any discomfort leaves.

Using the principles of color light therapy (see Chapter 15), shining a blue penlight directly on a point may also relax it, while a red penlight may stimulate it.

Not everyone reacts the same way to the points being stimulated and relaxed, so feel free to do the opposite if the above instructions do not seem to work for you and check if that makes a positive difference.

Acupressure point stimulation flows into massage

After checking for soreness in acupressure points, use all four fingers of both hands to massage your forehead and temples. Feel yourself letting go of any tension that is held there. You can continue massaging into the hairline and go over your skull. Go all the way to the back of the head, where the visual cortex is, and while you massage that area, open your eyes and be aware of seeing from the back of your head.

Next, go down to your neck and massage both sides. Squeeze into those neck muscles and let go of any tension that you may tend to hold there. Imagine the neck becoming soft and loose. Lastly, let one hand rest while the other hand massages the opposite shoulder. Notice any sore spots and spend extra time there. Imagine breathing into those spots and letting go of the tension on the exhale. Alternate and do the other shoulder. You'll probably feel a little more relaxed now!

Conclusion

Good vision is supported by a tall and relaxed posture, whether awake or asleep! A tall posture does not mean a military-type straight posture, because that involves a great deal of tension. What you are looking for is full-body dynamic relaxation. You want an ease of action without unnecessary strain that opposes your desired action; an effortless seeing without consciously trying to focus. Or, as Aldous Huxley put it:

> **Be active, and yet remain relaxed;**
> **don't strain and yet do your damndest;**
> **stop trying so hard and let the deep-seated intelligence of your body**
> **and the subconscious mind do the work as it ought to be done.**
> Aldous Huxley[8]

13. Breathe Freely

It will be obvious to you by now that the key to clear eyesight is dynamic relaxation of both body and mind. You see with your whole body. When all muscles are free to tense and relax as needed, your body works best. The more you approach vision holistically, releasing chronic tension wherever you find it, the sooner you'll see long-lasting results.

It was my eyesight teacher who first told me that breathing is important for clear vision, yet with his suggestions for deeper breathing, I was not able to transform my chronically shallow breathing pattern into something better. I could consciously breathe deeply for a few breaths when I thought about it, but three breaths later, I'd fall right back into my familiar, shallow pattern. I knew I ought to improve this aspect of my health and started looking for a breathing coach.

At a festival near Buffalo, New York, I met Mike White. I was there to teach about eyesight; Mike was there to teach about breathing. Unfortunately for me, we had been scheduled to teach our respective workshops at the same time in different locations, but at that event I took the opportunity to ask him my questions and concluded that this man knew what I needed to know. So I took the next opportunity to learn from him at an event we both taught at in Arizona a few months later.

I attended every one of Mike's classes there and invested in a one-hour private session. I distinctly remember the huge change this created in my breathing. I used to sleep in a fetal position, because tension in my upper body meant that sleeping on my back was simply uncomfortable. That night, I fell asleep on my back for the first time in as long as I could remember, with my breathing deep and steady. To my huge surprise, I woke up that way too: still on my back, very comfortable, breathing deeply and steadily. This unexpected major and fast improvement convinced me of the value of Mike's work, so I signed up for his teacher training course in North Carolina.

From Mike I learned that achieving better breathing was akin to achieving better eyesight – neither can be forced to improve; both only respond well to relaxation. I love that connection, and I expect you will too. Similar to eye exercises, breathing exercises tend to miss the point and can cause worse function through interference with what is supposed to happen naturally. Yogic breathing patterns such as "breathe in for four seconds, hold for two, breathe out for four" can never account for what the body actually needs in that moment, nor do you learn from such practices how to let go of tension that interferes with your natural breathing pattern.

Eyes need oxygen

Good breathing is an important element of good vision. That's because the retina is a large consumer of oxygen; it uses up oxygen more rapidly than many other parts of the body, including the brain.[1] Of course the brain requires lots of oxygen too, and because seeing is largely a mental process, it follows that if there is an insufficient oxygen supply, your vision will be negatively affected. Conversely, an abundant supply of oxygen to the eyes and brain will help you see better.

Dr. Bates wrote that many patients with imperfect sight are benefited by improved breathing.

> At one time I experimented with a number of patients, first having them hold their breath and test their vision, which was usually lower when they did not breathe. They became able to demonstrate that holding their breath was a strain and caused imperfect sight, double vision, dizziness and fatigue, while the deep breathing at once gave them relief.

> A man aged sixty-five had imperfect sight for distance and was unable to read fine print without the aid of strong glasses. After practicing deep breathing he became able at once to read diamond type quite perfectly, as close as 6 inches from the eyes. The benefit was temporary but, by repetition, the improvement became more permanent.[2]

Margaret Corbett mentioned in one of her books how one of her students, who had cataracts before the vision training, showed great improvement, which was observed by an eye doctor through his ophthalmoscope. In one eye, the cataract had entirely gone; in the other, a small amount of cloudiness remained – but only until the student was instructed to breathe deeply, at which point the eye doctor observed that this last remnant of cataract cleared up too. When the student held his breath, the cloudiness came back; when he practiced better breathing, it disappeared again. Margaret concluded: "If deep breathing will do this for a seriously affected eye, one can realize how great the benefit to normal or nearly normal vision."[3]

One of the first people who came to me for vision improvement after my training in breathing development, was a woman whose breathing seemed very restricted. She had been in a car accident and was still using crutches to walk. Her upper body showed a lot of tension. I decided to teach her how to improve her breathing before addressing her vision habits. After just a few minutes of helping her loosen up her breathing, she joyfully announced that she could already read an extra line on the chart behind me.

A pioneer in breathing development

Just as eyesight had a pioneer in Dr. Bates who was attuned to nature's ways, so breathing had a pioneer who was also attuned to nature's ways. His name was Carl Stough, and his work became known as "Breathing Coordination." Stough (1926-2000) was a choir director who was keen to improve his choir's performance by teaching the singers how to better support their voices with their breath. Through research and practical application, he became an expert on the function of the human breathing mechanism.

Stough's choirs became famous, and his expertise on breathing became so well known that he was asked to help emphysema patients in military hospitals. This request initially scared him, as he knew nothing about this lung disease. But as he began working with these patients, he found they were gasping for air using accessory muscles that are not meant to be part of natural breathing. With gentle touch, he was able to help them release this muscular tension and found they made steady improvements. This resulted in more requests to work in hospitals, at one point taking part in a medically supervised study where one group of emphysema patients was treated with a new intermittent pressure machine, while the other group was under Stough's care. The study was prematurely stopped because several of the group that used the machine had died, while several of Stough's group had recovered completely and were able to leave the hospital. Stough went on to work with athletes, and at the 1968 Mexico Olympics, he helped the U.S. Track and Field team win more medals than ever before in its history.

Stough said that, contrary to general belief, the most important phase of breathing is the exhale. If a container is to be refilled, it must first be emptied of its contents.[4] Dr. Robert Nimbs, chief of pulmonary medicine at the Veteran's Administration Medical Center in West Haven, Connecticut (the largest hospital for patients with respiratory diseases on the East Coast at the time), commented on Stough's work in the 1997 documentary, *Breathing, the Source of Life*:

> Many studies that have been done in the last five years have been done at the wrong end of the spectrum. They studied how forcibly the diaphragm can pull down in a respiration. That's not the important thing. The important thing is what Carl has shown, that the diaphragm can be gotten to relax and go up, to rise so that during respiration it can come down. It's got plenty of strength, so there's no need to measure the strength.

To me, that is the key. Like eye muscles that have plenty of strength to do their job despite being thought of as "weak" and in need of "strengthening," the muscles that control your breathing also have plenty of strength, and it is not weakness but undue tension that interferes with their natural function. Only in learning to release that tension can improvement and healing be achieved.

Stough wrote the following in his book, *Dr. Breath:*

> Because of the interrelationship of the respiratory system and the nervous system, the condition of one influences the condition of the other. Tension directly affects the breathing mechanism and tends to damage it, causing susceptibility to respiratory complaints and disturbing other systems of the body in turn. As tension mounts, muscles tighten and destructive air pressure builds within the lungs. Unless the pressure is released, nervous mannerisms are manifest and a disturbing interaction of one system upon another is established. Most people have become so accustomed to their tensions that they are unable to relax. Tension is accepted as a normal condition of contemporary life and is indirectly perhaps the greatest of the destroyers.[4]

Carl Stough said the muscles of your breathing system are designed to operate in a perfectly coordinated synergism to give you the maximum breathing efficiency of which you are capable and to give it to you with a minimum expenditure of energy. In other words, getting out of your own way and stopping any interference with what is naturally supposed to happen will bring your breathing back to its optimal function.

So, let's have a quick look at your main breathing muscle – the diaphragm – and then I will give you the one breathing practice that I find most effective for releasing undue breathing strain.

The diaphragm

The diaphragm is a dome-shaped muscle that divides the thoracic cavity (containing the rib cage, the lungs, and the heart) from the abdominal cavity. It is attached to the lower ribs.

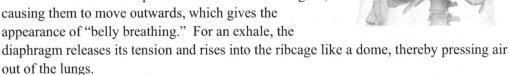

For an inhale, the diaphragm contracts, causing it to flatten and move down. It then pushes on the abdominal organs, causing them to move outwards, which gives the appearance of "belly breathing." For an exhale, the diaphragm releases its tension and rises into the ribcage like a dome, thereby pressing air out of the lungs.

Efficient use of the diaphragm

Imagine using a bicycle pump to pump air into a flat tire, but pulling the pump up only an inch or two before pushing it back down again. It will take a long time to fill the tire with air because this way of pumping is not an efficient use of the pump mechanism. In contrast, if you pull the pump all the way up before pushing it back down, you will transfer lots of air into the tire with every pumping action, thereby making more efficient use of the equipment. Your diaphragm works like that bicycle pump.

The higher the rise of the diaphragm on the exhale, the more stale air is expelled, and the more efficient the following inhale will be. The more you allow your diaphragm to relax upwards on the exhale, the more efficient your breathing becomes. Tension interferes with the upward movement of the diaphragm, resulting in a smaller range of motion for the diaphragm and therefore a shallower breath. To allow for bigger, fuller in-breaths, the diaphragm needs to rise higher on exhalation. This can be achieved by more relaxation, by better posture, and by practicing long, easy, slow exhales.

Natural breathing is a 360-degree motion

Natural breathing always fills the lungs from the base at the middle of the body, and the action of breathing occurs principally in this middle area. Sit or stand and lay your hands on your belly and lower ribs, feeling the motion of this area as you breathe. You should feel an outward motion when you breathe in, and an inward motion when you breathe out.

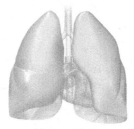

Human lungs

Now lay your hands on your sides at the lower ribs, and notice a similar motion happening there, albeit to a lesser degree. Lastly, lay your hands on your back at the lower ribs. Here too you ought to feel a slight outward motion when you breathe in, and an inward motion as you breathe out. The entire circumference of the mid-region should contract and expand with the movement of air into and out of the lungs.

Back motion in breathing is often neglected, but is important because your lungs are larger at the back than they are at the front. You may not even be aware that your back moves while breathing, or perhaps it simply doesn't move at all. If that's the case, it needs a little attention. If your back is not moving due to tight muscles there, the natural breathing pattern is lost and other muscles (such as the shoulders) will get involved in an attempt to "help breathe." You're then moving even further away from the natural breathing pattern.

If you simply lay your hands on your middle back and focus your attention on this area, it will sometimes be enough to return motion there. Once you have felt it, you can consciously use the awareness and sensation of the back motion to help maintain natural breathing at times where you otherwise might have tensed the back muscles.

If you do not feel any motion in the back while breathing, sit down on a chair and place your feet flat on the floor. Let your upper body bend forward from the hips, and let your hands slowly slide down from your knees toward your feet. If you can, let your upper body rest on your upper legs, and allow your head to hang down. Rest in this position and notice your breathing. You can move one or both hands to your lower back to feel if any movement is happening there now. Usually, due to the constriction of breathing space for the belly in this position, the back will release and allow for more breathing motion. If it does, enjoy the sensation of back breathing for a minute, then slowly come up and notice the change this back breathing makes to your overall breathing.

Other signs of a natural breathing pattern
Besides the 360-degree motion of natural breathing, the following are other indicators that you are breathing well.

- **Nose breathing**

In his book *Body, Mind & Sport*, John Douillard, D.C.,[5] writes about the importance of breathing through the nose. The nose filters incoming air through its hairs, and moistens and warms the air before it reaches the lungs. Douillard recommends breathing through the nose at all times, even during aerobic activity, where many of us have a tendency to breathe through the mouth instead. Although nose breathing under those conditions will likely slow you down at first, he says that, with practice, it will take you beyond your current ability and you'll experience quicker recovery times.

- **Resting breath rate is low**

The resting breath rate is three to eight complete breaths per minute (a complete breath is inhalation, exhalation, and pause). If you breathe faster, concentrate on slowing down your exhale with the practice given on the next page, while allowing the inhale to be what it naturally wants to be.

- **Exhale is followed by a pause**

A short pause follows each exhale, lasting from half a second to three seconds or more; this pause is a natural rest for the autonomic nervous system.

- **Yawn freely**

Yawning balances the levels of carbon dioxide and oxygen in the body. It helps to moisten dry eyes and it even pumps cerebral spinal fluids, so despite Western culture's frowning on this natural urge when done in public, please yawn freely because it's good for you!

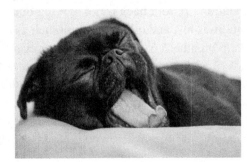

- **Dynamic relaxation and natural breathing**

Dynamic relaxation means doing more with less effort. We tend to try too hard. For example, many people tend to pull up their shoulders when asked to take a deep inhale. Your shoulder muscles are not part of your natural breathing mechanism, so if you have the tendency to pull them up as you breathe in deeply, pay extra attention to relaxing them down instead.

In *Free Your Breath, Free Your Life,* Dennis Lewis writes: "Our efforts are based on force, on will power, not on skill and sensitivity. The more we **try** to breathe naturally, the more tension we create in our minds, emotions and bodies, and the more we restrict the movement of our diaphragm and other breathing muscles. This unnecessary tension wastes energy... One of the main keys to learning natural, healthy breathing is a sense of effortlessness and comfort... Be sure to work slowly, gently and patiently... try less and enjoy more."[6]

The gentle number count

Working slowly, gently and patiently is the key to receiving the most benefit from this one breathing practice that I use most often with my students. It is based on the work of Carl Stough.

When you first practice the gentle number count, lie down on your back on a firm surface (like a yoga mat on the floor). For extra comfort you can place a pillow under your knees and one under your head. With full upper body support in this position it will be easier to avoid unnecessary tension. After you have experienced long, relaxed exhales and natural inhales when lying down, you can also practice the number count while sitting or standing.

The point of the gentle number count is to become able to extend your exhale naturally, through sound, not through effort. Because air is required to produce sound and your voice is created by an exhale, how well you are doing will be reflected by the length of time you can effortlessly sustain a sound and by the quality of your voice. To begin with, though, the practice starts in silence, counting numbers in your head only, not out loud.

 Practicing the gentle number count

Lie down and let's begin. First, check that you are very comfortable and that your jaw is loose (press on the back of the jaw and massage it if this area feels sore). Start to silently count numbers, but only while you exhale. Count smoothly and steadily without pausing between numbers. Let 1-2-3-4-5-6-7-8-9-10 take about three seconds. So, mentally take out those dashes between the numbers and treat them as one long word: 12345678910. If you are still exhaling at 10, instantly start the 1 to 10 count again; no pause. As soon as you feel your inhale wants to come, stop counting, let an inhale happen, and start counting again at the next exhale. If the inhale comes after having only counted to 3 or 4, that's fine, don't push to 10, that's not the goal! During the next exhale, again count silently. Keep counting silently on each exhale and notice what happens to your inhales when you let them happen by themselves.

If this is comfortable and you do not notice any tension in your body, you can start using your voice instead of the silent count. Begin with a low count (perhaps 1-2-3, or 1-2-3-4-5 at most) in your normal speaking voice and then continue to count silently as you exhale further. Wait for your inhale to come. Repeat this low audible count followed by silent counting on each exhale until it seems very easy to do.

You can then increase the audible count a little each time, taking care to do only as much as you feel you can do comfortably and effortlessly. For some that means an increase by two numbers at a time, while others may be able to increase by five. Feel free to lower your voice to a whisper toward the end of each count. With gradual rises in the count, your inhales will tend to deepen. If you feel the start of tension anywhere in your torso, or you notice a tendency to want to force the count, stop counting and wait for the inhale.

You will end up counting from 1 to 10 repeatedly, depending on the length of your exhale. As you get to the end of each exhale, say the numbers more softly, and let the last few numbers be silent; those are your breathing pause. Always allow each inhale to come in by itself, letting it be however big it wants to be.

During the exhale, you may let your knees move gently from side to side to help release any tension from your lower back. To help relax the upper back, raise your arms straight above you (keeping the shoulders down on the floor and relaxed), clasp your hands together, and let your arms swing gently from side to side while you exhale. You may find that you are able to count further while making these gentle, rhythmic movements.

When you first start practicing the number count, speak the numbers in a soft, smooth voice. As your ability increases over time, you can develop your breathing further by speaking louder or by singing, being sure to not pressure the sound but to keep a natural voice. A perfect natural voice is the result of effortlessly coordinated respiratory mechanics that allow the entire surface of the lungs to be compressed evenly so that air flows over the vocal folds, rather than being forced over them.

Stay relaxed throughout the practice, with your shoulders down and chest open. The inhale should always be a spontaneous response to the prolonged, relaxed exhale. Think of the inhale not as something you do, but as effortlessly "receiving" air into your lungs, similar to effortlessly receiving light into your eyes.

If you place one hand on your abdomen and one on your chest during the exhale, you may feel how smoothly the diaphragm rises on each exhale and how your abdomen smoothly sinks down toward the spine. If the diaphragm tenses at any time, you are likely to feel some pressure in your lower abdomen, and you know you are trying too hard at that moment. Let it go and start over. If the lower abdomen tenses or comes up during the audible count, stop counting audibly and return to silent counting.

If you have a serious respiratory condition, it is best to get guided through this process and it may be good to stay with the long, silent exhale.

Good times to practice the number count are first thing in the morning, right before any physical exercise, and last thing at night before going to sleep. The more you practice this number count, the faster your diaphragm will relax and move naturally. Let your comfort level guide you in determining the duration of your practice. Whether you do just a few breaths or as much as ten minutes at a time, it will help overcome shallow breathing and will keep you relaxed day and night!

Tips for the gentle number count

Practicing the gentle number count is one of the best ways of relaxing and reducing overall muscle tension. If the gentle number count has not gone smoothly for you, replace the numbers with a simpler sound, such as la-la-la-la-la or start with the sound of just one vowel, and learn to make this one vowel sound longer and longer, effortlessly of course. The more you practice this, and the gentler you allow it to be, the better your results will be.

For some people, it helps to imagine that they are still breathing in while they are exhaling. This "inhalation sensation" during an exhale cuts into any tendency to force the exhale, making the whole process effortlessly effortless ☺. Try it; see if it works for you.

Many people can reach a high count of about 100 on a single breath, which takes fifteen to twenty seconds. After the muscles have released chronic tension and developed tone, your high count may average thirty or forty seconds on a single breath.

Vision success through better breathing

George, my "laser swing" student who took lessons via email to overcome his -4 myopia, had a shallow breathing pattern. Through taking my course he came to realize how much breathing can affect vision. He thought about the connection between lack of oxygen, lactic acid fermentation and muscle tension and decided that perhaps relaxed breathing was a way of getting his eye muscles to relax too. He describes his little experiment:

I lay down and palmed. I usually start to feel some type of stiffness in my eyes when they are closed, even when they move. So, instead of paying attention to my head, I focused on my breathing. After doing what you said in the lesson on breathing, my eye muscles just loosened up. I did not even palm for five minutes. It probably wasn't three. I opened my eyes and could see 20/70 to 20/60. This better vision did go away, but it came back shortly. While riding in the car today, I had a flash that lasted longer than usual. Breathing is more important than I realized at first.

Compromised breathing indicators and some relaxation-promoting suggestions
If one or more of the compromised breathing indicators listed below affects your breathing ability, this may be a good time to make some changes to help you return to natural breathing. If you do, your whole life will be enriched, not just your breathing or your vision.

Compromised breathing indicators	Relaxation-promoting suggestions
1. Tense muscles	All your muscles are interconnected through the fascia surrounding them. To help release overall tension, go for a walk to warm the muscles, then stretch your body and massage any tense muscles. Do the same after stress. Give yourself plenty of TLC (Tender Loving Care!).
2. Tendency to hold the breath	Become aware of times when you hold your breath, whether during strenuous exercise, during stress, or periods of deep concentration, etc. When you catch yourself holding your breath, exhale, count silently while exhaling, and wait for a natural inhale to come by itself. (The natural 2 to 4 second pause after the exhale is not breath-holding.)
3. Forced breathing pattern	Let go of any ideas about how you should be breathing. Let your body lead you into a natural rhythm. Use the gentle number count to increase diaphragm relaxation.
4. Hyperventilation	Hyperventilation indicates that the blood pH is dropping below safe levels. If hyperventilation is common, dietary concerns will need to be addressed, because an overly acidic diet results in lower blood pH, which leads to shallow and rapid breathing as the body does its best to return the blood pH to its preferable slightly alkaline level.
5. Shallow breathing	Use all areas of lung expansion: belly, sides, back, chest (remember the 360-degree motion of the breath). Slow down or lengthen the exhale, gently let all air flow out, then wait for an inhale to come naturally, unforced. Repeat until you feel better and the breathing rhythm is down to less than eight per minute.

6. Slouched posture	Take the time for regular (outdoor) exercise and learn to relax habitually tense muscles. Check if sitting in your chair restricts your breathing pattern. If so, you may want to add a layer of foam to the back to improve its support of your posture. Experiment with layers of foam and their position until you feel you can sit comfortably *and* breathe freely.
7. Carrying bags	If you regularly carry a bag over one shoulder, start alternating with the other shoulder to balance out your spine. For a while I thought backpacks were the answer, but with regular use even those can cause breathing restriction as the shoulders tend to come forward. My solution is to carry less "stuff," and I use the hip strap on my backpack when I need it.
8. Tight belly muscles	Pay attention to letting your belly move out freely with each inhale. Learn to let go and relax. A good massage therapist may be able to help release habitually tight belly muscles.
9. Air pollution / Smoking	Use filter-masks whenever you must work in polluted air. Avoid tobacco smoke and other airborne pollutants as much as possible. Regularly visit a forest or beach.
10. Cosmetics	Be aware that perfumes and aftershaves tend to be full of toxic chemicals which the manufacturer is not obliged to show on the ingredients list. Avoid these products and use natural alternatives instead of the chemical cocktails, because the strong smell of the latter causes many people to hold their breath.[7]
11. Dehydration	Lungs use a quart of water every day to stay moist; drink water to quench your thirst.
12. Tight clothing	Allow room for the breath: allow for the 360-degree expansion of belly and chest areas. Wear loose-fitting pants/skirts and loosen up a tight belt, tight bra, narrow shirt-necks, neckties, etc.
13. Overweight	Being overweight makes it harder for the diaphragm to move down on an inhale. Also, high blood fat causes a decrease in oxygen uptake, which affects the body's pH balance, which in turn will affect the breath rate. Don't aim to "lose weight"; lost items are far too easily found. Instead, aim to "gain lightness": get more outdoor light, eat lighter foods, enjoy light exercise, and enjoy the new, lighter you.
14. Lung diseases / Asthma	Take care of all the above to ease the breathing. Check if you have any food allergies that could be contributing to mucus in your airways – common problem-causers are dairy products and wheat. You may want to drink only fresh fruit and vegetable juices for a week to help reduce mucus in the airways.

14. A Carrot a Day Keeps the Eye Doctor Away?

Dr. Bates seldom mentioned nutrition, probably because he believed that a change in diet does not relieve the symptoms of eyestrain.[1] This made sense to me, as my own myopia did not budge at all when I adopted a healthier diet, yet it disappeared as soon as I learned to see without straining my eyes. However, various people have told me they experienced a return to clear vision after a switch to more wholesome food and, as eye diseases are often linked to more than just eyestrain, it is wise to ensure you consume the nutrients that nourish your eyes.

Bates' wife Emily occasionally did give dietary advice – for example, to a young boy with red eyelids that she suspected were partially due to eating too much candy and other sweets that he was fond of.[2] Emily also wrote about a woman who complained of itching eyelids, which she treated mainly with sunlight. Yet, in the article, she added:

> We seldom advise patients about the amount of water they drink, or the kind of food they eat, but this patient had brought up the subject herself. My experience for many years with clinic patients has taught me much about the mistakes people make in eating the wrong food and not drinking sufficient water. I feel quite sure that my patient's assistance and intelligence about eating unseasoned foods and drinking a large quantity of water every day helped to cure the irritation and discomfort of her eyes.[3]

Studying health

I was a sickly child – in fact, my mother has often told me that she didn't expect me to live beyond age ten. Basically, health eluded me until I started studying it in my mid-twenties. For twenty-five years I relied on doctors for my health, because modern medicine leads us to believe that we are born with a deficiency of drugs and an excess of body parts. Since then I've learned that we mostly just tend to overdose on unnatural food and drink, and all we really lack is a thorough understanding of the laws of nature.

I don't claim to be a nutritional expert; I have simply delved into this topic fairly deeply, first for my own general health, and later to help my students find answers for various visual challenges. The research seems complex and at times confusing and contradicting. I do not have all the answers here and I trust there will be more extensive studies in the future to provide a clearer picture of how diet can help or hinder vision. Although as a species you'd expect that we all might thrive on one "perfect" human diet, I don't think we are all the same – what sustains a human living in the tropics may not sustain a human living in the Arctic Circle, and vice versa; what works for one doesn't necessarily work the same for another. So, pick and choose the foods that appeal to you, make small changes when you feel inspired to, discard what you don't like and continue with whatever brings the results you want. This chapter is mainly intended to help you make some better choices if you suspect your eyes could benefit from a dietary change.

> **Please live a healthy life; medicine is an imperfect science.**
> Hunter "Patch" Adams, M.D.[4]

Nutrition's role in eye health

If you study the causes of health, you are bound to spend a large portion of your time studying nutrition. If you study disease to become a medical doctor in the U.S. or Europe, nutrition turns out to be the subject of least importance, taking up less than one day out of four years of training. Isn't that odd? You cannot expect good dietary advice from most medical doctors – they simply don't know enough about it! Eye doctors are no exception to this. Unless they study ocular nutrition after their training, which very few do, the idea that carrots are good for your eyes is about as extensive as their nutritional knowledge goes, and your grandmother probably already told you that.

Now, especially if you have been diagnosed with any eye disease, you will need better advice than this. Your doctor saying "It's old age" or "Your eyes are genetically weak" isn't going to help you. In fact, thinking such comments are true puts you in a victim role, where you believe there is nothing you can do other than faithfully filling your doctor's prescription or subjecting your eyes to their recommended surgery. Until medical and optometry colleges catch up with reality, you must educate yourself on what your body and eyes need for optimal health.

Although myopia and astigmatism are typically symptoms of eyestrain, and releasing strain brings back clarity, tense muscles can remain tense if your diet contains too much sugar or lacks sufficient calcium or magnesium. This can keep muscles in spasm and cramps. So, even in cases of simple eyestrain, nutrition may play a role. In cases of eye disease, where relaxation can greatly assist recovery because it increases circulation, I believe nutrition ought to be seen as a major factor in bringing about improvement. If you have been diagnosed with an eye disease, also read Chapter 24.

Bad diet can lead to blindness

In 2014, a fourteen-year-old boy in Perth, Australia, was going blind and a variety of local eye doctors and hospitals could not help him. Eventually, his mother took him to a specialist in Sydney. The professor they met there had worked in Kenya and was familiar with symptoms of vitamin A deficiency. As it turned out, the boy's problem was his fussy eating habits since age five – nothing except chicken, potatoes, dry bread and Coke – which had left him so malnourished he was going blind. With vitamin therapy and a change in diet, his right eye mostly recovered after two years but his left eye sustained permanent damage.[5]

Most diets are not that bad, yet many of us could probably eat somewhat healthier than we do now, and if a small change can substantially help your sight, it is worth looking into! If you don't know what to add to your diet or what to leave out to help your eyes, the following pages aim to provide food for thought – some ideas and suggestions to consider.

From studies done in the past, many nutrients have been found to be important to your visual system. Your eyes' nutrient requirements are high, so a nutrient deficiency can show up in them before it affects other organs. Doing what it takes for your eyes to be healthy therefore also helps your general health.

Nutrients required for healthy vision

Based on a list of links which researchers found between certain nutrient deficiencies and specific visual challenges (see Appendix F), it is evident that the following nutrients are involved in keeping the eyes healthy:

> Vitamins: A, B-complex (B-1, B-2, B-3, B-5, B-6, B-7, B-9, B-12), C, D, E and K. Alpha Lipoic Acid, Amino Acids, Beta Carotene, Bioflavonoids, Calcium, Choline, Chromium, Copper, CoQ10, Enzymes, Essential Amino Acids such as Cystine, Essential Fatty Acids (EFAs), especially Omega 3 and 6 Fatty Acids including Alpha Linoleic Acid (ALA), Gamma-amino butyric acid (GABA), Glucosamine, Glutathione, Inositol, Iodine, Iron, Lutein, Lycopene, Magnesium, Manganese, Molybdenum, Para-amino benzoic acid (PABA), Phosphorus, Potassium, Quercetin, Rutin, Selenium, Taurine, Vanadium, Zeaxanthin, and Zinc.
> And not to forget these essentials: sunlight, water and clean air.

How exactly these nutrients work in the eyes or how much of each is needed, is beyond the scope of this book. But knowing they *are* needed leads to these obvious next questions: So where do you get all these nutrients? Do you have to use supplements or can you simply get them from your diet?

Sources of eye-essential nutrients

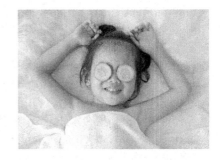

Luckily, getting these nutrients from your diet isn't as hard to do as supplement sellers would like you to believe... So rather than spending time and money on buying supplements, spend a little time learning which nutrients are in which foods, or what the body requires to make its own supply. In Appendix G you'll find a list of the eye-essential nutrients alongside some of their food sources. This can help you choose which foods to add to your diet if you are dealing with a deficiency.

Best food for your eyes

Most people instantly think of carrots when asked to name the best food for their eyes. You may be surprised to learn that this belief stems from a myth invented by the British Royal Air Force in 1940 to hide the fact that they were the first to successfully use radar. At the beginning of World War II, the U.K., the U.S., the Soviet Union, France, Italy, Japan and Germany each had explored and researched radar – but only the U.K. had developed a fully-functioning network. In the Battle of Britain, the British fighter pilot John Cunningham became the first person to shoot down an enemy plane at night with the help of radar. The RAF put out the story in the British newspapers that he and his fellow night pilots owed their exceptional night vision (and their suddenly improved shooting accuracy) to eating lots of carrots. A similar myth has been circulating about bilberry jam.

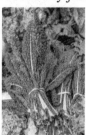

The number one food for the eyes is, in fact, kale, with spinach coming in a close second. Kale is highest in lutein and zeaxanthin, which are needed for a healthy macula and thus for sharp central vision, plus kale is a great source of vitamins C and K. It's high in beta carotene and contains vitamins B-1, B-2, B-3, B-6 and B-9, as well as alpha linolenic acid, calcium, copper, iron, magnesium, manganese, phosphorus, potassium, and zinc.

Lacinato kale

BEST FOOD FOR YOUR EYES*

LEAFY GREENS	**kale, spinach**, collard greens, Brussels sprouts, turnip greens, chard, mustard greens, dandelion greens, lettuce, beet greens, endive, bok choi, Napa cabbage, arugula, dock leaves
LEGUMES	**edamame/soybeans, lentils**, kidney beans, chickpeas/garbanzo beans, black beans, navy beans, white beans, green peas, roman beans, yellow beans, split peas, pink beans, adzuki beans, fava beans, mung beans, carob
OTHER VEGETABLES	**asparagus, broccoli**, carrots, sweet potatoes, potatoes, cauliflower, garlic, onions (red, yellow, spring), corn, red cabbage, garden cress, radicchio, leeks, watercress, butternut squash, acorn squash, summer squash, pumpkin, muskmelon, celery, alfalfa sprouts, sea vegetables, sauerkraut, okra
FRUITS	**citrus fruit, avocados, tomatoes**, bananas, apricots, sweet red peppers, hot chili peppers, mangoes, papayas, guavas, kiwis, figs, peaches, pomegranates, strawberries, prunes, pineapple, goji berries, raisins, raspberries, grapes, apples (unpeeled), cantaloupe melon, cranberries, currants, olives, pears, passion fruit, persimmons, elderberries, dates

NUTS	**almonds, walnuts, peanuts,** pine nuts, pistachios, cashews, pecans, hazelnuts/filberts, brazil nuts, chestnuts, macadamias
SEEDS	**sunflower, sesame, pumpkin,** flax, chia, mustard, squash, watermelon, poppy, camelina, perilla; cacao (unsweetened), coconuts
HERBS/SPICES	**parsley,** basil, coriander, spearmint, thyme, black pepper, dill, lovage
MUSHROOMS	**cremini,** maitake, shiitake, Portobello, white
GRAINS	**oats,** buckwheat, barley, brown rice, wild rice, quinoa

* = Not all foods are listed by their proper botanical classification. For example: peanuts are legumes, almonds and cashews are technically seeds, but most people think of them as nuts, so that is where I've listed them.

There simply is no better way to nourish your body and eyes than nature's way, i.e., to eat delicious fresh, whole foods such as those listed above. For the best nutritional value, your diet should include lots of unprocessed, whole, fresh, ripe foods that ideally are grown in nutrient-rich soil without the use of pesticides, herbicides or other toxins.

 Add a green smoothie to your diet

If possible, aim to include in your diet a daily smoothie made with fresh whole fruits and vegetables! My own favorite smoothie contains a few simple ingredients that are great for eyesight and it also tastes delicious. I simply blend two or three oranges with several leaves of dark kale or a handful of spinach, a stalk of celery, plus any extras that appeal to me in that moment, such as some frozen fruit on a warm day. Add a banana if you like a smoother texture. Sometimes I flavor it lightly with cinnamon, turmeric, kelp or dulse. Add a little water (or coconut water or watermelon) and blend it all together until smooth. Cheers!

 Chew well

Although smoothies are easy to swallow if you use a good blender, it is still important to chew and mix such drinks with your saliva so digestive enzymes can start their job before you swallow, resulting in better digestion and absorption of those much-needed nutrients.

 Healthy lifestyle

Good nutrition is important but cannot stand on its own. In addition to eating well, a truly healthy lifestyle involves getting sufficient exercise or play time, sunshine, fresh air, clean water, adequate rest and sleep, and having emotional poise, a sense of purpose, and loving relationships (which includes being kind and loving to yourself).

👁 Hydration – healthy alternatives to dehydrating options

A well-hydrated body is like a well-oiled engine, it simply works a lot better. If you prefer dehydrating drinks such as sodas, coca cola, coffee, alcohol or sugared fruit juices over water, you are basically dehydrating your body instead of hydrating it. In addition, sodas are highly acidic, creating a need for even more water as well as calcium to restore the pH balance. It's best to avoid such beverages.

How do you know you drink enough water? The answer is: when your urine is pale yellow. Certain medications and supplements with an excess of vitamin B-2 can cause deeper colors, but in general, if your urine isn't clear or pale yellow, you are dehydrated. Listen to your body's thirst signals (sometimes they resemble hunger signals, so drink before you eat) and choose plain water or fresh coconut water to quench that thirst.

Supplement caution

Supplements can easily provide too much of a good thing, thus turning into toxic excess. This is especially true for vitamins A, C, B-2 and E and for copper, zinc, iron and selenium.

Many vision-specific supplements have high doses of vitamin A and/or beta carotene. Both are nutrients the eyes need, yet they are far more beneficial for you when they come from your food and can actually be detrimental to your health in the form of supplements. An excessive intake of vitamin A and beta carotene is a potential health problem due to an increased risk of cancer and is a contributor to osteoporosis.[6]

Vitamin C is a common supplement and it too, in mega-doses such as 10,000 mg, can lead to visual problems, especially causing floaters and increasing the risk of vitreous detachment, retinal detachment, macular pucker, cellophane maculopathy, cataracts and macular degeneration.[7] In contrast, eating one or more oranges per day reduces the risk of macular degeneration by 60%.[8,9]

Typically, supplements are not as effective as their fresh food counterparts. Optometrist Benjamin C. Lane reported the following on the effect of diet on the quality of the tear-film, especially for contact lens users:

> We also found and reported that the food-obtained-folate (B-9) appears to be far more effective in protecting eye and visual function than the shelf-life-assured pharmacological form found in vitamin bottles.[10]

In general, be wary that most supplements contain synthetic vitamins or minerals to keep costs down. Ingredients such as Ferrous Fumarate, Chromic Chloride, Magnesium Stearate, Manganese Sulfate and Sodium Selenite are toxic and are best avoided. If you do choose pills, look for brands that are 100% natural, which means they are food-sourced. If they do not claim to be 100% natural, they likely contain cheap chemical or synthetic products that are not good for you.[11]

Proper nutrition is not difficult with a balanced, healthy diet, but if you feel off-balance, it may be a good idea to consult with a health counselor/nutritionist. The nutrient(s) you need may work best when taken together with other nutrients, and absorption may be hindered by some which should be avoided at the same meal.

Temporarily using supplements to overcome a deficiency can be helpful, yet it is smart to ensure that your new diet includes the nutrients needed so that the supplements can eventually be stopped. Obtaining nutrients from your food typically makes it much harder or impossible to accidentally overdose, but there are some exceptions. For example, one Brazil nut per day provides all the selenium your body requires, while eating a handful creates an overdose. Limit your Brazil nut intake to just one a day to be safe. Your goal is to get sufficient amounts of all healthful nutrients, in their proper balance, without overdosing on any one. In all health issues, use common sense, and gather as much information as you can.

 What to avoid

To promote health, it's not only important to consider what you eat but also what you leave out of your diet. If you currently have health or vision challenges, the following are best avoided:

- **All refined sugars and substitutes**: white, brown, beet, cane, raw, turbinado, fructose, dextrose, maltose, glucose, lactose, sucralose, aspartame, neotame, agave, molasses, corn syrup, rice syrup, sorghum syrup, barley malt, maltodextrin, fruit sugar, saccharin, stevia, truvia, xylitol, natural sweetener, and all artificial sweeteners. Fruit sugar, when listed as a separate ingredient, is also a refined sugar, so avoid it! Maple sugar and coconut sugar are only marginally better; they are still highly refined and far from healthy. Raw honey can be a substitute (except for babies) in sensible, small quantities. It is best to satisfy your sweet tooth by eating whole, fresh ripe fruits.

> **The more sugar in the diet, the greater the incidence of myopia.
> Refined sugar, while being processed inside the body, uses up
> huge quantities of vitamins and minerals, particularly calcium,
> sodium and phosphorus. The eyes need the whole gamut of these
> vitamins and minerals for good health.**
> Dr. Dhiren Gala, O.D.[12]

- **Alcohol** destroys many vital nutrients; regular alcohol drinkers will require a higher dosage of vitamins.

- **Caffeinated beverages** dehydrate you. These include coffee, soft drinks, regular tea and any herbal tea that contains caffeine.

- **Artificial colors, preservatives, artificial and natural flavors**, **including MSG***, **aspartame and table salt:** Check labels or buy fresh to avoid these timebombs that are hard on your body. *[Watch out for other names for Monosodium Glutamate (MSG): MSG Accent, Autolyzed Plant Protein , Autolyzed Yeast, Aginomoto, Calcium Caseinate, Citric Acid (when processed from corn), Gelatin, Glutamate, Glutamic Acid, Hydrolyzed Plant Protein (HPP), Hydrolyzed Vegetable Protein (HVP), Monopotassium Glutamate, Natural Flavoring, Natural Meat Tenderizer, Sodium Caseinate, Senomyx (wheat extract labeled as artificial flavor), Textured Protein, Whey Protein Isolate, Yeast Food or Nutrient, Yeast Extract.][13]

- **Dairy products** (especially pasteurized). Many physicians consider dairy products to not be a necessary part of a healthy diet and advise that, since most humans become lactose intolerant after age five, dairy products are best avoided.[14]

- **Refined grains**, **white flour, refined flours**. Replace these with whole grains and flours which still contain a large variety of nutrients.

- **Refined oils (especially hydrogenated oils and anything containing canola oil), fried foods.** In the refining process oils are denatured and stripped of the nutrients they are designed to come with and thus become a burden on the body, rather than a benefit. Instead, consume healthy fats from whole plant foods such as seeds, nuts, coconuts and avocados. These have an abundance of essential nutrients.

- **Smoking.** Smoking tobacco impairs night vision and increases the risk of developing eye diseases such as cataracts, macular degeneration and blindness.[15-18]

- **Drugs and antibiotics**. Check labels for side-effects that involve vision (see Appendix H). Consult with your physician about possible alternatives.

Why you crave sugar

Many people have a hard time giving up one of the biggest nutritional roadblocks to good vision – an addiction to refined sugar and artificial sweeteners. In a class with Hanna, a student in Wisconsin, I explained that her sugar addiction did not need to be hard to overcome. She had tried to quit sugar in the past, had felt deprived, and failed to stick to her good intentions. There is an easy solution! I explained to Hanna how I view the sugar issue:

Your body does need sugar, and a sugar craving is a built-in warning signal when you run low on this essential fuel. Yet what your body is truly asking for is sugar that comes with all the trimmings – a wholesome helping of fibers, vitamins and minerals – which are supposed to come along with the sugar! Fresh fruit is the real answer to a sugar craving;

fruit is what your body truly wants. When you answer that craving with empty calories from refined sugars, you are starving your cells of what they were hoping to get, so you stay hungry for sweets and you head for disaster instead of health.

Once you switch to using fresh fruit whenever the sugar craving pops up, you are feeding your cells what they truly need – sugar and an impressive line-up of additional nutrients. When you choose fresh fruit to satisfy the sugar craving, you will soon find it easy to stay away from artificial sweeteners. You may also find that cravings for sugar-laced junk foods lessen and then disappear as your body becomes truly nourished by the minerals and vitamins provided by wholesome foods.

With this perspective on the sugar issue, Hanna has found new inspiration to overcome her addiction. She finds switching to fruit makes total sense, and she does not feel deprived this time around.

If you are diabetic and have learned to "fear" fruit, please read Dr. Joel Fuhrman's book, *The End of Diabetes*.[19] When my dear friend Bonnie switched to Dr. Fuhrman's "Eat to Live" diet, her doctor took her off insulin within a few weeks and he declared she was completely cured from Type II diabetes within two months of making that switch!

Eliminating refined sugars is easier said than done, because pretty much every processed, packaged food is laced with one of its many forms. Even the deli in my local health food store lists coconut sugar in many dishes, including their kale salad, so what you expect to be healthy is not necessarily so… Read ingredient labels and, as much as possible, prepare your meals from fresh ingredients; then you won't need to worry about this.

"Sugar and Vision, an unintentional experiment" by Robert Lichtman
Here's a story from yesterday: I met an old friend for lunch and indulged in an old vice – sugary fizzy water, also known as soda. I haven't drunk soda in the longest time, and I was reminded why.

During the meal, I consumed a liter of soda. According to the label, there were 28 grams of sugar per serving and four servings per bottle. This means I took in 112 grams of sugar. At about 4.75 grams to a teaspoon, that means in about an hour I ate 23 teaspoons full of sugar! During the meal, my vision blurred and my strabismus came back. I also developed a whale of a headache.

It took a few minutes of practicing the short swing on a sign across the street, which unfortunately said "Donuts, Bagels, Sandwiches, Coffee" on it before I regained my vision and lost my headache.

Next time, I will be sure to wash my food down with water. I urge you to try this experiment for yourself: First, avoid sugar for a few days. Then throw down some soda or candy and see what happens over the next hour.

A note to parents and eye doctors: Since this product produces blur, it seems to me irresponsible to give a child an eye test unless this substance is first cleared from the child's bloodstream.

In fact, it would be more responsible to forbid this product the same way we forbid nicotine and alcohol consumption until the individual is considered old enough to make an informed decision. Further, to dose a child with sugar and then expect that child to sit still in a classroom is certainly inconsiderate of the poor child.

A healthy diet is required in order to gain optimal benefits from sunlight
Now that you know which foods to eat more of and which foods to avoid for a healthier you and healthier eyes, you can safely move on to the last chapter in this essential section of the book. Because a body filled with dietary toxins reacts poorly to sunlight, while a healthy body benefits from it greatly – and so do your eyes.

15. Sunlight: Friend or Foe?

Good nutrition doesn't come from food alone. Another important nutrient is sunlight. Creatures that live solely in dark, lightless caves do not develop eyes; eyes develop under the influence of sunlight. As such, eyes are organs of light, and they need the full spectrum of light for optimal health. Dr. Bates made extensive use of sunlight to successfully treat a wide range of visual conditions. He said sunlight is as necessary to normal eyes as are rest and relaxation.

Fear of sunlight

I am fully aware that warnings abound regarding the dangers of sunlight. The typical arguments I hear against exposure to sunlight are that ultraviolet (UV) light is harmful; the hole in the ozone layer has made it all much worse; the sun causes skin cancer and contributes to cataracts; it is dangerous for babies and children to be outside in sunlight; staring at the sun causes blindness; and if you have light-colored irises you are in double trouble due to higher light sensitivity. Then, of course, sunscreen and sunglasses will help you avoid all this, so you really ought to use them…

> **The fear that light will hurt the eyes actually produces sensitiveness to light.**
> William H. Bates, M.D.[1]

I will address these fears, because the band-aid of sunglasses will only make matters worse, causing an increase in light sensitivity and thus an unnatural dependency – even an addiction to "shades."

Many people are quite sensitive to bright light these days, and a number of students tell me about the "terrible glare" from the sun or from oncoming vehicle headlights while driving at night. You may tell me that sunglasses greatly reduce your eyestrain in bright light, which may be true in this moment, but if you know how easily you can eliminate your light sensitivity and how much both your eyesight and your health benefit when your eyes are comfortable in bright light again, I bet you will give your eyes a chance at overcoming their dependency on being shaded.

For example, Saskia in Sebastopol, California, used to wear her glasses all day long and was quite sensitive to sunlight before hearing about the Bates Method. A few weeks after learning how to safely sun her eyes she wrote:

> I have been LOVING the fact that I'm no longer sensitive to sunlight. Sunshine on my face is an instant happiness boost!

It is true that too much UV radiation is harmful, but so is too much oxygen, and you would never try to avoid all oxygen because too much is toxic. Too little oxygen is definitely hazardous to your health, and so is too little UV, even if the effects aren't instantly evident. Extreme tests show "the dangers of UV," yet exposing an anesthetized animal's eye under a full beam of high-level UV radiation for up to sixteen minutes without a chance for that eye to blink or look away is cruel and not a fair comparison to normal outdoor conditions.[2] Conclusions drawn from such unrealistic conditions should never be your reason to fear UV radiation or wear sunglasses.

The light spectrum

To understand why the fear of sunlight is unfounded, let's have a closer look at the spectrum of light coming from the sun. The image below provides a graph of all the solar rays that penetrate our atmosphere and reach the earth. Starting with the shortest wavelengths, the far-left shows trace amounts of cosmic rays, gamma rays and x-rays. Next are ultraviolet rays, consisting of UVC, UVB and UVA rays. Then follows the visible spectrum of colors: from violet through blue, green, yellow, orange and red, which occupy only a narrow band of the entire spectrum (from 380 to 750 nm). From there it goes into the extensive infrared spectrum including microwaves and radio waves which, like cosmic, gamma, x- and UV rays, are not visible to human eyes.

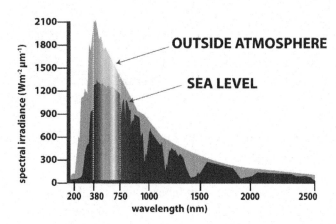

The solar spectrum at noon, both at sea level and at the top of the earth's atmosphere. The difference between the two (shaded) shows the energy absorbed by atmospheric gases which stop a portion of solar rays from reaching earth.

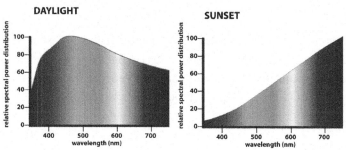

Zooming in on the 380 to 750 nm range only, these two charts show that the peak in the visible spectrum of sunlight shifts from blue/green at noon to red at sunset.

The solar spectrum is what your body and eyes are designed for and what they thrive under. The higher concentration of blues in daytime activate serotonin, dopamine and cortisol, which boost alertness. The lack of blues and higher concentration of reds at sunset triggers melatonin which gets you ready for regenerative sleep. Sleeping in darkness completes the cycle as the absence of light and solar radiation allows for cell renewal while you sleep. All life on earth existed under this natural cycle of light and dark, until first the discovery of fire and then the invention of the light bulb.

Artificial light

Fire and candlelight allowed humans to extend their evening activities. There is no standard spectrum map of light emitted by candlelight or a campfire; those depend on various factors, such as fuel used and temperature of the fire, yet it basically resembles the spectrum of sunset.

In the 1800s, artificial light evolved from candlelight to gaslights, kerosene lamps and incandescent light bulbs. These did more than simply extend our evening hours. They allowed us to spend our days indoors in windowless buildings and made night shifts possible, thus disrupting our natural lifestyle. Here is the spectrum map for the incandescent lamp. Light emitted by an incandescent bulb is nearly a copy of the natural spectrum at sunset. Using incandescent lamps at night extends your exposure to the red end of the spectrum, which isn't so bad. Yet if you spend all day indoors in windowless rooms with only incandescent lights, you will greatly lack exposure to blues and greens.

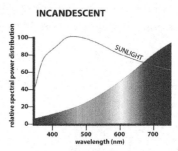

You may wonder why that is a problem, and I will explain that in a moment. But first, the enormous popularity of the incandescent bulb led to its widespread use, which became a huge burden on power supplies. So, in an effort to reduce the cost of lighting up the world, a variety of alternatives were invented, including fluorescent tubes, halogen lights, compact fluorescents and, more recently, LED and OLED lights. Take a look at their spectrum maps on the next page.

Fluorescent lamps are nothing like the sunlight spectrum. They have a few peaks of color intensity but lack a large part of the natural spectrum of sunlight. Halogen and LEDs show a slightly better representation of the spectrum, but they too have large areas missing compared to sunlight. The newer OLED light is somewhat better but also shows deficiencies in its spectrum.

Spectrum map comparisons

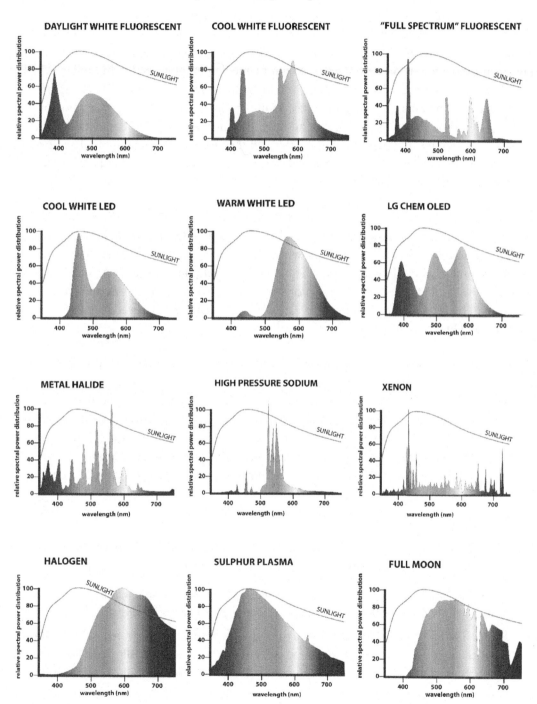

John N. Ott

It is time to introduce you to John Nash Ott (1909-2000), if you haven't heard about him already. John Ott's hobby was time-lapse photography. He loved to make videos of flowers bursting into bloom and created the illusion of primroses "dancing" to music. Walt Disney hired him to make a time-lapse movie of a pumpkin growing from seed to a new pumpkin for the movie *Secrets of Life*. So Ott planted a pumpkin seed in his cellar, which had fluorescent lights to supplement the limited sunlight from a skylight. He set up his cameras and filmed the growth of the baby pumpkin plant. However, the plant did not develop as it should. It produced beautiful male pollen-producing flowers, but the female pumpkin-producing flowers did not do well at all; they turned brown and fell off before the pumpkin could develop. Ott had to wait for the next season to try again and apologized to Disney for the delay.

That winter, his fluorescent lights burned out and Ott replaced them. The hardware store was out of his regular cool-white lamps (which are strong in the yellow-orange part of the spectrum) so instead he bought daylight-white fluorescents which are richer in the blue end of the spectrum. The following season he planted another pumpkin seed and waited for it to grow. This time the female flowers did well, but no male flowers developed – the opposite of his experience the previous year. The only difference between the two years was in the lights.[3]

At the time, Ott was also working on various other time-lapse photography projects with flowers and fruits that were showing abnormal problems. In searching for answers, all clues led to the influence of light on the healthy growth of plants. Ott found that certain parts of the spectrum influence different stages of plant growth – flowers blossoming, fruit ripening, etc. – and if any one part of the spectrum is missing, the corresponding part of the growth cycle will simply not happen. With the pumpkin, when Ott used both types of fluorescent lights side by side, both male and female flowers developed normally on the vine and a healthy new pumpkin grew.

Ott's research

Through various experiments with plants as well as collaboration with animal breeders, Ott made a series of highly interesting discoveries about UV light. Here are a few examples:

- Under artificial lights without UV, chloroplasts in the cells of a leaf slow down and clump together, rather than stream naturally as they do under light that includes UV.

- Under a red filter, the cell membranes of pigment epithelial cells from a rabbit's retina weaken and tend to rupture causing the cells to die; under a blue filter, the cells contort and become sluggish, stopping cell division. Adding a normal dose of UV light reverses these problems.

- Adding a small amount of UV to a fish tank eliminated a severe condition of exophthalmos (pop-eye) in several fish.

- Mice kept under sunlight were healthy and lived twice as long as mice kept under pink fluorescents. The latter developed lesions on the tail until they were brought back under sunlight when the tails would regain healthy skin.

Ott realized that the limited spectrum created by filters or artificial lights could be seen as the cause of the resulting growth and health challenges, yet he knew that the very same rays found in those artificial light sources are also part of the full spectrum of sunlight. He concluded that the *lack* of the spectral rays which are missing under these artificial light conditions was the real problem, not the rays of the reduced spectrum themselves. Ott's hobby had turned him into an avid researcher, which brought him many awards, including an honorary Doctor of Science degree from Loyola University in Chicago.[4]

Malillumination
Ott coined the term "malillumination" and compared it to malnutrition. In a 1986 interview for *Mother Earth News*, he stated:

> Malillumination [is] a lack of the necessary amount of sunlight, just as malnutrition is a lack of the proper nutrients in our diets. Malillumination occurs when wavelengths are missing in various types of artificial light or are filtered from natural light passing through window glass, windshields, eyeglasses (particularly tinted contact lenses or sunglasses), smog, and even suntan lotions.[5]

For example, if you only eat apples, and nothing else, and develop health issues from doing so, it is not apples that are to blame, but the lack of all other nutrients that are absent from apples. It is balanced nutrition that keeps you healthy. So it is with light. If you only receive pink light and develop tumors because of it, pink light isn't the culprit; the real problem is the lack of all other parts of the spectrum. This is a key perspective that needs to become common knowledge. Different parts of the spectrum influence different parts of human cellular life, same as they do for animal and plant life. Chronic lack of any one part of the spectrum will cause the corresponding cells in the body or plant to underperform.

Ott's research regarding eyesight
Other parts of Ott's research point to the health and vision challenges caused by wearing glasses, contact lenses, tinted lenses and sunglasses:[6,7]

- Native West Africans who lived in Lambarene, where Dr. Albert Schweitzer started a hospital, did not have cancer until the introduction of sunglasses. They did not have electric lights or glass windows in their simple surroundings and typically wore only loin cloths, so they received plenty of full spectrum light. But once sunglasses became a status symbol, and thus a popular addition to their limited wardrobe, cancer became a problem.

- Continuous exposure to light through a green filter led to retinal damage in various species of animals, causing Ott to suggest the need for further studies of the effects of placing colored filters in the form of sunglasses or tinted contact lenses in front of human eyes. Pink tinted lenses especially stop beneficial wavelengths from entering the eyes, thus causing an endocrine deficiency. I guess that ends the myth of happily viewing life through rose-colored glasses…

- An exceptionally high rate of pterygium, an abnormal growth in the eye that impairs vision, was found in a group of Cree Indians in northern Manitoba, Canada. This group of Indians had been issued specially designed wrap-around sunglasses that were trimmed with leather to prevent even the slightest bit of ultraviolet light from reaching the eyes. The sunglasses had been issued as part of a study on the problem of glare from snow and ice. They had been allowed to keep the glasses at the end of the study. When Ott checked on several other individuals who had developed pterygium while on military duty, he found that all had worn prescription sunglasses.

- A person was fitted with one UV-blocking and one UV-transmitting contact lens. Indoors, under artificial light containing no ultraviolet, the size of both pupils appeared the same, but outdoors, under natural sunlight, there was a marked difference. The pupil covered with the UV transmitting lens was considerably smaller. This indicates that the pupil constrictor muscle responds to UV wavelengths as well as to visible light. By blocking UV from entering the eye, the pupil remains larger than it otherwise would, and thus light will seem brighter. This, in turn, can cause a desire for and a dependency on darker glasses.
(Esther's note: The diameter of healthy pupils narrows down to 1-4 mm in bright light, whereas they dilate to 4-8 mm in dim light or darkness. Eyes that have little exposure to bright light do not narrow down as much as they should and may stay open with a 5-6 mm diameter, despite the bright light. This adds to light sensitivity.)

On the positive side:

- At Well of the Sea, a restaurant in a Chicago hotel basement, UV black lights for special effects were used continually for 20 years. The management reported that their staff was essentially still the same group of men hired 20 years ago. They had a consistently excellent health record, no flu absence, and were particularly happy, courteous and efficient. None wore glasses or had eye problems.

- Cancer patients who spent as much time as possible in sunlight without regular glasses or sunglasses and who mostly avoided artificial light sources (including TV) showed no further tumor development, and some showed reversal.

- Under regular cool white fluorescent lights in two windowless rooms in a school in Sarasota, FL, some of the first-grade children were hyperactive, unable to sit still or concentrate. Three children were about to be transferred to special schools. One of them, a boy, had extreme learning disabilities. After Ott replaced the fluorescent tubes with full spectrum lights, this boy became interested, calm and attentive, and learned to read within a few months. The entire class showed improvement in both behavior and academic achievement under the new lights, and no children needed to be transferred to special schools.

- Ott's own arthritis drastically reduced when he broke his glasses and spent considerably more time outdoors without glasses. When he purposely left his glasses off as much as possible for six months, he found that wearing them even for short periods caused eyestrain, so he had his eyes checked and was told that the rather strong prisms previously needed to correct a muscular imbalance were no longer required.

> **It is worth noting that old age, no cancer, and good eyesight are common factors associated with people living at high altitudes where the atmosphere is thinner and consequently the ultraviolet is stronger.**
> John N. Ott[8]

Support for Ott's research

Other researchers have come to similar conclusions:

- Research done in California in 2007 with 514 children (8 and 9 years old) who started out with healthy vision was aimed at finding a link between the onset of myopia and environmental factors such as parental myopia, reading time, sports and outdoor activities. During the study, 111 (21.6%) of the children became myopic. It turned out that time spent reading per week was not a significant factor. The strongest factor associated with myopia was the amount of time spent outdoors. The more time outdoors, the lower the chance of becoming myopic. Outdoor time was especially effective for children whose parents were myopic.[9]
A study with children in Australia came to similar conclusions.[10] But to the researchers' surprise, a follow-up study with children who were already myopic did not show this positive link to outdoor time.[11] This makes sense to me, as by then these children had developed strained vision habits and would need some education in releasing them.

- Ophthalmologist Hermann Cohn, author of *Hygiene of the Eye in Schools,* felt that parents had a right to demand that their children, who were compelled by law to attend school, should not suffer injury to their health by doing so. He believed good lighting in schools to be of the highest importance in preventing myopia and found the highest prevalence of myopia in schools where the least amount of sunlight entered through classroom windows.[12]

- Zoltan Rona, M.D., M.Sc., in his book, *Vitamin D, the Sunshine Vitamin,* writes that since 1940 the incidence of melanoma increased mostly in people who work indoors. Outdoor workers rarely get the disease (provided they avoid commercial sunscreens) and on average get nine times more solar radiation than their indoor counterparts.[13]

- Because cataracts are more common in countries near the equator, it was thought that sun exposure had to be the cause. Actual research repeatedly shows no validity for this hypothesis. John J. Harding, B.A., Ph.D., found that this hypothesis ignores all other differences between these countries and higher latitudes, such as diet, culture, poverty and prevalence of other diseases such as diarrhea.[14]

- Studies have shown that cataracts are less common at higher altitude where UV exposure is greatest, such as in the Himalayas.[15]

- Gwen W. Collman, Ph.D., and his colleagues in North Carolina did not find sunlight or working outdoors to be a significant risk factor for cataracts; nor were sunglasses associated with a protective effect.[16]

- The Beaver Dam study in Wisconsin (1995) showed that outdoor time in summer was not related to cataracts, while in men, outdoor time in winter turned out to be a protective factor.[17]

- ANSES in France (the French National Agency for Food, Environmental and Occupational Health Safety) issued a report with evidence that proves without a doubt that high-power LEDs can be detrimental to human health. It found that the human eye, in particular, may suffer serious damage due to the high blue content in white LEDs, because the intense blue-white light exerts "toxic stress" on the retina. Children's eyes are especially at risk.[18]

Light-colored irises

Some doctors may tell you that light sensitivity is related to light-colored irises, yet I have light-colored irises and am not sensitive to bright light, so am I an exception to the rule? The only time in my life when I developed sensitivity to light was when I joined the "cool crowd" in the 1990s wearing Ray-Ban® sunglasses. I mainly used them while sailing during summer weekends. Within a few weeks of using them, I found myself so sensitive to light that I needed sunglasses when driving home from the harbor on an overcast day! This was such a big contrast to my previous complete comfort in sunlight that I realized the sunglasses were the cause of my problem, and I weaned myself off them. I now have a high tolerance for light and have no trouble glancing up at the sun without a need to squint even at noon – and yet I have very light, blue-green irises.

So far, there is no conclusive research to support the hypothesis that light-colored irises are by definition more sensitive to sunlight. Richard A. Adler, M.D., says:

> Broadly speaking, one cannot decisively predict one's light sensitivity based solely upon iris color; we can all think of blue-eyed people without light sensitivity and brown-eyed people with such sensitivity. Nevertheless, it is theoretically possible that blue-eyed individuals, who have thinner irises may, in fact, have increased light permeability and thus increased light sensitivity. What people often forget, however, is that the backside of everyone's irises are brown! That back layer is usually enough to absorb light and prevent photosensitivity, whether the eyes are blue or brown.[19]

The cycle of light

Not only deficiencies in the spectrum but also anomalies in the level of illuminance create problems. Illuminance, or light intensity, is measured in lux. A bright, sunny day can reach around 100,000 lux outdoors, although that drops to 20,000 in the shade. A gloomy day may be 1,000 lux. Sunset is around 400 lux on a clear day and 40 lux on a cloudy day, while twilight comes in at 10 lux. A full moon on a clear night will be 1 lux at most. In contrast, indoors, a typical home in daytime will only reach between 100 and 300 lux. A classroom gets about 300 lux, an office may have 500 lux, while a surgery room is likely to have 1,000 lux and places where detailed work takes place may increase their light levels to between 2,000 and 20,000 lux. As such, most indoor light levels fall short of outdoor daytime levels.

At night, the opposite happens. While the forests go dark, the "civilized world" keeps its lights on and indoor light levels far exceed outdoor levels for many hours, if not all night. So instead of the natural cycle between bright days and dark nights, humans have created relatively dark days and relatively bright nights. This flattens the amplitude of our day and night light-level cycle and impacts the body's circadian rhythms, leading to insomnia and a host of other health issues.

Essential points to remember

You are susceptible to the effects of malillumination if you spend much time indoors under relatively low levels of artificial lights that lack part of the spectrum, if you habitually wear glasses or contacts that filter out UV, if you often use tinted lenses that filter out an even larger part of the spectrum, if you live in a city that's regularly shrouded in smog, if your nights are over-illuminated, or even if you paint the inside of your house all in one color and spend many hours inside it.

Because ultraviolet has been made out to be the bad boy of the spectrum, and fear of UV exposure is currently widespread, this logically has led to excessive protection from sunlight and underexposure to it, and thus all kinds of UV deficiency symptoms are common. Some UV deficiency symptoms are: low vitamin D levels, cancer (colorectal, breast, prostate, pancreatic), non-Hodgkin's lymphoma, hypertension, cardiovascular disease, metabolic syndrome, diabetes (both Type 1 and 2), obesity, Alzheimer disease, multiple sclerosis, rheumatoid arthritis, psoriasis, non-alcoholic fatty liver disease, statin intolerance, arthritis, allergies, attention deficit disorder, learning disabilities, depression, aggression, anxiety, irritability, restlessness, hyperactivity, sleep problems, lethargy, fatigue, loss of libido, loss of concentration, colds, flu, jet lag, feeling stressed, and headaches, as well as vision issues such as eyestrain, light sensitivity, macular degeneration, cataracts and myopia.[20]

Extensive exposure to artificial lights without any time spent in natural sunlight to balance that out will inevitably lead to vision challenges. Long-term, the stress on both your body and eyes adds up and leaves you wondering where you went wrong. Knowing the consequences of a lack of sunlight, and thus the importance of exposure to it, you will be less fearful of the sun. Regular exposure to sunlight is a necessary part of good vision and health. Yes, you can overdo UV exposure and cause sunburn and unpleasant side effects that are best avoided. A gradual increase in exposure and moving to the shade or covering up with clothing, rather than sunscreen, when your skin signals you've had enough, is a smart approach.

Some cautions
Here are a few reasons why some people may need to be cautious about increasing their exposure to sunlight:

- A healthy diet is essential, because without a plentiful supply of antioxidants in your body, sunlight can definitely cause harm to skin and eyes. Your eyes use antioxidants to compensate for the oxidation process that naturally happens with oxygen metabolism and exposure to sunlight. These antioxidants are: vitamins A, C and E, alpha lipoic acid, lutein, zeaxanthin, glutathione, CoQ10, selenium and zinc. (See Appendix G for food sources of these antioxidants.) If you choose to predominantly eat artificially sweetened or greasy junk foods it may be better to stay out of the sun, but then you will have to deal with the consequences of both malnutrition and malillumination.

- UV light can lower cholesterol levels, so if you take cholesterol-lowering drugs, consult with your physician if you choose to increase your sun exposure.

- Sun exposure lowers insulin requirements, so check with your physician if you use insulin and you want to increase your sun exposure.

- Some drugs and substances sensitize skin and cause easier sunburn. These include hypoglycemic agents used to treat diabetics, diuretics for high blood pressure, tranquilizers, antibiotics, anti-arrhythmic quinidine, PABA in sunscreen, halogenated antiseptic compounds used in soaps, cosmetics, and antihistamine for colds and allergies.[21]

- Research from 2016 on the Antarctic ozone layer [22] and a United Nations Report from 2018[23] indicates that the hole in the ozone layer is on its way to a full recovery. However, if you live in an area where this may still be an issue, do check local research and take precautions during the months when the ozone layer is thinnest.

- If using a brimmed hat or baseball cap to shade your eyes, the underside of the visor should be dull black or dark gray but not any translucent material such as dark green plastic.

- According to Dr. Bates, sunlight on the eyes improves vision to better than normal for people without eyestrain, yet people with eyestrain are likely to experience discomfort and some loss of vision when they look at the sun. Bates said this is not due to the sunlight but due to the strain.[24]

What about those yellow-tinted glasses?
Recently Joseph, a local farmer, showed up at the weekly market wearing a pair of yellow glasses. I asked him why he was wearing those, and he explained it was to protect his eyes from blue light. "Where is this blue light?" I asked. He seemed to think it was everywhere, that it was dangerous, and that he would save his eyes by wearing yellow-tinted glasses. I explained to him that the blue light itself is not a problem, that it's a part of sunlight, and yes, in that respect, it is everywhere. It is not blue light from the sun that is harmful, as that comes within a balanced, complete spectrum and boosts your alertness.

Using yellow glasses outside during the day creates an imbalance in the spectrum, and thus extensive use of such tinted glasses outdoors can only create problems for your eyes and health. However, blue light can become a problem at night, especially when the rest of the spectrum is chronically deficient, which is the case with computer screens. Yellow tinted glasses can be part of the solution under such conditions. For an explanation, see Chapter 19 where I cover eyestrain related to the use of light-emitting screens. Once Joseph understood the science behind it, he stopped wearing his yellow glasses outdoors.

Color light therapy
Color light therapy, also known as syntonics, is a form of therapy in which colored lights are shone into the eyes or on the skin to heal a number of ailments. The frequencies of various color bands elicit different responses from the cells, either relaxing or stimulating them. Some optometrists put this science to good use in treating their patients. After a six-week program of twenty minutes daily exposure to a range of colored lights, I scored

markedly better on a visual field test. So I support this work, yet I always keep in mind what John Ott wrote about it:

> Many biological responses are not to any light, but, rather, to narrow bands of specific wavelengths. When these are missing in an artificial light source, the biological receptor responds as if it were in total darkness, even though other wavelengths are present. If a particular ailment can be treated with certain wavelengths of light, we might logically assume that living under an artificial light source that lacks these wavelengths can contribute to causing the ailment in the first place.[25]

For this reason, I prefer to educate people about the benefits of sunlight exposure to balance out any deficiencies from indoor living, so the band-aid of color light therapy will not be required.

 Solutions

What can you do to minimize the problems of malillumination? With the following tips, you can turn the tide and reap benefits within a few weeks or months.

- Start with eating plenty of fresh foods high in antioxidants, so sunlight oxidation cannot age your skin or damage your eyesight.

- While indoors during the day, let as much sunlight as possible enter and, where necessary, supplement with bright, full-spectrum lamps.

- Spend more time outdoors and spend as much as possible of that time without glasses, contact lenses, sunglasses, and sunscreen.

- Take care to avoid sunburn. When the sun is high, it is better to briefly sun multiple times than to take one long sunbath. You do not need to be in full direct sunlight; even in the dappled shade of a tree you will benefit from UV rays. Because clothing blocks UV rays, do expose at least your face and arms to the sun.

- For your vision, a daily dose (ten to thirty minutes) of natural light, whether it is sunny or not, helps offset malillumination. How long to spend in the sun depends on latitude, season and skin or light sensitivity. For children, an average two to three hours per day of outdoor time provides protection from becoming myopic, while an average of just one hour per day outdoors does not.[10]

- Until your eyestrain is gone and your vision is excellent, do protect your eyes from extreme bright light conditions such as a snow-covered landscape on a sunny day.

- Consider getting UV-transmitting glasses, contact lenses and windows.

- Add full spectrum lighting in your home and office, or at least replace your worst lights and install lamps that emit a spectrum close to sunlight. Adding a black-light lamp to your home or workspace provides little actual light, but will at least fill some of the spectrum gap of regular lamps by emitting UVA.

- Limit nighttime exposure to light-emitting screens that emit mostly blue light. See Chapter 19.

- Last, but in no way least: Use the sunning routine on the following pages to overcome any light sensitivity.

Safely sunning your eyes

To gradually and safely overcome any light sensitivity you may have, and to increase overall health of the eyes as well as general health, Dr. Bates recommended doing lots of sunning. The more you sun your eyes, the more they get accustomed to bright light, and the less glare you will perceive from the sun.

Important: Please note that I do not ask you to look directly at the sun, although, once vision is back to normal, this can be safely done for brief periods. Dr. Bates did not think it was harmful to look directly into the sun with your eyes open once your vision had improved to normal, provided that you do not strain against the light and that you imagine the sun to be moving from side to side (the sun swing, page 164).

Depending on your current level of light sensitivity, there are various levels at which you can begin with sunning. Rob, a highly light-sensitive student in New York, started his first sunning session by standing with his back to the sun underneath a big shady tree, where, with eyes closed, he dared take off his sunglasses. Within half an hour he worked his way up to facing the sun with closed eyes. While turning his body from side to side he was able to open his eyes briefly at the sides, allowing sunlight to shine into his eyes from a 90-degree angle. At his next class a week later, he reported no longer needing sunglasses. He had practiced the sunning routine every day and loved it.

The key to sunning is to avoid straining against bright light. If at any time your eyes are uncomfortable with the level of light, either close your eyes, turn your head further away from the sun, or cover your eyes with your hands to give them a rest. It may be easier if at first you sun your eyes within an hour of sunrise or sunset when the sun is low in the sky. The light will be less intense, and it is also easier on your posture; no need to crane your neck. Do progress to sunning nearer to solar noon as your sensitivity decreases.

Important: Sunning the eyes is always done without glasses, sunglasses or contact lenses, and is preferably done outside. **Please always follow the guidance your eyes give you and let them close when they want to!!!** Straining to keep eyes open against too much light is not a good vision habit to develop.

Level 1 – Basic outdoor sunning for eyes that are highly light sensitive

If your level of light sensitivity is high, start by facing away from the sun and stand or sit with eyes closed. Notice the brightness of the sky coming in through your closed eyelids. Usually at this stage it is easy to feel comfortable with the light. If not, simply relax, think about something you love, and wait a few minutes until the closed eyes feel at ease in the light.

Once your eyes have adjusted for the light, start moving your head from side to side in an easy, slow motion, keeping the eyes closed. As your chin reaches a shoulder, the sunlight will be a little brighter on one eye. Pause there briefly, then gently move your head to the opposite shoulder and let the other eye have that brief sideways sunbath. Repeat this until you are very comfortable with the amount of light and your eyes do not tense up against it.

Now you can begin opening your eyes in the center, looking away from the sun. If that feels comfortable, move your head gently from side to side, allowing the eyes to blink regularly, and always close your eyes whenever you sense that the sunlight coming over your shoulder is too bright. Play with this until you find you can easily keep your eyes open (accompanied by regular blinking) as your chin moves from shoulder to shoulder. You may find it only takes a few minutes to acclimate to the light, or you may want to repeat this several days in a row before you move on to the next level.

Level 2 – Basic outdoor sunning for eyes that are mildly to moderately light sensitive

Once your open eyes are comfortable with your back to the sun, close them and slowly turn around to face the sun. You can stand, sit or lie down; whichever you prefer. Point your nose to the sun and feel the warmth coming through your closed eyelids. You will likely see bright red, orange and yellow colors, which is normal.

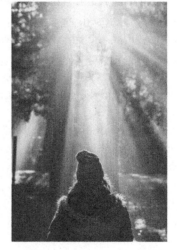

Begin turning your head gently and slowly from side to side in at least a 90-degree arc. As your head turns to the left, you'll notice your right eye receiving most of the sun and warmth while the left eye gets a little shade from your nose. When your head turns to the right, the left eye receives most of the sun and warmth. Just be aware of those sensations, let the warmth relax you, and continue to slowly and easily turn your head from side to side. Imagine the sun swinging through the sky opposite to your head motion. Be sure to have a loose neck, a relaxed posture and breathe freely.

Any initial discomfort will usually disappear in a few minutes. Your very first session of facing the sun can be one minute, five minutes, half an hour or longer of just this gentle head movement with closed eyelids. When you are done, keep your eyes closed and turn away from the sun. Softly cover your eyes with your hands for a minute or longer, then uncover them, open your eyes, let them blink, and notice how your eyes feel.

This basic outdoor sunning should be done as often as possible, and for as long as you are comfortable in the sun without burning your skin. You can completely forget about your eyes while you sun and just think of something you love. Do remember to gently turn your head from side to side, because this varies the light intensity on each eye, which naturally stimulates the pupil muscles to contract and release. They get a workout while you relax!

Level 3a – Advanced outdoor sunning: eyes open sunning

If basic sunning feels good to you and your eyes are comfortable with the sun on your closed eyelids, then it is time to advance. Begin your next session as above. Gently move your head from side to side with closed eyelids, until you feel totally at ease in the light. At that point, you can start turning your head further (in a 180-degree arc) with your chin turning all the way to your shoulder. (If your neck is tense, move your upper body along too.) When your chin is aligned with a shoulder, allow your eyes to open briefly, like a flash. Simply take a quick look at something in line with your shoulder, then close your eyes again and turn your head gently to the opposite side. Do the same there; very briefly open your eyes to look at something in line with your shoulder. Repeat this until it feels comfortable and it is easy to open your eyes briefly with the sun at a 90-degree angle. Gradually allow your eyes to remain open longer while you continue to look at things in line with your shoulder.

Level 3b – Advanced outdoor sunning: approaching the sun

The next step is to allow your eyes to stay open (with blinking) while you slowly move your head back toward the center. Pay close attention to how your eyes feel and allow them to blink as much as they want while your nose slowly approaches the sun. At some point before you reach the sun, the light will feel too bright for your eyes, causing them to want to close. Always close your eyes at that point; avoid squinting your eyelids. Continue the movement past the sun with closed eyes until your chin is back over the opposite shoulder. There you open your eyes again, blink, and repeat this procedure in the opposite direction. Do not be in a hurry to look near or at the sun. Take your time; be sure to let your eyes close as soon as they want to and do not strain at all to keep them open. At first, you may want to make an arc underneath the sun, with the sun in the top of your peripheral field, yet as you progress you can point your nose higher and let your arc move right through the sun, blinking all the way. For some people it is easier for the first few days to sun one eye at a time, keeping the other eye covered with a hand.

You will find that the more you repeat these increasing levels of the sunning routine, the less sensitive to light your eyes become. If you can sun your eyes for five minutes or more every day for a couple of weeks, you will likely overcome any light sensitivity. You can expand the basic sunning routine with a few useful extra techniques.

Additional sunning technique 1: Sunning-palming sandwich
Point your nose to the sun and alternate five seconds of letting the sun shine on your closed eyelids with five seconds of palming your closed eyes. This will alternately activate and release the pupil constrictor muscles, giving them a gentle workout, which increases circulation and eye health. Enjoy the "sandwich" for about a minute at a time, or as long as you like.

Additional sunning technique 2: Strobing
For strobing you also face the sun with closed eyelids. Spread the fingers of both your hands and hold your hands in front of your eyes with palms facing you. The fingertips can overlap slightly. Wave your hands up and down in front of your closed eyes. The spread fingers will create a dark-light-dark-light-dark-light strobing effect on your eyelids. Keep your hands close to your face for the best effect. If you do it right, you'll see a kaleidoscope of colors created by the strobing pattern on your retina. This light show is like a massage for the retina, and it has the wonderful effect of causing your eyes to start

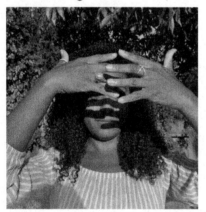

moving in a natural way. To encourage natural shifting while strobing, also move your head gently from side to side, up and down, or in a circle. This additional head movement greatly encourages more eye motion in an effortless way. Enjoy strobing for a minute, or until your arms get tired. At that point, cover your eyes with your palms and rest your eyes (and arms) for half a minute. Then return to the waving of hands to create the strobing effect once more. Another minute or so will be fine; do more if you like.

Caution: You may want to avoid strobing if you are prone to seizures.

Additional sunning technique 3: Sclera sunning (optional)
Sclera sunning (the sclera is the white outer layer of the eye) involves covering one eye and letting the sun shine on the white of the other eye while the pupil is safely tucked behind an eyelid. Not everyone can roll their eyes up or down far enough to hide the pupil, but those who can tend to love the sensation of bright sunlight on the sclera and may find they see better immediately afterwards. It also helps reduce light sensitivity and can lessen inflammation.

To find out if you can successfully roll your eyes up or down far enough, start with your back to the sun (or indoors if you prefer) and test each eye for both directions as described below. You want to be sure you only see the inside of your eyelid, nothing else. If you do see anything in front of you, part of your pupil is not yet covered! From an onlooker's point of view, the pupil disappears completely behind your eyelid, even though some of the iris will still show. Only proceed to facing the sun if you can successfully roll your eye so the pupil is hidden behind your eyelid. It is okay to do only the up or down direction if you can't do it both ways. If you can't roll your eyes far enough in either direction, simply skip this optional practice.

Sclera sunning is done one eye at a time. Start with both eyes closed, point your nose to the sun, and cover your right eye with your right palm. Keep your head in this position and now look as far down as you can, as if looking at your chin. While looking far down, use the pinky of your left hand to gently raise the upper eyelid of the left eye. You should only see the inside of your lower eyelid at this point. Using your pinky to pull the upper eyelid up reduces the chance that you accidentally shade your eye with your hand. You can move your eyes a little from side to side; look low-left to low-right a few times, or move your head slightly from side to side while the sun shines on the upper white part of your sclera. About three seconds of this is plenty. Then release the upper eyelid and let the eye close.

With closed eyes, switch from looking down to looking up as far as you can; it's like looking into your forehead. Now gently pull the lower eyelid of the left eye down with the tip of a finger. As before, the pupil should disappear from view, this time behind the upper eyelid. All you see is the inside of your eyelid. Look top-left to top-right underneath your upper eyelid a few times or move your head gently from side to side while letting the sun shine on the sclera below your pupil for a few seconds. Then release the lower eyelid to close the eyes, relax the eyes back to center, then blink rapidly or squeeze-blink to re-moisturize your eyes as needed.

Repeat both ways for the right eye.

Sunning duration

Once you are familiar with the entire sunning routine, you can forget about your eyes while you sun. Imagine the sun swing, think of something that makes you smile, or let your mind drift from one happy thought to another. This will relax the mind as well as the eyes.

If possible, practice the basic and advanced sunning routine daily for at least five minutes, and include one or more of the optional techniques as desired. This time can be increased as much as you like. Enjoy the sun at every opportunity; make sunning something that you habitually do as soon as you walk outside. Dr. Bates recommended sunning for half an hour or longer three times a day, or more often when possible. He said: "The more sun treatment, the better, as it rests and strengthens the eyes." Several short periods of sunning are just as beneficial as one long period.

When you end your sunning routine, close your eyes, face away from the sun and palm a while, if you like. Then open your eyes, blink, and notice if the light conditions now seem less intense.

The Sun Swing
It should be no trouble to look up at the sun to estimate time or general direction. A quick glance is all that is required for this. If your vision is not yet 20/20 or better, use the level 3 sunning routine described above until you are comfortable blinking through the sun before you attempt looking near or at the sun for longer periods. If you want to look directly at the sun for longer than a glance, initially pick a time when the sun is low in the sky, be sure to blink often and look from one side of the sun to the other, which will create the illusion that the sun is gently swinging in the sky.

On overcast days
If the weather isn't cooperating with your sunning endeavors, a bright (preferably full spectrum) lamp can be used indoors instead. The type of lamp often used to treat Seasonal Affective Disorder will work well, as will a theater spotlight or bright work lamp (for examples see my website).[26] Sit close enough to feel its warmth and ideally use it in the mornings to help set the circadian rhythm for the day.

Even on heavily overcast days, the light intensity outdoors easily beats any light indoors, so you may choose to use the brightest part of the sky instead of the sun for your sunning routine. If the sky isn't too heavily overcast, you may even still get some UV benefits from being outside.

Instead of sunglasses
Initially when you go out in bright sunlight without sunglasses or photochromic lenses, pay close attention to how your eyes feel. If you experience discomfort or eyestrain, you may be trying too hard to keep your eyes open. This is counterproductive. To overcome such strain, let your eyes blink rapidly until the light becomes more comfortable. Rapid blinking can be used any time when you move from a shaded area to a brightly lit area, or when you turn toward the sun after looking away from it. Let your eyes blink rapidly until they adjust to the light. When you combine this little trick with regular sunning, you will soon wonder why you ever needed sunglasses.

Once your eyes have become used to sunlight, you will no longer need sunglasses or photochromic lenses. It is best to not use those again; however, if you still feel any eyestrain under extremely bright light conditions and rapid blinking isn't helping enough, it makes sense to shade your eyes. For most circumstances, a wide-brimmed hat with a dull black or dark gray underside will adequately shade your eyes, if needed.

A note on sun-gazing

There is a practice called "sun-gazing" which is often confused with Dr. Bates' way of sunning the eyes. At first Bates also used the term sun-gazing, but in 1925 he dropped the term completely and only used "sun treatment" from then on, perhaps to avoid confusion. Dr. Bates' sun treatment is very different from sun-gazing. Bates taught sunning to increase the comfort of the eyes under bright light conditions and to improve their overall health.

In contrast, sun-gazing appears to be done mainly for spiritual reasons, with little regard to eye health. It is a daily practice that requires looking directly at the sun in its first or last hour of the day. The first day this is done for no more than ten seconds, and each day thereafter this time is increased by at most ten seconds until, after about nine months, the goal of forty-four minutes total sun-gazing in one session is reached, at which point the practice is discontinued.

As Dr. Bates stated that someone with eyestrain should not be looking directly at the sun, I do not advocate sun-gazing. I prefer Bates' methods, which can safely be done by anyone, regardless of the level of eyestrain or light sensitivity they start with.

The use of a "sun glass"

Dr. Bates often used an 18-diopter magnifying glass, which he called a sun glass, to increase the beneficial effect of the sun, once a basic light tolerance was regained by his patients with the sunning routine (progressing from closed-eye sunning to sclera sunning). A sun glass concentrates the light of the sun and was first used on closed eyelids (while the patient keeps their eyes pointed down). After some days or weeks, depending on the individual case, Bates would progress to focusing the sunlight on the sclera for a few seconds at a time. The results were amazing: It cured inflammatory conditions and dissolved scar tissue, while it also proved beneficial to myopia, astigmatism, presbyopia, itchy eyelids, glaucoma and cataracts.

It is awkward to use a sun glass on your own eyes, so it makes sense to have an experienced instructor help you. I will therefore skip giving directions for its use. It is best to start with the regular sunning routine anyway, and if you feel you could benefit from the sun glass, contact a teacher who has been trained in the traditional Bates Method.[27]

Conclusion

- Sunlight is good for you; sunburn is not, nor is staring at the sun.

- For optimal eyesight you need regular exposure to the full spectrum of light.

- Gradually increase exposure of your eyes and some skin to the sun.

- Once your eyestrain has gone and your vision is good, you will not need to shade your eyes from bright sunlight. Until then, use the sunning routine to help you get to this point, blink more in bright light and use a wide-brimmed hat to keep eyestrain at a minimum when light still feels too bright.

- To avoid or recover from conditions caused by spectrum deficiencies due to artificial lights and light-emitting screens, you need to spend sufficient time outside. (See also Chapter 19.)

- Better indoor lighting will help your vision: brighter and/or full spectrum in daytime, while dimmer and reduced blue spectrum in the evenings. Limit your screen time at night and use nighttime adaption of screen colors.

- As lamp and screen manufacturers continue to work together with health scientists to improve lighting technology, and when all buildings are optimized for receiving sunlight, many health issues will be resolved. In the meantime, go outside and enjoy the sun!

> *The best six doctors anywhere,*
> *And no one can deny it,*
> *Are sunshine, water, rest, and air,*
> *Exercise and diet.*
> *These six will gladly you attend,*
> *If only you are willing.*
> *Your mind they'll ease,*
> *Your will they'll mend,*
> *And charge you not a shilling.*
> Anonymous[28]

Part IV

–

How to Apply the Relaxation Methods

16. Seeing Effortlessly All Day Long

Now you know the essence of the Bates Method, or the way nature intends your eyes to be used. In every moment, all day long, you can choose to see effortlessly, receptively, blinkingly, to remain open to all light, with curiosity and interest in details, with your attention in motion and allowing apparent motion as a result. You can have a relaxed, tall posture so your eyes don't need to compensate for a head out of balance or a neck that is overly tense. With a relaxed, tall posture comes easier breathing: effortless motion of your diaphragm all the way up on the exhale allows for effortlessly deep inhales. You can use your memory and imagination to create better images in your mind of what you perceive, letting current blurriness be a gentle reminder to no longer try so hard to see. With each meal you provide the nutrition your eyes need from wholesome, fresh foods, while letting water quench your thirst. And you can choose to spend more time outdoors, giving your eyes the sunlight they have been craving. None of these are "eye exercises," not a single one. This is a way of seeing, and a way of life.

> **While there are many strains, however, there is only one cure for all of them, namely, relaxation.**
> William H. Bates, M.D.[1]

In order to adopt nature's way of seeing, go back and forth a few times between trying to see and simply receiving light. Between staring and blinkingly receiving images without judging the blur. Between a rigid stationary world and perceiving your surroundings as constantly being in gentle motion. Become more and more aware of the difference between these ways of seeing. How does it feel different to you? Regardless of current blurriness, the feeling of receptive seeing is what's most important at first.

Do the same with your breathing: Take a few forced, deep inhales and notice how this feels in comparison to inhales that happen after relaxed, long exhales. What is the difference? Become familiar with how effortless a deep inhale can be.

Why not also apply more movement instead of rigidity? More letting go, rather than forcing? Vision improvement can impact your life on many levels, if you let it. Truly, you see best when you forget about your eyes and simply let images come to you; when you stay receptive and accept any blurriness as a friendly reminder to let go of effort or fear. Whenever blur bothers you, check in with your posture, your blinking, your breathing, your peripheral vision, your interest in what you are doing. If that's not enough to bring about a change, close your eyes or give them a deeper rest with some palming and/or sunning. Repeat this formula until clarity has returned. By then, the receptive way of seeing will have become a habit and vision is likely to remain good.

In every moment, regardless of what you are doing, you have a choice as to how you see: with or without ease, with or without blinking, with or without interest. Effortless vision does not take time; it simply takes awareness and a willingness to relax. Now that you know how to achieve this, the choice is yours to make, in every moment of the day. To build your awareness, ask a friend to give you gentle reminders when you stare, squint, tilt your head or are in any way straining to see. Stick little notes on a bathroom mirror, a computer screen or a fridge, with text that, for example, reminds you to always blink instead of squint, or to keep peripheral vision open, or to let the world swing.

> **So many people with imperfect sight say that they have not the time to practice relaxation methods, as their time is taken up at business or in the performance of other duties. I always tell such people, however, that they have just as much time to use their eyes correctly as incorrectly**.
> William H. Bates, M.D.[2]

Students nearly always want to know what someone else did to overcome the same challenge they have. Knowing how someone else succeeded may inspire you to try the same methods, yet copying those methods does not guarantee similar results. In Bates' many years of teaching, he found that "what was good for one patient was not necessarily a benefit to other patients suffering from the same trouble, and that various methods must be tried in each case in order to determine which is the most beneficial for each particular case."[3] He also left the responsibility for finding the most beneficial treatment with the patients themselves: "All the methods I recommend have relaxation for their object. It is for the patient to determine which treatment is most beneficial and to continue its practice faithfully. Some patients tire easily when one thing is done continuously. For this reason, several methods are suggested in order to vary the practice."[4] He pointed out that: "when one method is found which improves the vision more than any other method, it should be practiced until the vision is continuously improved."[5]

 Find your optimal daily routine

To help you find what to practice most on a daily basis, the following list provides some guidance. Check which items in the left column apply to you and start using the solutions provided in the right column. To begin with, pick just one applicable item per day. Work on releasing that particular strained vision habit through increased awareness and replace it with the opposite relaxing habit. Work most on whichever technique brings you the best results. Move on to the next item once your progress levels out.

Note: Some of the solutions offered are discussed in chapters to come, and are indicated as such.

IF – THEN LIST
Pick one per day or use as needed!

IF... (What to be aware of)	THEN... (The habits to relax into)
You have blurry vision.	Accept it, look for what you *can* see, imagine details, use your foundation memory, and *refuse* to use strain to clear the blur.
You tend to try to see.	Practice flashing, receptive seeing and seeing from the back of your head. Imagine you have no eyes.
You have a staring habit.	Build awareness of it, ask others to point it out to you, blink rapidly each time you catch it.
You squint to see.	As above, plus become open to your peripheral vision.
Your eyes are tired.	Close them. Palm for a few minutes. Get more sleep.
Your eyes are dry or itchy.	Practice thirty seconds of rapid blinking. Squeeze blink. Improve your nutrition.
You tend to diffuse or try to see a large area clearly.	Find the interesting details in all you see.
You have tunnel vision; you get lost in a book or screen.	Open your periphery, notice apparent motion.
Your distance vision is blurry.	Use your foundation memory, accept blur, enjoy shapes and colors you do see, imagine what it would look like if your distance vision was clear and you could see things easily.
Your near vision is blurry.	Read: *"Read Without Glasses at Any Age."*
You often close one eye.	Close both eyes when you notice it; sense and release any strain from the eye you closed first. Open that eye first, then blink and continue with both eyes open. (Use a patch if needed to engage the eye that tends to close. Chapter 23)
Your world stands still.	Sway and become open to your peripheral vision.

You "sketch" or use a "nose feather" or in any way move your head consciously regardless of where your attention goes.	Switch to letting your interest lead your eyes and simply let your head follow as needed.
You read without head motion.	Release neck tension with some gentle neck stretches and allow your head to follow along as needed, even if only slightly.
You read while consciously moving your head.	Stop that. Close both eyes and relax the neck, then open your eyes and continue reading while letting the head follow only as needed.
You tend to tilt your head to one side.	Temporarily tilt it to the other side and massage the tense side of your neck. (See Chapter 18.)
You tend to have your head down or you gaze up.	Temporarily practice doing the opposite and release neck tension until level feels best.
You tend to have your head up or you gaze down.	Temporarily practice doing the opposite and release neck tension until level feels best.
You turn your head to one side.	Temporarily turn your head to the opposite side and massage the side of your neck until center position of head feels best.
Your work or school demands specific scanning habits. (See Chapter 18.)	Allow the head to follow your eyes, stay relaxed in motion. If possible, rearrange your work space regularly (monthly) to avoid developing astigmatism.
You spend many hours at the computer.	Take breaks (use break-reminder software), get more outdoor time to balance this out. (See Chapter 19.)
Your posture is slouched or tense.	Relax "up" - work on releasing the muscles that pull you forward into a slouch.
Your breathing is shallow or forced.	Practice the gentle number count.
You are light sensitive.	Build tolerance with gentle sunning every day. Create a brighter environment indoors.
Your night vision is bad.	Delay switching on lights, enjoy night walks, do the glow-in-the-dark practice (page 202).
You have sore spots around your eyes.	Massage these spots until no longer sore.
You lack 3-D vision.	Use a half-patch, use the Eyeport, close both eyes and imagine using the suppressed eye. (See Chapter 23.)

You have double vision (due to an eye-turn).	First, learn to control the muscles by making the double vision worse. Then learn to relax the extraocular muscle(s) that pull(s) the eye out of alignment. (See Chapter 23.)
You use an alarm clock to wake up.	Go to bed earlier so an alarm is not needed.
You sleep with your face pressed into the pillow.	Release postural tension so that you can sleep comfortably on your back.
Your eyes strain during sleep and you wake up with worse vision.	Practice the long swing for a minute, palm your eyes and imagine emptying your eye sockets before going to sleep and upon waking.
You are thirsty.	Drink plain water.
You have a sugar craving.	Eat fresh fruit.
You lack motivation.	Remind yourself of progress and goals and imagine how you will feel when you reach your goals.
You use a chart at 20 feet where it appears very blurry.	Use the chart mainly at your optimal practice distance (slightly blurry) where improvement will be seen much faster.
You find a technique difficult to do with eyes open.	Close your eyes and imagine doing the technique successfully.
You are not sure what technique to work with.	Practice several techniques with the letter chart at your optimal practice distance. Work most with any techniques that bring greater clarity.
You find a technique works really well for you.	Repeat it often!

If for any reason, like a highly stressful time, tension returns to your eyes and brings back blurry vision, you know what to do to reverse it. Blurry vision is not a life sentence, it is simply a message for you to let go of strain. Keep practicing this letting go, keep building your awareness of tensing habits, and keep replacing the tension with the easy, receptive way of seeing, over and over, until optimal, effortless eyesight becomes a habit that serves you well for a lifetime.

> **The cure of imperfect sight, then, is to stop all effort.**
> **It is not accomplished by doing things;**
> **it can only come by the things that one stops doing.**
> William H. Bates, M.D.[6]

17. A Bold View of Letter Charts and Small Print

Using letter charts to improve distance vision

Eyecharts, or letter charts, which is a more appropriate name, tend to be mainly associated with visual acuity tests, and as such, many people have developed a strong dislike for them. The chart reminds them of eye doctor visits where they "failed" to live up to expectations, causing some to feel they were "sentenced" to wearing glasses. So now, looking at a letter chart creates instant eyestrain; many fear it and would much rather avoid it than look at it. This negative association is unfortunate, because letter charts are an extremely useful tool in vision improvement.

Dr. Bates tells of a champion rifle shot who had unusually good vision when looking at a bull's eye, but when he looked at an eyechart, he had compound hyperopic astigmatism with a drop in visual acuity to 20/80. "Glasses in such a case would have been a crime," Bates commented.[1] Some people are therefore better off improving their sight using anything but a letter chart. However, if you can become friends with your blurry vision, you can probably also get on friendly terms with a chart and let it give you instant, impartial feedback about your eyestrain and how to release it. It can be a great teacher and helpful friend when you use it intelligently and stop viewing it as a "test."

First of all, remember that a chart is just a piece of paper with bits of ink; it won't harm you. Secondly, eyecharts were first created by Herman Snellen, a Dutch eye doctor, who presumed that the smallest detail a human eye can see covers one minute of visual angle. This turned out to be a wrong assumption; many people with good sight can see details half that size, but the charts are still based on this old standard and thus having "20/20 vision" does not actually represent good eyesight, but rather a refraction of a quarter diopter, or very mild myopia. My advice: Don't take eyecharts too seriously! And yet, charts are totally fine and useful when used as a feedback tool for how well the visual relaxation practices work for you, and as a tool to track your progress. So don't throw them out just yet.

You cannot effectively change something unless you are given appropriate feedback, and a letter chart is your primary biofeedback tool on your path to clear vision. When you practice relaxed ways of seeing, and letters become sharper and easier to distinguish, you know you are doing something right and your brain will register this as positive action – something worth repeating. More blur on the chart indicates that you are straining to see, and what you are doing in that moment obviously does not work well for your vision.

When Dr. Bates placed letter charts in classrooms with the simple instruction to the teachers to let the children become familiar with the chart and let them read it every day with each eye separately, the prevalence of myopia among 2000 students dropped from 6% to only 1%.[2] The chart taught the children how to keep their eyes relaxed, and its familiarity helped avoid eyestrain.

The numbers on the chart explained

Most charts will have a number associated with each line of letters. These numbers represent the distance from which the letters on that line can be read by someone who is considered to have good visual acuity. In the U.S. the numbers are given in feet while many other countries use meters. (This book uses the imperial system common to the U.S. For a comparison with other notations, please see Appendix D.) In the U.S., many charts start with a large letter at the top which may have the number 200 next to it, indicating this letter can be read from 200 feet by someone who sees well. Visual acuity is written as a fraction: the numerator of the fraction indicates your distance from the chart; the denominator denotes the number associated with the smallest line you can read from that distance. So, if you stand 20 feet from the chart and can read as far down as the line that has 40 next to it, your visual acuity is written down as 20/40.

> **A vision of 20/10 would mean that the ten line, which the normal eye**
> **is not ordinarily expected to read at a greater distance than 10 feet,**
> **is seen at double that distance. This is a standard commonly attained**
> **by persons who have practiced my methods.**
> William H. Bates, M.D.[3]

 Basic instructions for using charts

Various charts are provided at the back of this book and on my website. Hang the largest chart on a wall where you can stand 10 feet or more from it and where you are likely to glance at it often. Place the center of the chart at eye level.

Generally, vision is better when the light is good, but a person who is highly sensitive to bright light may do better in conditions of lower light. So, use the chart under the amount of light that allows for your best vision. Under such optimum conditions, your vision will become better sooner and, once you see well under the best light, you can practice with the chart under less than ideal light conditions.

Establish your optimal practice distance. This is where the chart isn't overly blurry and you can easily read most of it (see Appendix A.) Make a note of the last line that is easy to read.

Use the chart often. If you have not used glasses yet, half a minute per day with the chart will likely be helpful. If you have used glasses, five minutes or more each day (in multiple sessions) may be more effective. The more familiar the chart becomes, the more useful it is as a tool to improve your vision.

> **There are at least ten million children in the schools of the United States who have defective sight. Practically all of these cases could be cured and the development of new ones prevented by the daily reading of the Snellen test card.**
> William H. Bates, M.D.[4]

Look at the chart with one eye at time (cover the other with your hand without putting pressure on the covered eye) and **only read letters that you recognize with ease**. Repeat with the other eye, then use both eyes together. Once a week (using similar light conditions) make a note of the lines you can read with ease to track your progress.

Often the biggest challenge is to read the chart as far down as you can *with ease*. I do not want you to make any effort to clearly see a blurry letter or a line that is hard to read. Avoid all strain by sticking to what is easy for you to read right now. If none of the letters are easy, get closer! If you squint, you may read an extra line, but that is a false improvement created by strain which will only lead to worse vision in the long term. As one of Dr. Bates' patients put it: "Ain't no use trying."

Let it be easy
David is a student who, like many others, tends to subconsciously make an effort to see the letter chart clearly. He really wants his vision to clear up right now. I notice that his blink rate reduces drastically, or each blink is very slow and looks laborious, when he tries to see the chart better. When I remind him to relax into seeing, to let the light and images simply come into his eyes, he lets go of the effort he's been making. Then, without even being conscious of blinking, his blinks automatically become swift, easy and regular again. His vision fluctuates between 20/80 and 20/20 as his mind alternates between his habitual strain to see and his letting go of that effort.

Tips for using letter charts
With all following suggestions for using letter charts, it always pays to close your eyes often and let go of any strain that may have crept in. Check for strain in your posture, neck, breathing, and facial muscles too.

You can intersperse these practices with some rapid blinking or, if your eyestrain is severe, only flash each letter and close your eyes or palm after glancing at the chart.

Allow for natural shifts of attention. Notice if your attention begins to wander away from the chart. Whenever a distraction occurs, don't fight it. You are not a prisoner of the chart, so simply let your eyes follow your attention away from the chart and come back to the chart when your interest returns.

Remember: The chart is a friend, not a judge; allow it to give feedback.

 ### What to do with the chart

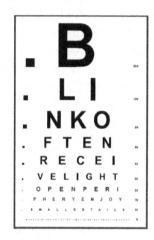

All the relaxation practices described in Chapters 5 to 15 can be evaluated for effectiveness with the chart. You simply note the last line you can easily read before and after you apply the technique(s) of your choice and compare the results. Although it can be useful to start with one technique at a time to build your awareness of how you use your eyes, you will get better results when you start combining various techniques.

Here are a few suggestions:

- **Let your eyes be closed more than open at first**

  With the chart at your optimal distance under your preferred light conditions, first spend a little time with eyes closed or palm your eyes. Then flash your eyes open a few times to remind yourself of receptive seeing. Whenever you play with letter charts, take plenty of breaks with eyes closed and keep eyes-open time to a minimum until you feel comfortable and can avoid straining to see the letters.

  If charts tend to cause a stress response in you, initially glance at things away from the chart, and slowly approach the chart until you can take brief glances at its white edge while staying relaxed. Then continue glancing at the letters. If you notice any eyestrain, close your eyes to release it and start over.

- **Relax with white spaces**

  Notice the chart has many more white spaces than black. And that looking at those white spaces is infinitely easier than trying to recognize the black shapes. So, whenever you notice strain come back in, go explore some white spaces to relax with.

- **Notice central clarity**

  Within your large field of vision, be interested in small details on the chart and notice that you cannot see a whole line clearly all at once. Use the small squares to the left of each line to give you an indication of the size of detail to look for in each letter on that line.

- **Keep it easy**

  Remember that there is no use in trying to clear up blurry letters! You may take brief glances at blurry letters, but return quickly to letters that are easy for you right now.

- **Imagine bright white halos**

  Notice where white and black areas touch each other. Does the white seem a little brighter right there where it touches black? Although the paper isn't actually whiter there, the contrast provided by the black does make it appear that way. So, each letter has a thin, bright white outline – a halo. Imagine you can see these halos; it will help the black stand out. Compare the whiteness in the center of a letter with the memory of a brighter white, such as sunlit snow on a mountain top. It may help to paint the chart with magic white paint – an imaginary paintbrush dipped in bright white paint that magically doesn't ever stick to anything black. Paint the chart abundantly in this magic white paint to help the white halos become more obvious.

- **Blink instead of squint**

  Are you still blinking easily and often? If not, do the 30 second rapid blinking technique!

- **Shift your attention**

  Many people stare when they look at a letter chart, and they often don't realize it until I gently move the chart from side to side a bit to break the stare – and then their vision instantly improves. Only briefly look at each letter. When a letter is seen clearly, you will get bored with it quickly and automatically shift to something else to look at. When a letter isn't seen clearly, there is a tendency to stare, to look at it longer hoping for more clarity, but this is counterproductive. So, dodge any blurry letter and move on to another.

- **Have fun with a boomerang ball**

  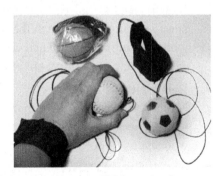

  One way to help keep your attention in motion is to use a boomerang ball.[5] I let students of all ages use a boomerang ball if they habitually look at letters too long! Throwing a ball toward or alongside the chart – a ball that must be caught as it bounces back to you – is a great way of distracting you from the chart. When you keep a steady rhythm of throwing the ball, you can only take quick glances at the chart between a catch and the next throw. With each glance, go to the next letter. Return to the top when it gets too hard, and repeat the game until you can read the whole chart.

- **Let the chart swing**

  Does your chart happily move around as your attention shifts around? If not, sway your body from side to side and let your attention pick up the same rhythm as your body. Look to the left of the chart when you sway left; look to the right of the chart when you sway right, and notice the chart responding with an apparent opposite motion. Once you can imagine the larger motion, practice smaller motions and let the chart swing just the width of a small letter. If the swing is not happening yet, close your eyes and imagine the swing. Open your eyes and gently sway your body from side to side, while remembering the imagined swing.

- **Use optimum letters to your advantage**
  You may find that one letter on a line is easier to see than others on the same line. Bates would call this letter an optimum, one that likely has some extra familiarity or a positive association for you, like your initials. You can use that letter to help the others on the same line clear up. Close your eyes and remember the easy letter. Remember its shape, whether curved or straight or some of both; remember how black it is; remember the white spaces around it. When you have created a good mental image by remembering parts of the letter, open your eyes and remember the clarity and ease of that letter when you glance at other letters on that line. Pretend those other letters are just as easy to see, and you will likely find they begin to clear.

- **Use your memory**
  Memorize the chart's words: "Blink often, receive light, open periphery, enjoy small details." Your memory of the words will reduce any tendency to strain or squint when you come to a letter that is not yet seen clearly. You already know what the letter is and are just looking to recognize its shape. The better you remember the shape of a letter, the easier it will be to see it. Memorizing the chart is not cheating; it simply helps you learn how to see effortlessly. If you find it hard to remember this chart, make your own, or simply use the alphabet in chart format.

- **Take advantage of your foundation memory**
  What is your foundation memory? Close your eyes and recall it. Enjoy this memory, relax into it, then open your eyes, blink, and keep thinking about it while you let your eyes roam across the chart. My students often find that suddenly they see the chart with perfect clarity! And all they did was relax by recalling a favorite memory.

- **Set up multiple charts**
  Another great way to play with charts is to set up several charts at various distances and align them so you can easily glance from one to another. Multiple charts do not need to be of the same size, but it does make sense to use charts that have the same sequence of letters. Hold the medium or smallest chart in your hand, while others can be leaning against books, hanging on a wall or window, or even pinned to a tree

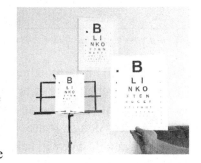

outside your window. This way you can use all the above suggestions at various distances, but you can also use the clarity of the nearest chart to increase your relaxation when you look at the same letter on a chart further away.

When you come across a letter on a far chart that is readable but not quite clear, instead of straining to improve on it, simply "cheat" and look at that letter on the chart in your hand, where it is much clearer. Notice every part of its shape, notice how black this letter is, and how white the background. Then close your eyes and remember the details of this easy-to-read letter. While keeping your eyes closed, imagine that letter is just as easy to see on the farther chart. When you can pretend that you see it easily at that distance too, open your eyes and remember the clarity of the near letter while you glance at its distant twin. Does that clear it up a bit? If so, repeat for other letters on the same line until all are easy to read, then progress to the next line or a greater distance.

Simply practice pretending you have great eyesight at all distances. Which of the other charts provides the most flashes of clarity? Practice mainly at that distance for quickest improvement. When you can pretend you see well at greater distances than you are used to seeing clearly, your vision is likely to follow suit because you are taking the effort out of seeing.

General chart advice

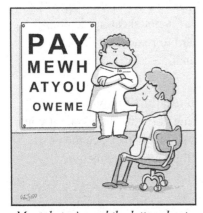

Mental strain and the letter chart

- If you have a dislike for the chart you are using, change to a different chart![6]

- There are no failures, there is only feedback! If you see more blur instead of more clarity, don't let it discourage you. This is not the time to quit; it is time to ask yourself some questions. What is this teaching me? What not to do? What can I change here? What good habit did I forget? Am I straining to clear the blur? How can I make this easier?

Clarity may only happen in brief flashes at first, but with practice these flashes will last longer and eventually the clear vision becomes permanent. Be careful not to try and "hold on" to a flash of clarity, because that attempt will instantly bring back blurry vision. Bates recommended "dodging" the clarity. When a flash of clarity occurs, look somewhere else, because a smooth shift will help keep your vision relaxed and can therefore prolong the clarity.

Using small print to improve distance vision

Nearly everyone with myopia finds that reading small print is the easiest thing to do, especially when doing so without glasses. When glasses for distance vision are used for reading at the near point, the eyes must overcome the diopters of the distance prescription in order to focus up close, which is a big additional strain that leads to higher levels of myopia. The usual reason I'm given by people who do this, is that their eye doctor said to wear the glasses all day long in order to get used to them. Yes, you will get used to that added strain, but do you want to? If you can read with perfect clarity when print is held close to the eyes, feel free to do so!

Because of your near clarity, your eyes shift effortlessly over text when you read. There is absolutely no inclination to stare or strain when text is seen clearly. Notice this easy, rapid shifting of your eyes when they scan over the words. Isn't it enjoyable? This is how they are supposed to move all the time! Now, if you read small print instead of regular print, you will also add a higher degree of central fixation, effortlessly noticing smaller details. This is why reading small print is good for your sight and a great tool on your path to clarity.

When you enjoy reading small print, notice how relaxing this is for your eyes when done in your range of best vision. You can use the awareness and memory of this easy eye motion to improve your vision when reading outside your range of clarity.

> **It is impossible to read fine print without relaxing. Therefore, the reading of such print, contrary to what is generally believed, is a great benefit to the eyes.**
> William H. Bates, M.D.[7]

Use the thin white line when reading outside your range of clarity

When you look at blurry print, it is helpful to imagine a thin white line beneath the lines of text. This thin white line is only imagined, because the line is not really there. The paper isn't made with thin, bright white strips placed neatly under each line of text, yet it does seem that way when you pay attention to it.

If it doesn't yet seem that way, close your eyes and imagine the white line as white as possible; as white as freshly fallen snow sparkling under a winter sun. Then open your eyes and continue imagining that bright white line touching the line of black letters. Alternate a few times between eyes open and closed until you can easily imagine a thin white line that the line of text rests on.

When you hold text in your blur zone, it helps to imagine the letters as really black even though they may appear gray or blurry. However, imagining the thin white line underneath the letters to be brighter white is usually easier to do and has the happy side effect that the letters clear up too.

Don't imagine you see the white line when you look directly at the letters – you can't achieve clarity of both the letters and the thin white line at the same time, but you can certainly alternate between the two.

Use microscopic print

Dr. Bates found that practice with microscopic type is most helpful in nearsightedness. His wife, Emily, recommended holding the fine print as close as you can and looking at the white spaces between the black lines of type while blinking, then looking out of a window or at a far corner of the room.[8]

Fine Print (9-point font)

The photographic reduction of the fine print can be used with great benefit to patients suffering from high degrees of nearsightedness. At first it has to be held at a certain close distance from the eyes and cannot be seen so well if placed an inch further or an inch nearer. When read easily or perfectly, the white spaces between the lines appear much whiter than they really are and the card seems to be moving from side to side or in other directions, if one takes the trouble to notice it. The eyes are blinking frequently and this is also usually an unconscious act.

More perfect rest or relaxation of the eyes is obtained by reading this fine print perfectly than by doing some other things. By alternately looking at the large letters of the Snellen Test Card at 5 or 10 feet or further and reading the fine print close to the eyes, one can obtain flashes of improved vision at the distance. By practicing, these flashes become more frequent and the letters are seen more continuously. The method is to be highly recommended because it seems to be one of the best methods of improving the distant vision.

William H. Bates, M.D.[9]

On the next page you can practice with the same text in progressively smaller print, including diamond and microscopic size fonts (5 and 2-point fonts respectively).

Fine Print (7-point font)

The photographic reduction of the fine print can be used with great benefit to patients suffering from high degrees of nearsightedness. At first it has to be held at a certain close distance from the eyes and cannot be seen so well if placed an inch further or an inch nearer. When read easily or perfectly the white spaces between the lines appear much whiter than they really are and the card seems to be moving from side to side or in other directions, if one takes the trouble to notice it. The eyes are blinking frequently and this is also usually an unconscious act.

More perfect rest or relaxation of the eyes is obtained by reading this fine print perfectly than by doing some other things. By alternately looking at the large letters of the Snellen Test Card at 5 or 10 feet or further and reading the fine print close to the eyes, one can obtain flashes of improved vision at the distance. By practicing, these flashes become more frequent and the letters are seen more continuously. The method is to be highly recommended because it seems to be one of the best methods of improving the distant vision.

Fine Print (5-point font – Diamond size)

The photographic reduction of the fine print can be used with great benefit to patients suffering from high degrees of nearsightedness. At first it has to be held at a certain close distance from the eyes and cannot be seen so well if placed an inch further or an inch nearer. When read easily or perfectly the white spaces between the lines appear much whiter than they really are and the card seems to be moving from side to side or in other directions, if one takes the trouble to notice it. The eyes are blinking frequently and this is also usually an unconscious act.

More perfect rest or relaxation of the eyes is obtained by reading this fine print perfectly than by doing some other things. By alternately looking at the large letters of the Snellen Test Card at 5 or 10 feet or further and reading the fine print close to the eyes, one can obtain flashes of improved vision at the distance. By practicing, these flashes become more frequent and the letters are seen more continuously. The method is to be highly recommended because it seems to be one of the best methods of improving the distant vision.

Fine Print (4-point font)

The photographic reduction of the fine print can be used with great benefit to patients suffering from high degrees of nearsightedness. At first it has to be held at a certain close distance from the eyes and cannot be seen so well if placed an inch further or an inch nearer. When read easily or perfectly the white spaces between the lines appear much whiter than they really are and the card seems to be moving from side to side or in other directions, if one takes the trouble to notice it. The eyes are blinking frequently and this is also usually an unconscious act.

More perfect rest or relaxation of the eyes is obtained by reading this fine print perfectly than by doing some other things. By alternately looking at the large letters of the Snellen Test Card at 5 or 10 feet or further and reading the fine print close to the eyes, one can obtain flashes of improved vision at the distance. By practicing, these flashes become more frequent and the letters are seen more continuously. The method is to be highly recommended because it seems to be one of the best methods of improving the distant vision.

Fine Print (3-point font)

The photographic reduction of the fine print can be used with great benefit to patients suffering from high degrees of nearsightedness. At first it has to be held at a certain close distance from the eyes and cannot be seen so well if placed an inch further or an inch nearer. When read easily or perfectly the white spaces between the lines appear much whiter than they really are and the card seems to be moving from side to side or in other directions, if one takes the trouble to notice it. The eyes are blinking frequently and this is also usually an unconscious act.

More perfect rest or relaxation of the eyes is obtained by reading this fine print perfectly than by doing some other things. By alternately looking at the large letters of the Snellen Test Card at 5 or 10 feet or further and reading the fine print close to the eyes, one can obtain flashes of improved vision at the distance. By practicing, these flashes become more frequent and the letters are seen more continuously. The method is to be highly recommended because it seems to be one of the best methods of improving the distant vision.

Fine Print (2-point font – Microscopic size)

The photographic reduction of the fine print can be used with great benefit to patients suffering from high degrees of nearsightedness. At first it has to be held at a certain close distance from the eyes and cannot be seen so well if placed an inch further or an inch nearer. When read easily or perfectly the white spaces between the lines appear much whiter than they really are and the card seems to be moving from side to side or in other directions, if one takes the trouble to notice it. The eyes are blinking frequently and this is also usually an unconscious act.

More perfect rest or relaxation of the eyes is obtained by reading this fine print perfectly than by doing some other things. By alternately looking at the large letters of the Snellen Test Card at 5 or 10 feet or further and reading the fine print close to the eyes, one can obtain flashes of improved vision at the distance. By practicing, these flashes become more frequent and the letters are seen more continuously. The method is to be highly recommended because it seems to be one of the best methods of improving the distant vision.

The last paragraph is in microscopic print (2 point-font). If reading fine print benefits your vision, create your own! Print your favorite texts in tiny fonts and enjoy relaxing with them.

A note on speed reading

I am often asked whether speed reading courses are good for the eyes. I have never felt the need to take such a course but have looked at a few to see what they are about. My impression of these courses is that they teach you to take in several words, a whole line, a whole paragraph or even a whole page at one glance. This leads to diffusion of the eyes, which is a major strain and may lead to headaches as well as visual problems. Nearly all of my students who have tried speed reading tell me it gives them a headache. If you experience problems while attempting to speed read, you are probably straining your eyes!

Dr. Bates did not recommend such strained methods of rapid reading and explained his thoughts:

> In my writings, I have remonstrated against the methods employed to teach rapid reading. The usual procedure was to encourage the student to see all of the letters of a word at once, or to see all the letters of a paragraph of words at the same time. This was accepted as the correct method and very intelligent scholars have recommended it. My research work has proved that there is nothing more injurious to the eyes than to make an effort to see a whole letter or a whole word, all parts equally well. If one looks at the first letter of a word, the last letter is not seen perfectly at the same time. If an effort is made, the whole word becomes blurred and may not be distinguished. The stronger the effort that is made, the more injurious it is to the mind and eyes.

> With perfect sight, no effort is made and the eyes and mind are at rest. There is no fatigue, and one can read with great rapidity for many hours continuously, without being conscious of having eyes.[10]

My own experience is that I can read quite rapidly while using my eyes the way Dr. Bates suggests, by scanning over the white spaces in the text. This keeps the eyes moving swiftly and easily, there is no effort, and there is no conscious thought about my eyes. It is this ease of reading that allows for fast reading.

18. Clarifying Astigmatism

It took me several years to understand astigmatism. Dr. Bates wasn't very specific about it, and eye doctors I asked were typically just as confused as I was on this topic. You, if you are a lay person, are even less likely to have any clue what astigmatism is or what causes it.

Recently, when I was talking about my work with a small group of people in the street, one man interrupted me and said: "But I have 'stigmatism,' so it won't work for me." Not only did he not know how to say or spell the word, he had no clue what it really was. He believed it had to be something very serious, and definitely incurable. I know he isn't alone in his belief. He isn't to blame either; his eye doctor likely contributed to this fatalistic point of view.

What is astigmatism?

So, I will answer this question first: What *is* astigmatism? As a picture is worth a thousand words, let's take a look at some images. The human eye is not quite shaped like a perfectly round ball – it has a "bulge" on the front: the cornea. It looks like part of a smaller diameter ball that has been attached to the front of the main eyeball.

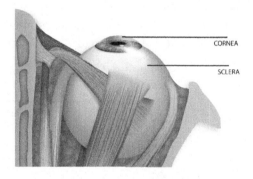

In a relaxed, healthy eye, the corneal curve is spherical, and if you make a topographical map of that healthy cornea it will show evenly spaced, symmetrical rings like this:

In an eye with astigmatism, the cornea looks different. Instead of being spherical it has more of a rugby-ball shape, which results in a steep curve in one direction and a flatter curve in the opposite direction. If the axis is at or near 90 degrees, its corneal topography map can look like this bottom image:

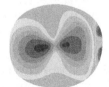

What causes astigmatism?

A quick search on the internet reveals that many eye doctors provide a poor explanation on their website as to "what causes astigmatism." They mainly point to the asymmetrical curvature of the cornea as "the cause." That asymmetrical curvature, however, is just a *symptom* of astigmatism, not its cause. Similar to Dr. Bates' conclusion that the elongated shape of a myopic eye is not due to the eye having grown that way but due to it being squeezed into that shape by the oblique eye muscles, the two teams of recti muscles (one side-to-side team and one up-and-down team) can have an uneven tension and thereby pull differently on the sclera (the white of the eye) in one meridian compared to the other. With the cornea attached to the sclera, it follows that this thin tissue is also affected by these forces pulling on it. So if, for example, the nasal and temporal recti muscles have more tension than the superior and inferior recti, the resulting uneven pull will lengthen the cornea horizontally, thereby flattening it somewhat in the horizontal axis and curving it relatively steeper in the vertical axis. Basically, astigmatism is related to muscle tension, and once you know what causes that tension, you have found the true cause of astigmatism. And that is something you can work with.

Astigmatism compensation in prescription numbers

An eye doctor measures the corneal curvature and adjusts the prescription accordingly – adding a cylinder to the glasses or contact lenses with a corresponding diopter (depending on the corneal curvature) at the appropriate axis (in this example, horizontal: 180˚). In a lens prescription, the astigmatism compensation (always a cylinder at a certain axis) may show as follows:

Sample prescription	Sphere	Astigmatism	
		Cylinder	**Axis**
Right Eye (OD)	-1.00	-0.75	180
Left Eye (OS)	-1.00	-0.75	180

The number under Sphere represents the power of the overall lens in diopters; it has either a minus sign for nearsighted eyes or a plus sign for farsighted eyes. The cylinder is also given in diopters. It has a similar – or + sign in front of it, and this diopter is tied to the axis number, which represents the angle at which the lens will be ground into a different curvature. This results in a rugby-ball-curved lens (the least-curved axis of which is called the cylinder) to compensate for the rugby-ball-shaped cornea. So, astigmatism is always represented by two numbers in a prescription: the cylinder and the axis.

It's easy to get confused by these numbers. I have been asked more than once if it is okay to reduce the astigmatism part in a prescription by reducing the axis number from, for example, 180 to 120. No; that will not work at all. Altering the axis number merely changes the angle of the cylinder but does not reduce its power. Rotating an axis to an angle where your eyes do not have a corresponding pull will result in glasses that greatly distort your vision and thus will only increase your eyestrain! So, don't mess with the axis numbers when you want to reduce your dependency on an astigmatism cylinder. Instead, lower the diopters of the cylinder. See Chapter 5 for suggestions for reducing the diopters.

Corneal versus lenticular astigmatism

A point of contention that eye doctors raise when I talk about my view on astigmatism, is that there are two places where astigmatism can manifest in the eye. One is the cornea, called corneal astigmatism, which I've discussed so far; the other is the lens inside the eye, which is called lenticular astigmatism. The lens is encircled by the ciliary muscle, and I suspect that uneven tension in various parts of this muscle can create a similarly uneven pull on the lens, thus creating an uneven curvature there too. Dr. Bates wrote that both corneal and lenticular astigmatism respond equally well to his relaxation techniques, so it doesn't matter which astigmatism you have or if you have both. Learn to release eyestrain and either one can be overcome.

Astigmatism fluctuates

The tension that creates astigmatism can be highly variable; cylinder and axis numbers can easily change from day to day, hour to hour, and even from minute to minute. This is especially true if you have not yet used glasses with a cylinder compensation. It also explains why it can be a challenge for an eye doctor to prescribe glasses that an astigmatic person is happy with, especially at first.

Once you do start using glasses or contact lenses with a cylinder, your eyes are likely to adapt to this static cylinder that they now get to peer through, which results in your astigmatism becoming more ingrained, and the tension that created it becoming chronic.

If your astigmatism numbers have been fairly steady, you can compare your axis numbers with the examples given below, so you can draw your own conclusions and begin to work more specifically on changing the habits that contribute to your astigmatism. If you don't know your axis numbers, the following chart will help you make an educated guess – whether you have astigmatism and at what axis.

This astigmatism chart (for a larger version, see page 285) shows axis degrees the way you see them. Your doctor uses a mirror image of this, with 180 degrees on the left, as he/she is looking at your eyes. Using one eye at a time (cover the other), look at this image in

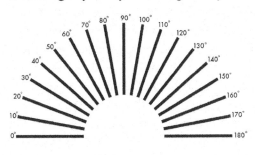

your blur zone and check for lines that look less black than others. If all lines look equally black or gray, chances are that you do not have astigmatism. If some lines look less distinct than others, you may have astigmatism and the axis is likely to be at the angle of most blur if you are myopic (this can be different for far-sighted eyes). Astigmatism can appear at any angle and each eye can have a different axis.

187

What an astigmatic eye sees

Astigmatism can cause some lines of the astigmatism chart to look perfectly black and clear while others, often 90 degrees away from the clearest line, look gray, fuzzy or doubled. Here are a few examples of how astigmatic vision can appear:

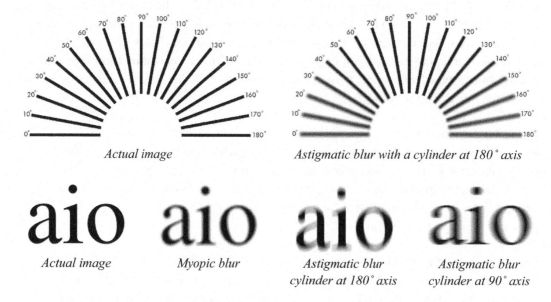

Actual image   *Astigmatic blur with a cylinder at 180° axis*

Actual image   *Myopic blur*   *Astigmatic blur cylinder at 180° axis*   *Astigmatic blur cylinder at 90° axis*

If the cylinder has a 180-degree axis (horizontal), the eye's strongest curvature is at 90 degrees (its vertical axis), which creates a double image that is pulled apart vertically. A horizontal line will therefore appear doubled or with gray edges, while a vertical line will seem clear, except at its top and bottom, where some blur may appear. Astigmatism can also create multiple images, such as seeing several moons – one bright, clear moon with one or more ghost-like moons to the side.

👁 Dr. Bates' advice regarding multiple images from astigmatism

Dr. Bates knew that strain causes these double or multiple images and said that palming your eyes will clear them. He also felt that learning to create multiple images on purpose would go a long way in overcoming the strain required to do so. Plus, he recommended imagining things perfectly, i.e., ignoring any additional images, and, knowing there is only one moon or one top letter on the chart, paying attention to and perfectly imagining the one main form that you know is reality. The less time and attention you give to any ghost images, the less prominent they become. The more you relax about the presence of such multiple images – not analyzing, judging or worrying about them – the sooner they disappear. Remember that instead of imagining a letter as perfectly black, it may be easier to imagine the white spaces in and around it to be perfectly white, which can help clear up the letter.[1]

Sometimes it can be difficult to tell which of the multiple images is the "real" one. In that case, one of my colleagues, Anna Bambridge from Scotland, suggests to totally accept however many images you see and give equal attention to every one of them. This is impossible to sustain, but it will elicit a natural shifting response which, in turn, may lead to a collapsing of all the images into one.[2]

Deeper understanding of the cause of astigmatism

It wasn't until I found Dr. Elliott Forrest's research with its clear explanations, that astigmatism began to make sense to me. After a four-year study,[3] Forrest, an optometrist in New York, found that astigmatism is an imbalance in the extraocular muscles caused by ingrained habits that disturb the natural relationship between eye motion, head motion, and posture. He found that repeated eye movement without head movement, which he termed "eye scanning," can cause astigmatism to set in along the same axis as the direction of the eye movements. Forrest realized that he could predict a person's typical posture or eye scanning habits simply by looking at their astigmatism cylinder and axis numbers.

Once I understood Forrest's work, I checked his conclusions on my astigmatic students and, like Forrest, I found I could quite accurately predict someone's postural and eye scanning habits based on the astigmatism numbers of their prescription. For example, I asked a student in Amsterdam if he tended to hold his head still while reading, because his astigmatism axes were at 180 degrees in both eyes. He emailed back, describing that his head was actually resting on his fist as he read my email, and yes, he had to admit that, his head didn't move along with his eyes as they scanned the text.

Paul Harris, O.D., a student of Forrest's work and a researcher and teacher at Southern College of Optometry in Memphis, Tennessee, used Forrest's findings and conducted his own research with symphony musicians.[4] Symphony musicians tend to play their instrument in specific, long-held postures, while often having to keep the head still as their eyes scan from music to instrument to conductor and back. Harris' findings support Forrest's conclusions: that habitual scanning habits without head motion contribute to astigmatism and often create a stronger astigmatism in one eye.

Dr. Forrest's research

One of Forrest's patients, a 43-year-old female with long-standing, stable astigmatism of -6.00 diopters at axis 90, showed a dramatic improvement to -1.25 diopters at axis 90 within two months. This led Forrest to believe that "under specific conditions, the visual system, at least in respect to astigmatism, might be sufficiently plastic in nature to be capable of alteration regardless of age."[5] The woman in question had experienced eight weeks of bedrest with her head immobilized, resulting in extensive side-to-side eye scanning, which counterbalanced her previous habit of vertical eye scanning that had led to her astigmatism.

What followed was a four-year clinical investigation with hundreds of his patients with astigmatism. These patients were questioned about their prolonged visual tasks – how they did these tasks, how they sat, how they held their head, where they placed their work, and how they moved their eyes. This study revealed that "most astigmatism, regardless of magnitude, was functionally related to visual task habits and that it developed or changed in a consistent manner."[5]

The research findings

Forrest concluded that many cases of astigmatism are functional – caused and altered by use, based on the interrelationship of three factors: eye scan, head scan, and head posture. An eye scan, as a reminder, is eye motion without the head following, while a head scan refers to the naturally yoked motion of the head following the eyes. Head posture reflects the head's habitual angle (chin up or down), tilt (ear to shoulder), and rotation (chin to shoulder) relative to the direction of gaze.

Your head and eyes need freedom to move in all directions. If you persistently limit free motion in one direction, but not in the direction 90 degrees away from that, you start to develop an imbalance in the eye muscles which will result in astigmatism within a few months. For example, if you typically let your head follow when you look up or down, but along a horizontal axis the eyes move while your head stays centered, you are likely to develop a minus cylinder astigmatism along the horizontal axis – in the meridian of greatest eye scan. The relatively greater tension in the medial and lateral recti muscles (compared to the inferior and superior recti) pulls the cornea flatter in the horizontal meridian, creating a cylindrical shape.

Don't worry if any of this is hard to wrap your mind around. Just knowing that unbalanced interplay between the three factors of eye scan, head scan and head posture can lead to astigmatism, tells you that changing this interplay can return balance. And with the release of habitual tension, you bring back non-astigmatic sight.

Examples of astigmatism axes and likely contributing causes

In the following images the black line across the eye represents the astigmatism cylinder, shown at various axes. With each example, you'll find a description of the correlation of the axes shown with the likely causes, as found by Forrest.

Important: All examples of axes shown represent *minus* cylinders, and the axes seen best are applicable to myopic eyes (*minus* sphere). For farsighted eyes (that have a *plus* sphere) the axes seen best can be the same as the axes of the cylinder – not rotated by 90 degrees. If your prescription shows a *plus* cylinder, you can convert it to an equivalent *minus* cylinder by turning the axis 90 degrees, either adding or subtracting 90 from the original number to stay within 180 degrees. For example, if your prescription shows a +1.50

cylinder at axis 80, this equals a -1.50 cylinder at axis 170. If it shows +0.75 cylinder at axis 110, the conversion will be -0.75 at axis 20. (Do *not* use this simplified conversion when ordering glasses; it is only useful here to find possible causes of your astigmatism.)

Let's start with two common examples. Horizontal eye scanning (such as holding the head still while reading) is likely to cause 180-degree (horizontal) astigmatism, while vertical scanning will trigger 90-degree (vertical) astigmatism.

Astigmatism axes as seen from an observer's point of view   **Axes seen best**:

R Axis 180/L Axis 180   R 90/L 90
Horizontal eye scan, vertical head scan.

R Axis 90/L Axis 90   R 180/L 180
Vertical eye scan, horizontal head scan.

Another of Forrest's observations was that if the head is held still and the eyes are turned in one direction for an appreciable length of time, the eye that crosses the midline of vision (the one that gazes across your nose) will be more astigmatic than the other, i.e., it will have a higher cylinder diopter.

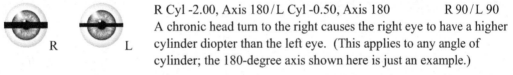

R Cyl -2.00, Axis 180/L Cyl -0.50, Axis 180   R 90/L 90
A chronic head turn to the right causes the right eye to have a higher cylinder diopter than the left eye. (This applies to any angle of cylinder; the 180-degree axis shown here is just an example.)

The angle at which you tend to hold your head (tilted to one side or leaning forward or back) will also influence astigmatism development, as can the angle at which reading material is held. For example, if your head typically tilts to your left by 20 degrees, both eyes are likely to show astigmatism with an axis of 70 degrees in case of a vertical eye scan, or 160 degrees in case of a horizontal eye scan.

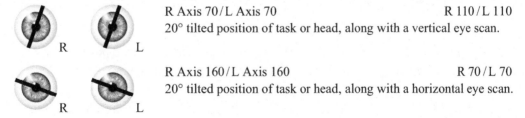

R Axis 70/L Axis 70   R 110/L 110
20° tilted position of task or head, along with a vertical eye scan.

R Axis 160/L Axis 160   R 70/L 70
20° tilted position of task or head, along with a horizontal eye scan.

People who have developed a habit of keeping the chin down while they gaze up at the world tend to have obliquely intorted axes, as shown below.

Astigmatism axes as seen from an observer's point of view   **Axes seen best**:

R L

R Axis 45/L Axis 135   R 135/L 45
Chin down, gaze up.

Combine the upward-gaze habit with either a vertical or horizontal eye scan and the intorted axes will either approach more vertical or more horizontal angles.

R L

R Axis 80/L Axis 100   R 170/L 10
Chin down, gaze up, vertical eye scan.

R L

R Axis 10/L Axis 170   R 100/L 80
Chin down, gaze up, horizontal eye scan.

If you tend to tilt your head back or gaze down a lot, the axes tend to point away from each other at the top, known as obliquely extorted.

R L

R Axis 135/L Axis 45   R 45/L 135
Chin up, gaze down.

This too can be combined with either a vertical or horizontal eye scan, which causes the extorted axis to either come closer to vertical or horizontal angles.

R L

R Axis 100/L Axis 80   R 10/L 170
Chin up, gaze down, vertical eye scan.

R L

R Axis 170/L Axis 10   R 80/L 100
Chin up, gaze down, horizontal eye scan

If the axes oppose each other as shown here, you either use different head positions for different planes of work, or you may have binocular fusion problems or an oblique scanning preference.

R L

R 180/L 90   R 90/L 180
Binocular fusion problem and/or oblique scanning preference.
Different head position for different planes of work.

Astigmatism overview

The obvious point in Dr. Forrest's research is that the head not following the eyes freely and equally in all directions is the underlying factor in astigmatism. Releasing tension and returning to the natural relationship between eye motion, head motion, and neck/postural balance addresses this imbalance and is the way to eliminate astigmatism.

Forrest noted that the actual level of astigmatism a person develops depends on the level of **tension and rigidity** with which a task is done. Rigidity and tension become astigmatism. If the same task is done with the same head tilt or same eye scan, yet the person remains relaxed, then vision tends to return to normal and astigmatism does not develop.

Forrest also stated that if there is equal eye movement along all the axes, no astigmatism forms. He therefore suggested that someone with a horizontal astigmatism in both eyes practices eye-scanning at the vertical axis to balance the muscles and overcome astigmatism, yet he found that those exercises did not always bring the desired result, especially when they were done with tension. That makes total sense to me, and I recommend that, rather than adding opposing eye-scanning habits to the strained habits you already have, it is more effective to release the strain of your current postural and scanning habits and return to the smooth, easy, natural order of motion in all directions, as described in Chapter 9.

19. Computer Screens: Look Beyond the 20/20/20 Rule

Since the invention of television, followed by computers, smart phones and tablets, the average amount of time adults in the U.S. now spend looking at light-emitting screens has risen considerably over the past few decades. Nine hours per day is the new norm.[1] This number is likely to rise, and the habit is spreading among children too. This doesn't seem like a healthy trend, considering the predominantly indoor, sedentary lifestyle that typically comes along with all this screen time.

What does so much screen time do to your eyes?
Along with the increasing screen time came a new condition: Computer Vision Syndrome, with a variety of symptoms experienced by those who "stare" at their screens too long. Headaches, fatigue, eyestrain, pain in or around the eyes, increased blurry vision, dry and irritated eyes, slow refocusing, inability to maintain near focus, neck and shoulder issues, backache, sensitivity to light, double vision and color distortion are among the unpleasant effects. In response to these issues, eye doctors often recommend "computer glasses," and they may also tell you to pay attention to good posture and better lighting, or to take breaks and follow "the 20/20/20 rule": Every 20 minutes, take a 20-second break and look at something 20 feet or more away. This advice is somewhat helpful; however, computer glasses do not solve the underlying problem of eyestrain, nor do they reduce the time you spend staring at these light-emitting screens. And the 20/20/20 rule is not enough to balance out the excessive use of screens.

Why are screens such a challenge to your eyes?
Part of the issue is the gross distortion of the light spectrum due to the use of LEDs in the screens. LEDs produce a lot of blue light and are grossly deficient in other parts of the spectrum (see Chapter 15). During the day, this distorted spectrum from the screen is not a big issue when natural light comes in through windows to balance it out. However, after sunset, this blue light inhibits the production of melatonin, the hormone needed to help you sleep. Even looking at relatively dim light from screens will delay melatonin production and messes with your circadian rhythm. Nighttime over-exposure to blue light is becoming more common, as more and more homes are lit by LED lights and so many people spend their evenings looking at screens. Without melatonin your circadian rhythm gets disrupted, which can lead to insomnia and health issues. According to the ANSES study I mentioned in Chapter 15, the retinas in your eyes, and especially in children's eyes, are at risk from over-exposure to blue light.

Another big part of the problem is that your eyes are designed to work with reflected light; they were not intended to look directly into light for extended periods. When you look at the pixels that make up a screen, it is very different from looking at a piece of paper held at the same distance. The piece of paper provides a clear focal distance: there is no ambiguity about where in space this paper is and thus where you need to focus. On the other hand, when you look into pixels of light in a screen, it is not as easy to discern the exact focal distance. Similar to an autofocus camera that zooms in and out trying to find the best focus on something not well-lit, your eyes also strain to find the right focal point when looking into pixels of light. Exactly how far away are these pixels?? Like that autofocus camera, your eyes will make many tiny focal adjustments back and forth to find the right focus, which can be an exhausting process if your vision isn't perfect anymore.

Although the blur often starts as a temporary condition, it will likely get worse if you don't learn how to not strain your eyes under these unnatural circumstances. Wearing computer glasses does not solve the problem; it only adds to the visual strain by encouraging the straining (and the long hours at the computer) to become a habit. Instead of those glasses, use some common sense and moderate your use of screens.

 Solutions

Use a screen projector instead of a screen. Until screen technology improves to something that is easy on your eyes, probably the best interim solution is to project your screen to a wall or a portable projector screen. This eliminates the problem of looking into pixels of light; your eyes can look at reflected light for which they are designed and thus eyestrain reduces drastically. Examples of screen projectors that you might consider using are provided on my website.[2]

If you can switch to using a projector, it will likely make a big difference to your eyes, yet this may not be a feasible option for everyone. For people who still have to deal with light-emitting screens, the following tips will likely help reduce strain resulting from too many hours looking into pixels of light.

Peripheral vision awareness. It will relax your eyes a lot if you make it a habit to stay aware of your peripheral vision when you use a screen. So often when viewing a screen, people fall into a tunnel vision mode, where the screen becomes all there is and the rest of their surroundings go unnoticed. This habit is often accompanied by squinting. Excluding the periphery makes it extra challenging to determine the correct focal distance of the screen. If, at the same time as seeing the screen, you release that squint and open your peripheral vision, you may notice the outer edges of the screen, the keyboard, items on your desk, the wall behind the screen, etc., and your brain can use these items as reference points to determine the actual focal distance of the screen itself. You will feel physical strain release as soon as you open to your peripheral vision. Your attention obviously is with the screen, and the peripheral items are not seen clearly, but they are there, and their exclusion can only cause strain, so let them be present.

Attention to small details and imagining the swing. While your interest is with the screen, practice continuously shifting your attention. You can't see the entire screen clearly all at once, so find the smallest details for extra clarity. With a computer, you can push the cursor around and follow its movement as an example of how your attention can shift easily across the screen. While your attention moves from one point on the screen to another, imagine the screen to be swinging. Actually, with peripheral vision open, everything around the screen will be swinging too. If you also set the font size to the smallest you can comfortably read without glasses, your eyes will make many small shifts that contribute to their relaxation.

Blink! It is amazing how blinking seems to be the first thing to go "out the window" when you look into any computer "window"... You may need lots of rapid blinking breaks, and it may help to stick a small label on the edge of your screen with the word "BLINK!" to remind you.

Reminders. That reminds me of another tip: Stick one or more narrow labels on the edge of your screen with your favorite (or most needed) vision hint written on it, such as: "Always Blink instead of Squint," "Peripheral Awareness," "Receive Light," "Effortless Central Clarity," or "As Attention Shifts, the World Swings." Make at least one of them in tiny print. Let your attention and eyes shift to one of those labels on a regular basis for a joyful mini-break. Besides serving as a reminder, it's a rest from the unfathomable pixels!

Look away. Deliberate shifts in focal distance are also restful to the eyes. Look up regularly, preferably out into the distance. If you don't have a window near your computer, a mirror on the wall behind the computer will provide the illusion of seeing into the distance (behind you). A well-placed mirror will also allow you to notice when your eyes begin to look strained or whether they remain relaxed.

Break-reminder software. I suggest you download software that reminds you to take breaks from your computer. On my PC, I currently use EyeLeo,[3] a free program that reminds me to take ten-second breaks every ten minutes to rest my eyes, while every hour the screen goes black for five minutes with a recommendation to get away from the computer for a while. For Mac screens, TimeOut[4] (also free) does the same thing.

These reminders and breaks are extremely good for me! I return to the screen with relaxed eyes and a fresh mind and thus can work more effectively. The reminders EyeLeo provides are not always in line with the Bates Method, but you can replace any of their "move your eyes" suggestions with relaxed alternatives. For example, each time a break-reminder box appears on your screen, check your posture and do some rapid blinking until the box disappears. TimeOut allows you to customize the reminders so you can target your own biggest strain issues and write reminders that increase awareness and promote a faster transition to relaxed habits.

Both these programs allow you to delay or cancel the hourly break, yet I highly recommend you resist the temptation to do so. Make this break a new healthy habit. Go outside, if possible, and you'll soon find it pays off in happier, healthier eyes; a happier, healthier you; and lots of little off-screen tasks that suddenly get done!

I suggest that you regularly schedule a day that is free from television, computer, and all your other light-emitting screens. Even better: enjoy a week-long screen-free holiday!

Smart use of light-emitting screens at night. Limiting your exposure to backlit screens at night is the best option, but if you do need to use them at night, use the pre-installed software that reduces the blue peak in their spectrum, such as Night Light (for PC/Android) or Night Shift (for Mac/iPhone/iPad). You can also download software such as f.lux, Iris, Redshift or Sunset Screen.[5-8]

The use of yellow-tinted glasses when using screens at night will also reduce the excess of blue light reaching your retinas, while orange or red-tinted glasses will get rid of all the blue and some of the greens too, which may be needed for anyone with insomnia, especially in the last hour or two before bedtime.

Another software solution is to invert the colors on your display so that you read white text on a black background. Look for the "Dark Mode" option in the device's settings. There is also software called "Dark Reader"[9] that lets you read white letters on black background on various internet browsers. You may find this white-on-black reading is easier on your eyes, and it also cuts down on blue light.

Keep at least one light on in the room when you watch light-emitting screens at night so you can stay aware of peripheral vision. It helps if that is an incandescent lamp, rather than a lamp that also spikes in the blue range of the spectrum.

Screen brightness, distance, height and your posture. Adjust the brightness of the screen to your liking. Whenever possible, place yourself at a distance from the screen at which you are most comfortable. Check your body posture for balance and overall relaxation. I sometimes teach at a student's home and have found more than once that the computer screen was placed too high in relation to their eyes. When you have to look up toward the screen, your neck muscles tense and your vision is affected, adding to astigmatic issues. Lowering the screen to where its top edge is level with your eyes takes much of that tension away. When you look slightly down toward the screen your neck and eyes will be more at ease. Laptops may have to be raised for comfort – there are special stands available to make that easy.[10] One thing to test is whether you breathe as easily and freely while sitting at your computer as you do when standing. If you notice less ease of breathing, support your middle back with some cushions until you find you are very comfortable and can breathe freely. A standing desk may be a good alternative.

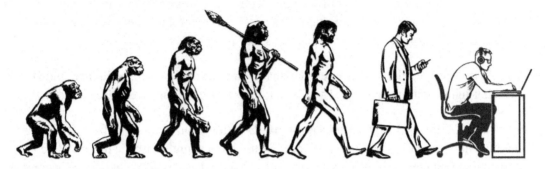

Use a plain wall or familiar picture to release eyestrain. If eyestrain remains an issue when using screens, look at a plain wall behind the screen or hang a favorite picture (or letter chart!) on a wall near the screen. Look at that wall, picture or chart, and notice if your eyes feel different when not looking into pixels. Do your eyes relax? Can you keep this feeling of relaxation while you shift your atttention and eyes to the edge of the screen? You are not even looking at the screen yet, just looking at its solid edge. Then back to the wall or picture. Then venture a little further into the screen. Continue going back to a plain wall or familiar picture where your eyes are able to relax, then gradually increase the amount of time viewing the screen, but only for as long as you can keep the eyes relaxed.

Play a 'Tele-Vision' game. If watching television tends to cause you to forget about your own vision habits or you regularly find yourself staring at the screen, you can make a game out of noticing the eyes of people on TV. Count their blink rate – how many seconds before they blink? Notice if they squint, and if so, do they squint both eyes or just one? Do you spot any head tilts? Let any bad habits you notice inspire you to use good habits, and if you happen to see a person whose face and eyes look relaxed and who blinks regularly and easily, copy their good habits! Basically, instead of worrying about your own vision habits, start noticing other people's habits. As a happy side-effect of this game you may find that awareness of your own habits increases.

20. Peering into the Night

It is common for people with blurry eyesight to complain of having their worst vision at night. The reason you see better in daylight is because bright light narrows down your pupils to a small opening and this smaller aperture, like a camera, provides a greater focal distance – greater clarity over a longer range, thus reducing myopic blur. In dim light or darkness, the pupils stay open wider, which makes blurry vision more obvious. So, until your daytime vision clears up, you can't expect nighttime vision to be perfect. But there are a few things you can do in the meantime to help your night vision.

 Wait a while

Your retinas contain a pigment known as rhodopsin, or visual purple, which helps your night vision. When exposed to light, rhodopsin bleaches and becomes opsin, which changes back to rhodopsin in the absence of light. This transformation takes a little time, causing you to be momentarily blind when going from light to dark, and momentarily sensing extra brightness when going from dark to light. Some people adapt from one to the other fairly quickly, while others take longer. In fact, it takes an hour for vision to fully adjust to true darkness, but luckily, 80% of the night adaptation is done in the first fifteen minutes, and it doesn't take very long to see reasonably well at night. A little patience, along with avoidance of artificial light, goes a long way in your ability to see in the dark.

 Get more dark exposure

The more you experience darkness, the better your eyes adapt to night vision. It is therefore beneficial to sleep in a dark room where artificial lights are excluded. The darker the better for your eyes, as even small amounts of light can come through closed eyelids and interfere with the production of rhodopsin.

In Europe during World War II, nighttime blackouts were the norm, as streetlights or house lights would attract the attention of aerial bombers. In *Improve Your Eyes at Home*,[1] Robert Brooks Simpkins relates an experience of improved night vision during these blackout periods in England:

> Many of us making our way about in the black-out of the last war found that our ability to see in the 'dark' progressively improved in an almost astonishing manner – while when we returned to a lighted room our sight was noticeably keener. One of the disadvantages of modern civilization, with our lighted streets in the towns, is that mainly we do not use our eyes enough in the dark – and many villages have adopted some form of outdoor lighting.

Gary, an American man I met in Costa Rica, told me about his night vision experience during an extended exploration in a remote, forested area on his property near Uvita. He did not even use as much as candlelight, so in the first three months he would settle into his campsite at dusk, wait for darkness, and then simply go to sleep, as there wasn't anything useful he could safely do from that point onward. Early in the fourth month, however, he found his eyes adjusted. To his surprise, dusk did not give way to darkness one night. He assumed it was a full moon, got up, and carefully moved around in this unusual greenish-tinged light. When he looked up through a break in the canopy, he saw the crescent of a waning moon, barely visible through the thick cloud cover! He expected this "unnatural" night vision would disappear as mysteriously as it had come, but it did not. From then on, even on new moon nights, he found he no longer went "blind" at night and was able to explore and move around as easily as he did during the day.[2]

Regular exposure to darkness clearly is a major component of improved night vision adaptation. So before bedtime, go take a walk under the stars, or if you live in a city where darkness is hard to come by, sit in a dark room and make plans for a vacation to the forest. When you go on your night walk (with a group of friends for safety, if needed) leave your flashlight off and give your eyes time to adjust. Notice how blackness soon gives way to shades of gray and different levels of shimmer. A well-trodden forest trail will appear lighter than the soil next to it; a starry sky will contrast clearly with the outline of trees. When you regularly explore in the dark to the edge of your level of comfort, you will soon find yourself going well beyond old perceived limitations.

If you would like to get involved in reducing excessive light pollution at night, contact the international Dark-Sky Association.[3] They work on changing policies that regulate outdoor lighting at night. A dark sky conserves energy, is better for your eyes and health, and also benefits wildlife.

Use Dr. Bates' advice on night vision

Bates' advice for improving night vision was to practice the imagination of perfect sight, not only in the bright light of daytime when that is easier to do, but also in dim light. Use a favorite letter on the chart, or use any object you enjoy looking at, and after looking at it in your area of best vision, move it into your slight blur zone. Close your eyes, then imagine seeing it with perfect clarity, one detail at a time. Let your eyes open in flashes while you continue using your imagination of perfect vision and notice how, gradually, this will improve your vision in low light.[4]

Dr. Bates once described how a patient had found relief from night blindness when he straightened his spine to improve his posture.[5] In addition, staying mentally relaxed results in a smaller pupil than being fearful does, so relaxation also improves clarity in dim light.

Plus, regularly enjoying the sunning-palming sandwich (Chapter 15) can aid your ability to adapt to dim light and darkness.

 Use your peripheral vision

In true night vision conditions, there is not enough light to stimulate the cones of your central vision, while the rods that provide peripheral vision continue to function quite well. Driving at night is not an example of true night vision, because car headlights provide enough light for the cones to function. Walking in nature (away from city lights) on a moonless night does provide the right conditions for true night vision. During such a night walk, stop for a minute and look up at the stars. Pick the dimmest star you notice up there, then look directly at it. When you look directly at it, you'll find the dim star disappears, as if someone flipped off its light switch. That's because the cones in your central vision are not triggered by the star's dim light. As soon as you look slightly away from it, your peripheral rods will be triggered by the dim light, so the star will "magically" reappear.

A successful experiment in using peripheral vision at night

In the late 1980s in Northern New Mexico, Nelson Zink and Stephen Parks wanted to explore the difference between seeing with the eyes versus seeing with the mind. Looking for references on this topic they found texts from Taoists of early China, books by Carlos Castaneda, and advice from Miyamoto Musashi, the legendary swordsman of fifteenth century Japan, all mentioning the power of peripheral vision. Having studied the difference between rods and cones, they decided it would be a nice experiment to get out of tunnel vision and practice opening to their peripheral vision. They started this practice in daytime, but soon moved it to nighttime, realizing darkness would drastically reduce the tendency to use the cones of central vision.

On the bill of a baseball cap they mounted a metal rod welded to a binder clip, which extended about a foot in front of their eyes. On the tip of the rod they glued a small bead of plastic resin, about the size of a baby green pea. This created a fixed point on which to focus. For night vision practice they added luminescent paint to the beads. Making sure the bead was at eye level and directly in front of their nose, they would go out at dusk in an area where no city lights would interfere.

They started walking, with their central gaze relaxed on the bead, navigating the trail relying only on their peripheral vision. They soon found their feet seemed to know where to step: obstacles were avoided without consciously seeing them. They could shift their attention to any object in their peripheral vision without needing to shift their eyes. As they became proficient at seeing in the dark, they

---

found that they could run down arroyos and climb steep banks in the dead of night, all while focusing on the luminescent beads.

They found that anxiety and fear of the dark, so common in our culture, were effectively eliminated. Instead, they experienced relaxation, exhilaration and delight, which increased their sense of safety and happiness. An optometrist they consulted to make sure they were not harming their eyes, gave them a clean bill of health, and after joining them for his first night walk speculated about the value of night walking in treating myopia.[6]

You don't need to go to the extent of using a small bead extended out from a baseball cap, but it does improve your ability to relax and see in the dark when you stop looking for details and instead increase awareness of what is visible in your large peripheral field.

A "glow-in-the-dark" practice to improve night vision and peripheral vision
In the 1950s, Robert B. Hagmann of Daly City, California, developed vision improvement techniques to reduce myopia and to improve binocular vision and night vision. Hagmann recommended the following practice in a dark room to help improve night vision.[7,8]

Requirements: Two glow-in-the-dark items (available from toy stores or make your own with glow-in-the-dark paint) and a dark room after sunset, or a windowless room during the day. When the light is off, the room should be pitch black.

Place the two glow-in-the-dark items under a bright light for a few minutes to "charge" them. Then sit or stand within easy reach of the light switch and pick a point to look at straight ahead of you. Notice what the limit of your peripheral vision is to your left and to your right while you look at this point. Place the two items in those areas, one on each side of you, about 5 feet away. If placed correctly, they will be just visible at the edge of your peripheral vision while you look at your chosen point straight ahead.

Once these items are placed on each side of you, gaze at the point straight ahead, and keep your attention there while you switch off the light. As soon as the light is off, count softly to yourself while you wait for your eyes to adjust for night vision.

How long does it take before you are able to distinguish the two items glowing in your peripheral vision? Is one eye faster in picking it up than the other? Once you can see both items glowing in your periphery, switch the light back on and let them charge up again. Repeat this several times, switching the light off and counting numbers until you can see the glow, then switching the light on again. Notice if your eyes get quicker at picking up the glow of these items in the dark. Regular peripheral stimulation like this will help your eyes adjust faster to night vision.

Detriments to night vision

Lastly, here are a few possible detriments to night vision:

- Being in "fight or flight" mode causes pupil dilation, as does mental strain and strong emotional stimulation.

- Some drugs cause pupil dilation (including some antidepressants, amphetamines, psilocybin, LSD, ecstasy, cocaine and mescaline).

- Smoking affects the production of rhodopsin.

- High cholesterol levels.

- Deficiencies of vitamin A, vitamin B-complex, lutein, zeaxanthin, and zinc.

21. Drive the Road to Clarity

Natural Vision Habits for Driving

Driving often has a positive influence on vision because it requires constant shifting, and it stimulates peripheral awareness with its near-constant apparent motion. Even though you sit still and may even have a staring habit, the car's motion creates apparent motion, which will keep breaking that tendency to stare. For this reason, many students report their first flashes of clarity while driving. My own first 3-D experience came while driving. Yet in my nearsighted days, I used to not be able to drive for more than an hour before I'd have to stop and allow my eyes a few minutes of total rest. Ever since I improved my sight back to clarity, I can easily drive for hours, with toilet breaks now being a first reason to stop, not tired eyes. I have driven from coast to coast across the United States several times and have created the following vision tips for driving from my own experience.

 Afore ye go…

- Regularly clean windshields, mirrors and headlights. Don't forget the insides of front and rear windshields, especially if you like to drive with open windows. You'll be surprised at how much clearer things look when you get rid of the "road haze" that has accumulated!

- Sit behind the wheel in a tall, relaxed posture, with adequate support to allow for easy, deep breathing (no collapsed chest). Use a small cushion for extra back support, if necessary. In this relaxed posture, adjust your rear-view mirrors to optimal angles. This way your mirrors will remind you to lengthen or adjust your posture when the view from them becomes less than ideal due to slouching, tensing or leaning forward while trying to see better.

- Loosen any restrictive or tight clothing (belt, necktie, bra, etc.).

- Be safe on the road: Use 20/40 glasses if required (see page 33) and keep full-prescription glasses in the glove compartment, in case you feel a need for them

- Smile. ☺ Smiling relaxes your face muscles as well as your mind.

- Remind yourself of good vision habits to be used while driving. (See below.)

- Have a relaxed grip on the steering wheel.

- Start the engine, check gauges, and enjoy your trip.

As you drive:

- Remember: You cannot control other drivers, but you can control the distance between you and the car in front. A little extra distance is a lot more relaxing.

- Relax by imagining that all other drivers are your friends traveling with you today, and it is not a race…

- Release your neck muscles so your eyes and head can move freely. Move and flex your body occasionally; a mini "twist dance" in your seat helps blood circulation.

- Glance frequently at gauges and mirrors.

- A relaxed awareness of your peripheral vision greatly enhances your safety and relaxes your central vision. Rear-view mirrors are excellent peripheral vision practice tools – can you stay aware of all of them while looking at the road ahead?

- Imagine that the center stripes and the road surface are rolling toward and underneath you like a conveyor belt. Notice that everything outside moves opposite to your movement. Consciously allowing that movement is far more relaxing than unconsciously trying to stop it. Motion sickness happens when you try to not see movement. One of my students had a friend with great eyesight; this man would never just "go for a drive." Instead he would suggest "let's go make the world spin!" thereby demonstrating his innate awareness of apparent motion while driving.

- Occasionally check that your grip on the steering wheel remains relaxed.

- Blink frequently and effortlessly, especially when using the heater or air-conditioner, as these tend to dry out the eyes. Point the air vents away from your face to reduce the drying effect of air blowing onto your eyes.

- Breathe abdominally. If something tenses you, exhale fully by blowing that tension out and then allow your natural abdominal inhale to return by itself.

- Shrug shoulders when tired for extra circulation to the eyes and brain. Pull your shoulders up to the ears, push them back, then relax and let them drop down.

- On long trips, stop and rest at regular intervals, especially when your eyes feel tired. When parked, close your eyes for a while – just five seconds will help. Then get out and move around: stretch out, swing your arms, twist your spine, jog in place. Do anything to increase circulation!

- If you're driving into a rising or setting sun, use the visor to shield your eyes and let them blink as much as they want. I prefer to not use the visor, but as soon as I turn the car toward the setting sun my blink rate instantly changes from once every two or three seconds to two or three times per second! With that rapid yet relaxed blinking, I have no need to squint and remain quite comfortable and able to see the road ahead of me with ease.

Night driving

I did not take naturally to learning to drive; I had to overcome a fear of being hit by other cars. This fear, which probably stemmed from a few accidents my dad had while I was a small child in the back seat, was especially present at night. It was the time when my vision became slightly blurry, and I now think that learning to drive may have been a contributor to my initial blur. I found headlights of oncoming traffic to be my biggest challenge, and I really did not like the night-driving lessons I had to take to prepare for my test. To help me be more at ease, my instructor told me to not look into those oncoming headlights and instead look away to the side of the road. I realize now that his advice caused more strain than it solved – I cowered away from the lights even more and strained to avoid them.

Eyes are naturally drawn to light. To demonstrate this, close your eyes outdoors at night, then open them briefly and quickly close them again. What were your eyes drawn to while they were open? It was likely an area of light, not an area of darkness. This is totally normal, because your eyes are designed for light and they naturally seek it out in the dark. So, any avoidance of looking at light is a strain. This includes headlights of oncoming traffic. While I learned to avoid looking into the headlights, my stress level only increased, and my discomfort with night driving stayed.

When I improved my vision and did a lot of sunning, I found that those oncoming lights were no longer a problem. They no longer seemed overwhelmingly bright. In fact, I have learned to allow my eyes to look into these lights, and I do not fight that natural tendency any more. Looking into these lights does not blind me at all; dipping my eyes into them is actually very relaxing! A brief dip into the light is all that I need; it satisfies my eyes' natural tendency and it puts my mind at rest to see that this vehicle is not on a collision course with mine. I then return my attention to the road and continue to drive with ease.

If oncoming headlights seem blinding

For some people, oncoming headlights seem particularly "blinding." My student Albert had this problem. He had severe light sensitivity after episodes of sudden blindness. Albert was unable to drive at night because oncoming headlights blinded him and bright lights in general hurt his eyes.

I helped him relax his way of seeing, got him out of his habitual and chronic squinting, and taught him the basic sunning practices to become more comfortable in the bright sunlight of the Southern California desert. After a few sessions, he wasn't so sensitive to light anymore and was able to drive at night. If someone with such a severe case of light sensitivity as Albert can accomplish this, then I think almost anyone can.

Night driving

- Pay attention to what you CAN see, rather than what you can't see. Notice how the center stripes seem to move toward you and pass you by.

- Keep a relaxed awareness of your peripheral vision. It will serve you even more at night than during the day.

- Happily glance into oncoming headlights and road lights; don't strain to avoid them. This will become easier after regular closed eyelid sunning during the day.

- All of the daytime vision habits for driving apply equally at night. So relax to see; use attention to detail within the area lit up by your headlights; let your attention shift continuously and effortlessly; blink often and breathe easily.

- On dark, rainy nights, besides lowering your speed and increasing the distance between you and the car in front of you, it is even more important to use relaxed vision habits. It is normal to see much less under these conditions, so avoid straining to see more. Bring greater awareness to your peripheral vision instead, without staring of course.

- Keep your full prescription glasses within easy reach so they are available if you need them. If you're wondering whether to use them or not, it probably is time to put them on. Don't hesitate to do so, especially on rainy nights. Your safety is far more important than any worries about the temporary loss of vision improvement.

- Use your common sense as much as your natural vision habits!

22. Help a Child to Better Sight

When a parent calls to ask for my help because their child has just been diagnosed as needing glasses, they typically express deep concerns for their child's future eyesight. They sense something is wrong about making a child wear glasses and are looking for a better solution. They understand what Dr. Bates meant when he said: "As for putting glasses upon a child, it is enough to make the angels weep."[1]

I know how they feel. When I first saw my fun-loving niece Emma after she was given glasses for hyperopia (farsightedness) at age five, I noticed a big change in her demeanor. It seemed to me that the outgoing, carefree and playful little girl I knew had suddenly become introverted and serious. This is not surprising; glasses affect a child in many ways. The child knows they "failed" a test; that something is wrong with their eyes, and that somehow their life is permanently changed – their gaze is no longer free to roam, their body is more tense than before, their confidence is shaken, and their vision is permanently impaired. They have been sentenced to a life behind glasses.

Often children experience headaches, fatigue or discomfort from their glasses. They may get teased about their changed appearance, feel inadequate, have low self-esteem, and they can no longer play freely without fear of breaking their glasses. That's a lot to deal with for a child, and they will carry these issues with them into adulthood – unless they are shown how to let vision be effortless again.

Vision varies greatly in the first year of life

For some years, Dr. Bates tested the eyes of newborn babies and kept records of their vision over their childhood years.[2] He found that babies get eyestrain too and that their vision varies tremendously in the first six months, changing from normal to hyperopia, to myopia, to astigmatism and back to normal on a regular basis. Various forms of eyestrain, including strabismus (such as "cross-eyes"), can also occur while the child sleeps and can persist for some time when awake. Bates found that only after six months or by one year old do the eyes become more continuously normal. An optometry journal from 2011 shows that refractive errors at birth typically range from -1 myopia to +5 hyperopia and this tends to level out by three or four years of age.[3] Bates agrees, saying that at four to six years of age, just before children begin school, their vision is usually normal. After a year or more in school, hyperopia tends to start and increases every year. Myopia tends to appear around age ten or twelve and increases, while hyperopia gets less by then. Bates noticed some children change from hyperopia one year to myopia the next, then back to hyperopia, and then to normal.

Glasses are not a good solution

Due to these fluctuations in children's vision, it really does not make sense to try fitting them with something as static as glasses. Glasses only reinforce the strain and create worse vision over time. If the child has headaches or symptoms of eyestrain, it makes more sense to let them rest for a few days or a week to give them a chance to recover without ever needing glasses. Dr. Bates guaranteed that he could cure any child under the age of sixteen if they had not yet worn glasses. He said they would usually be cured within a few days, weeks or months, and always within a year.[4]

Determining a young child's prescription is challenging

Schools are not the only problem in the current global myopia epidemic. The protocol used by eye doctors who are quick to prescribe glasses for minor visual problems needs to change too. Eye doctors can end up writing inaccurate prescriptions for young children, especially when they use pupil-dilating eye drops and when the diopters are plus numbers. Tania, the mother of a two-year-old boy, told me her son's examination before eye drops showed +2.00 hyperopia, but after the doctor put drops in her son's eyes it increased by two whole diopters to +4.00. Those two additional diopters are *caused* by the eye drops; this is not representative of how the boy sees in normal daily life when his eye muscles are not numbed by eye drops. Making him wear +4.00 glasses will only worsen his problems. The original +2.00 diopters measured for this boy under artificial light and stressful conditions are unlikely to be accurate to begin with.

Blindly trusting the eye doctor may not be in your or your child's best interest. In 2013, I visited Tara in Arizona, whose seven-year-old son Adam was very reluctant to wear his glasses for astigmatism that had been prescribed six months earlier. He only put them on if his mother insisted on it, and then only for short periods. When I asked Adam to read the chart without his glasses, he did fairly well; his right eye read 20/20, his left 20/60, but when I asked him to put on his glasses and read the chart again, we found the glasses did not improve his left eye's vision at all – still 20/60 – while the right eye could suddenly only read 20/160. His vision was much worse with glasses than without! This young lad was unable to explain to his mother that the glasses made his vision worse; he was just trying to please her. And she was just trying to follow doctor's orders... Tara was mortified when she realized that the glasses made his vision worse and that she had admonished him to put these glasses on, despite his protests. Moral of the story: Listen to your child and your instincts more closely than you listen to an eye doctor.

Children's eyes adapt to the power of the glasses given

If children who have normal sight are made to wear reading glasses continuously, they become farsighted and able to see with these glasses. In fact, many people with normal sight can, by wearing glasses continuously, become able to see well at a distance with plus lenses, even though they are not farsighted. Just as there are children who can wear minus lenses and see with them, although their vision may be perfectly good without the glasses.[2] Luke's story is an example of a young child's eyes adapting to the glasses he used.

Luke's story, written by his father, John C.

My wife, Roxana, and I had often wondered about our then three-year-old Luke's eyesight. He often did not seem to be able to see things. When we tried to test him, he would usually agree that he could see something we pointed out, but I wasn't so sure. Then, the day we went to the wild animal park and Luke asked us where the elephants were that we were talking about, my wife and I knew the poor little guy couldn't see. The elephants were about 30 yards from us, in plain sight, in the middle of the day and Luke appeared not to be able to see anything at all.

A visit to the optometrist confirmed what we suspected: Luke had bad vision, very bad vision: +6.25 in each eye. Practically, he couldn't see anything. At first, even with full prescription glasses, Luke could not see better than 20/40 on the eyechart.

The optometrist was a bit surprised to find a little guy with such poor vision. She recommended that we "work up to" his full prescription, as it could be difficult for his eyes to jump from no glasses to full time +6.25 prescription glasses. We started at +4.25. The optometrist said eventually Luke's eyes will relax into the glasses and that full +6.25 prescription glasses should eventually allow him to achieve 20/20 vision without strain.

Six months later, Luke had a somewhat discernible "lazy" eye. The optometrist recommended we start patching his eye for two hours each day. Now, asking a three-year-old to put a patch over his "good" eye every day for two hours is about as easy as asking my cat to jump into the pool every day for a bath. I couldn't even wear a patch myself for more than twenty minutes without getting nauseous.

We tried, and three months later, Luke's vision was a little better. His lazy eye was less lazy and his vision had improved somewhat, so we stopped patching. However, six months and another disappointing trip to the optometrist later, I started to wonder what else could be done. The two optometrists we had seen could not suggest any other options for improving Luke's eyes, other than wearing his glasses and patching his good eye to make his "bad" eye stronger.

That's when I found a Vision Therapy Optometrist. After a thorough examination, the vision therapist told us Luke had amblyopia and strabismus. Even while wearing full prescription lenses, his "bad" eye could not see any more than 20/40. Thus, we began vision therapy.*

After about three once-a-week sessions of vision therapy, a couple things became clear to me: 1) vision therapy was going to work great and 2) we needed to do the vision therapy primarily ourselves at home. We bought the home vision therapy software and we did it religiously for five or ten minutes almost every day.

After about eight weeks of vision therapy, Luke's vision started to improve, his eye turn was more difficult to detect, and his eyes started working together somewhat better. What was also interesting to me was that his "refractive error," or basically his eyesight, had improved dramatically to +4.25, exactly equal to his glasses prescription. How did that happen? Had he "grown into" his glasses? Did his eyes adapt to the glasses?

Surely this was not a coincidence. I asked the doctor if she would lower the prescription a little to see what happens. She lowered his prescription from +4.25 to +3.50 and three months later, we found that his vision had adjusted, again, to match the new prescription. That's when I knew we were on to something potentially very significant. That is also when I was blessed to have found Dr. Marc Grossman in New York.

Based on Dr. Grossman's guidance, we reduced Luke's lens prescription again by a small amount, +0.25 diopters. After two months with the new lenses, his eyes had adjusted again to exactly match the new prescription. Thus began the long, steady journey of reducing Luke's lenses by 0.25 diopters every two months and finding that his vision was indeed tracking the improvement exactly. From +4.25 to +3.50 to +3.25, to +3.00, to +2.75, to +2.50, to +2.25, to +2.00, to +1.75, to +1.50, to +1.25, to +1.00, to +0.50. Thirteen new lenses over two years. We were also still doing vision therapy the whole time to support his eyesight and the transition to the new lenses, though we had cut the practices down to just a couple minutes each morning.

At six years old, in May 2016, Luke threw away his glasses for good and currently has 20/20 vision without glasses. His strabismus and amblyopia have both been corrected. He has a slight refractive error, +1.50 in each eye, and one eye is still slightly more strained, but we are hopeful these last bits will naturally correct over time. He is an avid participant in physical activities and an eager student in school.

* Esther's note: Vision therapy involves doing eye exercises using a variety of equipment. It is usually combined with wearing glasses. It can be beneficial, yet progress is often slow, the exercises are tedious, and it typically requires weekly office visits.

Parents influence children's sight

Although myopia is not inherited (see Chapter 3) children do imitate their parents, including their visual behaviors. If you have relaxed habits and blink often, your child has a good example to follow. Similarly, if you habitually stare, strain, squint or tilt your head, chances are your child will copy that strained example. The environment you provide for them can help or hinder their visual development, so where possible provide them with more outdoor time, good visual examples, and less stress.

Of course, parents cannot control all the factors that determine a child's vision. For example, a difficult childbirth can cause vision problems at a very young age. In this case gentle massage of areas traumatized during the infant's birth (e.g. its head or neck) is likely to be helpful. When accidents happen and an eye is injured, besides the medical treatment the child may need, it will likely also be useful to teach the child how to keep their eyestrain at a minimum, so healing can happen faster.

Schools and children's eyesight

For most myopic eyes, the problem started during school years. This is no surprise, as at the age when school starts, outdoor time diminishes. By age eight, learning to read turns into reading to learn, expectations rise, pressure increases, outdoor time diminishes even further, indoor time is often under poor artificial lighting – and thus the eyes typically respond by straining for the first time. This eyestrain is closely followed by a first pair of glasses, which are to be worn all day long. The glasses create even more eyestrain and less relaxed motion, and so the child ends up joining the crowd in the myopia epidemic with gradually increasing prescriptions. Glasses have become the norm, rather than the exception they used to be. Millions of children are burdened by this, both physically and mentally. Yet Dr. Bates knew that practically all cases of poor eyesight in school children can be cured – and the development of new ones prevented – in a simple way.

Children usually improve their vision faster than adults

If children have not yet worn glasses or developed chronic habits of strain, they often return easily and quickly to clear vision. Even when they already have worn glasses, children tend to be quicker at overcoming vision challenges than adults.

> **Eyestrain can be cured so easily in the average child by Dr. Bates' method that it should be against the law to fit children with glasses.**
> Paul Hotson, O.D.[5]

Here are a few examples of children who were quick to respond to the Bates Method:

Zoe's double vision

In the fall of 2013, Bianca, the mother of ten-year-old Zoe, asked for my help. Zoe had been experiencing some blurry vision and double vision that year, at first intermittently, but during the last few months it had become a chronic problem. An eye doctor they consulted felt the blurry vision was mild and that Zoe didn't need glasses, while the double vision was mainly caused by her left eye turning outward. This turn was not yet deemed stable, so Bianca was asked to return with Zoe in two months to talk about the option of surgery to straighten that eye. The doctor did mention that Zoe needed to learn to strain less to see, without explaining how to achieve this. Bianca researched this topic on the internet and found a book on the Bates Method written by my colleague Saskia Naber.[6] From the book, she taught Zoe how to palm her eyes. Palming helped Zoe overcome her mild blurry vision, but the double vision was still a problem. Bianca was eager to avoid surgery for her daughter, so they came to see me.

My first aim was to help Zoe increase the distance between the objects she saw double. With some effort she was able to do so, and by releasing the effort she noticed the distance between the two images reduced again. At this point, Zoe began to realize she had some control over her left eye's position, but tension in the lateral rectus muscle of that eye prevented it from straightening completely. When she looked at the tip of her nose to encourage the left eye to come in, it would come to center, but not to her nose.

As Zoe began to grasp that undue tension in one muscle was her main problem, I talked her through a palming meditation which focused on releasing the tension in that specific muscle. When she opened her eyes, at first in flashes, her vision was single. I allowed her to keep her eyes open longer, yet I instructed her to close them as soon as images started doubling again. She promised she would do so, but she didn't close her eyes other than for blinking. I reminded her to close them at the first sign of doubling, but she joyfully assured me she saw everything single, and to my own and her mother's surprise, it stayed that way. We had only spent one hour together.

I kept in touch with Bianca in the following months and was delighted to hear that by the summer of 2014, the eye doctor no longer saw a need for regular check-ups, the surgery plans were cancelled, and although on rare occasions Zoe's eye would still wander out a bit, she knew how to release that strain and maintain her single vision. What a fantastic and speedy result! It was, of course, fortunate that Zoe had not yet worn glasses and that her mother had brought her to me soon after the problems started, but it did show how easily and fast children can be saved from a lifetime of vision challenges if they are shown how to help themselves.

Overcoming reluctance
Sometimes children are reluctant to work with me. I distinctly remember two girls – Jen, a teenager in California, and Tanya, an eight-year-old in Arizona – who each felt that coming to see me was their mother's "stupid idea," and neither was inclined to cooperate with me. With both girls I found palming was an effective way through their armor – as soon as they finished palming and saw distinctly better, reading several lines more on the chart, their attitudes improved delightfully.

Of the two, it was Tanya's resistance that lasted a little longer, perhaps because she had already read several "stupid books with weird, silly eye exercises." I told her that I used to think just like she did – that eye exercises were boring and stupid, and that I was not willing to do them for the rest of my life either. I then calmly explained that I eventually learned that exercises were not the right answer, and that vision can only improve through relaxation. Well, she had tried palming (for five minutes) and "it did not help, and it was a stupid thing to do."

I managed to convince Tanya to try "my way" of palming, as I expected it would be different from what she had done before. Sure enough, this palming session doubled her vision from 8/30 to 8/15 in her left eye. (Her right eye already had excellent vision, seeing 8/7.) However, she still balked at it all.

"Am I now supposed to do palming all day?" she asked.

"No," I explained in a soft, friendly voice, "because palming is passive relaxation, and it's not very useful in regular daily life. For that, you need dynamic relaxation. You need to learn how to relax your left eye while you are using it."

"Oh great, I don't know how to relax it, so I can't do that," she responded.

"I understand," I said, "but I can teach you how to relax it. Would you like to know how?"

Tanya reluctantly decided that maybe I could teach her something that was different from all those "stupid books"… And so I did, and she took to it, loved it, and her left eye improved to 8/10 in that session. What worked beautifully for her was the eye-balancing practice, helping her left eye see with the same clarity that the right eye had just given her (see Chapter 23, Step 1D). I was so warmed by her turn-around in attitude and by her sweet hug at the end. It was immensely satisfying to see a girl like Tanya start to relax and learn to love the Bates Method.

Children helping others

In his monthly *Better Eyesight* magazines, Dr. Bates related endless stories of children improving their sight, some quickly, some taking more time. In the second issue,[7] he relates the most wonderful story of Emily, who helped other children in her class improve their vision after she had been taught by Dr. Bates:

The story of Emily

The efficacy of the method of treating imperfect sight without glasses has been demonstrated in thousands of cases, not only in my own practice but in that of many persons of whom I may not even have heard; for almost all patients when they are cured proceed to cure others. At a social gathering one evening a lady told me that she had met a number of my patients; but when she mentioned their names, I found that I did not remember any of them, and said so.

"That is because you cured them by proxy," she said. "You didn't directly cure Mrs. Jones or Mrs. Brown, but you cured Mrs. Smith and Mrs. Smith cured the other ladies. You didn't treat Mr. and Mrs. Simpkins, or Mr. Simpkins' mother and brother, but you

---

may remember that you cured Mr. Simpkins' boy of a squint, and he cured the rest of the family."

In schools where the Snellen test card was used to prevent and cure imperfect sight, the children, after they were cured themselves, often took to the practice of ophthalmology with the greatest enthusiasm and success, curing their fellow students, their parents and their friends. They made a kind of game of the treatment, and the progress of each school case was watched with the most intense interest by all the children. On a bright day, when the patients saw well, there was great rejoicing, and on a dark day there was corresponding depression. One girl cured twenty-six children in six months; another cured twelve in three months; a third developed quite a varied ophthalmological practice and did things of which older and more experienced practitioners might well have been proud. Going to the school which she attended one day, I asked this girl about her sight, which had been very imperfect. She replied that it was now very good, and that her headaches were quite gone. I tested her sight and found it normal. Then another child whose sight had also been very poor spoke up,

"I can see all right too," she said. "Emily" – indicating girl No. 1 – "cured me." "Indeed!" I replied. "How did she do that?"

The second girl explained that Emily had had her read the card, which she could not see at all from the back of the room, at a distance of a few feet. The next day she had moved it a little further away, and so on, until the patient was able to read it from the back of the room, just as the other children did. Emily now told her to cover the right eye and read the card with her left, and both girls were considerably upset to find that the uncovered eye was apparently blind. The school doctor was consulted and said that nothing could be done. The eye had been blind from birth and no treatment would do any good.

Nothing daunted, however, Emily undertook the treatment. She told the patient to cover her good eye and go up close to the card, and at a distance of a foot or less it was found that she could read even the small letters. The little practitioner then proceeded confidently as with the other eye, and after many months of practice the patient became the happy possessor of normal vision in both eyes. The case had, in fact, been simply one of high myopia, and the school doctor, not being a specialist, had not detected the difference between this condition and blindness.

In the same classroom, there had been a little girl with congenital cataract, but on the occasion of my visit the defect had disappeared. This, too, it appeared, was Emily's doing. The school doctor had said that there was no help for this eye except through operation, and as the sight of the other eye was pretty good, he fortunately did not think it necessary to urge such a course. Emily accordingly took the matter in hand. She had the patient stand close to the card, and at that distance it was found that she could not see even the big C. Emily now held the card between the patient and the light and moved it back and forth. At a distance of 3 or 4 feet this movement could be observed indistinctly by the patient. The card was then moved farther away, until the patient became able to see it move at 10 feet and to see some of the larger letters indistinctly at a less distance. Finally, after six months, she became able to read the card with the bad eye as well as with the good one. After testing her sight and finding it normal in both eyes, I said to Emily:

"You are a splendid doctor. You beat them all. Have you done anything else?"
The child blushed, and turning to another of her classmates, said:
"Mamie, come here."
Mamie stepped forward and I looked at her eyes. There appeared to be nothing wrong with them.
"I cured her," said Emily.
"What of?" I inquired.
"Cross-eyes," replied Emily.
"How?" I asked, with growing astonishment.

Emily described a procedure very similar to that adopted in the other cases. Finding that the sight of the crossed eye was very poor, so much so, indeed, that poor Mamie could see practically nothing with it, the obvious course of action seemed to her to be the restoration of its sight; and, never having read any medical literature, she did not know that this was impossible. So she went to it. She had Mamie cover her good eye and practice the bad one at home and at school, until at last the sight became normal and the eye straight. The school doctor had wanted to have the eye operated upon, I was told, but fortunately Mamie was "scared" and would not consent. And here she was with two perfectly good, straight eyes.

"Anything else?" I inquired, when Mamie's case had been disposed of. Emily blushed again, and said: "Here's Rose. Her eyes used to hurt her all the time, and she couldn't see anything on the blackboard. Her headaches used to be so bad that she had to stay away from school every once in a while. The doctor gave her glasses, but they didn't help her, and she wouldn't wear them. When you told us the card would help our eyes I got busy with her. I had her read the card close up, and then I moved it farther away, and now she can see all right, and her head doesn't ache any more. She comes to school every day, and we all thank you very much."

This was a case of compound hypermetropic astigmatism. Such stories might be multiplied indefinitely. Emily's astonishing record cannot, it is true, be duplicated, but lesser cures by cured patients have been very numerous and serve to show that the benefits of the method of preventing and curing defects of vision in the schools which is presented in this number of *Better Eyesight* would be far-reaching. Not only errors of refraction would be cured, but many more serious defects; and not only the children would be helped, but their families and friends also.

Solutions to use at home

Children essentially need the same method as adults, and all relaxation techniques described in this book apply equally to children's eyes. Yet children need a more playful approach. Rather than telling a child they need to "relax their eyes," it makes more sense to them when they're told that we'll do some fun things to help their eyes "be happy." Theoretical explanations may not be useful, and children may respond best when they don't even realize an activity is designed to improve their sight. After all, vision games are simply games, and fun is the main goal to help induce visual relaxation.

During the visit with my cousins after my niece Emma was given glasses, I started teaching her to release eyestrain. Her mother at first did not appreciate my help because she felt I was contradicting the doctor's orders, which was confusing the girl. But at every visit Emma would ask me, "Esther, can we please do an eye lesson today?" So she and I would sneak off to her bedroom, where she had my chart hanging on the door, and we would do a few vision games. By age nine, their eye doctor told them that Emma's eyes were fine and she no longer needed glasses. She was delighted about that, and it was a huge relief to me.

Depending on the child's age, a letter chart may not be useful, so "Tumbling E", "Rolling C" or picture charts can be used instead. These charts typically have numbers on the side and come with instructions to use them at 10 or 20 feet. Feel free to ignore this distance advice unless you want to check the child's acuity. Let the child decide what distance they like best. They will naturally stand where the entire chart can be read easily. Then encourage them to stand slightly further from (or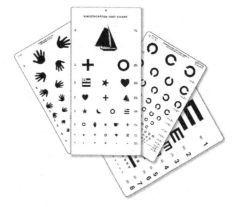
closer to) the chart where they can still read most letters but not (or not easily) the last line. Measure that distance and make a note of it, then have them demonstrate the negative results of strained ways of seeing, such as staring (which will likely create more blur). Next, encourage them to only read letters that are easy to read and skip any that are hard. Then have them practice some relaxed vision habits that counteract their typical strain, so they learn what does and does not work for clearing the last line. They can try blinking more, side-to-side motion, taking glances away from the chart and back at it, looking at the white spaces, etc., any of which will likely create more clarity.

 Looking at familiar versus unfamiliar objects

While working with school children in North Dakota for several years, Dr. Bates observed that when they looked at an unfamiliar object on the blackboard, seeing something new that they had not seen before, the retinoscope always showed that they were myopic at that point, even though their vision would be normal under other circumstances. When they looked at familiar objects, they were able to look at them without strain and therefore with normal vision.

If a child first looks at a familiar object and can relax with it, and then looks at an unfamiliar object at the same distance, the strain of looking at the unfamiliar object will be less. Children soon become able to maintain the relaxation they gained from looking at the familiar object and then look at unfamiliar objects without strain too.

 Become familiar with the letter chart

Due to this difference in reaction to familiar and unfamiliar images, Bates found that it was easier for children to read a letter chart when they became familiar with it. If he left a chart up on the wall at school, next to the blackboard, the children would use it as their familiar object. They would learn to relax their eyes with it. Then they could look back at the blackboard and keep that relaxation to see the board better. Reading the eyechart regularly improved their vision, both for the chart and other things as well.

Children whose vision was below normal improved, in most cases, to normal vision. Children who already had normal sight, 20/20, became able to read 20/15 or 20/10. This was regardless of the light conditions in the room.

 Keep a letter chart in a classroom permanently

Before this system was introduced in one particular classroom, the teacher had noticed that during the fifteen years she had been teaching, at the start of the school year the children had no trouble reading the blackboard from their seats, but by springtime they could not read it beyond 10 feet away. She then kept the eyechart in her classroom and let the children read it every day. The result was that since then, none of the children in her class developed vision problems.

Because of this success in one school, the system of using an eyechart was introduced into all the schools of Grand Forks, North Dakota. These schools used charts continuously for eight years, with as many as 2,000 school children. At the beginning of that period, 6% of the children were nearsighted, while only 1% were nearsighted at the end. All the others had improved to the point of normal vision, and new students generally avoided myopia.

Letter charts helped both nearsighted and farsighted students

With his retinoscope, Dr. Bates could show that when children learn to read – or write, draw or do anything that requires them to look at unfamiliar objects up close – their eyes would always show hyperopia or hyperopic astigmatism. In these school experiments, not only was myopia cured, but hyperopia improved also with use of the charts.

Sonya learns to use a letter chart

Eight-year-old Sonya from Arizona had been given glasses for -2.50 myopia with -0.25 astigmatism in both eyes. Sonya didn't like the glasses much, so her parents decided to give the Bates Method a chance and scheduled three sessions in a row for her. In her first session I placed a chart one foot beyond Sonya's clear zone and asked her to only read the letters that were easy for her to read. She stopped after correctly reading all letters on the 15 line. I let her palm her eyes for a few minutes, then reminded her to blink and asked her to think about her favorite doll. When I directed her attention back to the chart, she read all letters on the 10-line with ease too.

In her second session the following day the chart was placed nearly 2 feet further away, and Sonya was keen to read the last line again but was trying too hard to succeed. To stop her from making such an effort, I let her hold a smaller version of the same chart in her hand, so she could first look at the letter on the near chart to become familiar with it before looking at that same letter on the large chart 5 feet away. Alternating between the clear letters up close and the blurry letters on the far chart, she began to recognize the shapes of the letters on the far chart with more ease. She soon read the entire last line without needing to refer to the near chart. On day three she avoided strain by throwing and catching a ball before reading any letter, and a happy memory of pink lipstick on her doll made her smile and allowed her to read an extra line.

 What children need most for their vision

So, what children need more than anything is to learn how to keep their vision relaxed when looking at unfamiliar things. Only after they become able to look at the near point without strain, can they expect to make much progress with their studies. In every case that Dr. Bates worked with, he could always reach that goal by getting the children to practice daily with a letter chart. Once they can stay relaxed with the chart at a distance, it can be brought closer and they can learn to do the same for their near vision.

As happy "side effects" of improved vision, the children experienced fewer headaches, were less fatigued, and had better attitudes.

After Dr. Bates moved back to New York in 1910, he introduced his methods into the schools there and teachers and children alike were enthusiastic about the results. But unfortunately, despite this success, in 1912 the Board of Education of the City of New York decided that the use of letter charts in classrooms was "unscientific and erroneous" and they forbade the use of these charts in schools – other than for the stated purpose of occasionally testing the children's sight.[8]

Dr. Bates felt that if New York had led the way, the whole country would have followed, so he was saddened that his method was "condemned without trial" and that the children were deprived of the blessing of perfect sight.[9] If we can bring charts back into classrooms and provide basic instruction to both teachers and children, much eyestrain can be avoided.

Improving your child's vision – some cautions and positive actions

It isn't difficult to help a child see better, especially when they haven't worn glasses yet. The following may be useful reminders for you as you help your child to clarity.

First three cautions:

- Don't be harsh with children – they tense up instantly. Forcing them to do anything simply does not work well. As an example, eight-year-old Becky's mother was my biggest challenge during a private class for her daughter. She verbally lashed out at Becky with razor-sharp "Listen!" commands, as well as "Sit up straight!" and "Pay attention!" Hearing my gentle reminders for her daughter to blink more, she soon expanded her repertoire with a regular whipping of "Blink!" I had to tactfully let her know that this was not helpful. It took several of these hints before she got it. By the end of the day she'd made quite a turn around and spoke much more lovingly to her daughter.

- Don't let children play with anyone's glasses! Toddlers' and young children's eyes are very fast at adapting to the prescription in those lenses, which is not what you want. At age 1¾, Grace developed strabismus right after she played with her grandmother's glasses, which had a prism in one lens. I helped her parents understand the cause and gave tips on how to release the girl's resulting eyestrain. It worked, thankfully. Glasses are not toys; please keep them out of children's reach.

- Don't give up too soon... Until a child actually sees better, even if just for a moment, they may not understand what you are doing for them and may be uncooperative. Be inventive and find different ways of helping them to relax. As soon as one method works, you will have their attention and cooperation.

Many positive actions to build upon:

- Be kind and gentle with children. Abundant love and praise will help their eyes relax.

- Let the child sleep in a dark room at night, especially in the first two years of life. This reduces the chance of developing myopia in childhood from a grand 48 to just 9 percent.[10]

- Gently swing a baby in your arms when it shows strain in its body or eyes. A rocking chair can benefit both parent and baby.

- Let babies get a daily dose of sunshine, including on their eyes, whether awake or asleep.

- Allow children lots of outdoor play; get them into fresh air and sunshine at every opportunity. Aim for a minimum of two hours outside per day (preferably glasses-free), including some time during UVB hours if possible (see Chapter 15).

- Allow children to take glasses off as much as possible.

- Encourage a healthy diet. Supply fruit instead of candy bars, sweets, or any product with refined sugars (see Chapter 14).

- Place a picture chart or letter chart in the child's bedroom and let them become familiar with it. Let them read it daily, but only as far down as is easy for them, with both eyes together and also using each eye separately. Give them stories in small print to practice with too.

- Write down their progress with the chart every week.

- Have FUN and play games, especially ball games (with progressively smaller balls). Play search games too: Hide small things for them to find, call their attention to a certain color to find around them, or any small but doable targets that you can make them curious about. For children with high myopia, ball games are challenging and frustrating, so they tend to avoid them. A wrist-ball (Chapter 17) can help them overcome their fears. Peekaboo games involve both palming and flashing and are ideal for your child's sight.

- Teach the child to sway and imagine apparent motion. Playground swings are great vision relaxers!

- Play games that use and improve memory and imagination.

- Involve other kids in the games, especially friends of the child.

- Let kids be as noisy as they like.

- Find subjects that the child is particularly interested in; this makes everything flow so much easier!

- Teach children to regularly rest and palm their eyes. Let them describe their favorite toy while palming, which they can also use as their foundation memory when playing with charts. For babies, gently cover their eyes with your hand(s) while you tell them a story, sing a song, listen to soothing music, or sway them in your arms. An e-booklet, *Fairy Tales for Better Eyesight,* contains 26 fairy stories which were originally published in Dr. Bates' *Better Eyesight* magazines. These are great for reading to your child while they rest their eyes. The e-booklet is available on my website.[11]

- Teach the child the negative effects of eyestrain and the benefits of letting the eyes simply receive light and blink often. Help them become aware of times they stare.

- Get children hooked on rapid blinking competitions instead of staring competitions!

- Ask children what they worry about or what they are sad about and help them work through emotions (see Chapter 11).

- Work on reducing your own eyestrain, if you have any, so you set a good example for the child to follow.

- Take some lessons from an experienced Bates Method teacher and learn how to help your child at home.

- Consult an eye doctor when needed. Ask for references and find one who is kind and patient with your child.

23. Two Points of View for 3-D

When both eyes work together as a team, the brain receives two slightly different images (one from each eye) and fuses them into one image for three-dimensional (3-D) vision. The slight difference in viewing angles of the images from the left and right eye helps you determine where objects are in space. When only one eye is used, a limited perception of depth will be created by the brain. Objects in the visual field are then judged by their relative size to create a rough idea of where they are in space. Although this one-eye view of depth is useful, it is not as accurate as depth perception created by using both eyes together.

When one eye sees significantly better than the other, or when one eye is highly dominant, or when one eye points in a different direction than the other, a variety of visual challenges can arise, including suppression, double vision and a loss of depth perception. These are often considered permanent issues, yet they are forms of eyestrain which can be reduced or overcome with visual relaxation.

The practices covered in this chapter are related to:
Anisometropia – a difference in acuity of each eye.
Suppression – partial exclusion of one eye's visual field.
Amblyopia – total suppression of one eye's visual field, also known as lazy eye.
Strabismus – misaligned eyes, also known as squint or cross-eyes.

Anisometropia, suppression, amblyopia and strabismus all lead to a loss of depth perception; there is limited or no fusion of the two images from the eyes. I'll explain the four terms a bit further.

Anisometropia and Suppression
It is normal for one eye to be dominant; that is the eye you use to look through a telescope or microscope or to peer through a hole in a fence, and it is the eye that your finger lines up with as you point at a distant object. Suppression happens when the dominant eye becomes overly dominant, at the expense of not fully using the other eye. It can develop due to anisometropia, when one eye sees distinctly better than the other, allowing for clearer images in the brain from the better eye's input.

Amblyopia and Strabismus
Amblyopia is the term used when images from one eye are not used at all. There isn't necessarily anything organically wrong with the amblyopic or suppressed eye, that is, nothing wrong that an eye doctor can see; but the person who is dealing with an amblyopic

eye doesn't see through it and is considered blind in that eye. An amblyopic or suppressed eye is not used, or only partially used, unless the other eye is closed or covered, at which point the brain has no choice but to use the suppressed eye. When that happens, it sees with it, although the image may be of lower quality. The brain basically can learn to ignore the input from one eye, thereby foregoing binocular vision in favor of clearer vision from the better eye.

Amblyopia can develop when one eye points in a different direction than where the attention and other eye are focused (strabismus). This creates two very different images that cannot be fused into one. The brain doesn't like this "interference signal" from the wandering eye, and, rather than deal with double vision, it may learn to suppress the second image by ignoring it, or by "switching that eye off."

Strabismus is also known as squint or cross-eyes. A strabismic eye can point in any direction, not necessarily crossing to the nose, and it is also possible for the eyes to alternate in wandering off-center. Strabismus often leads to amblyopia of the wandering eye, because if the brain keeps using the image from that eye, there is double vision, which is a big visual challenge. Over time, therefore, the brain will likely start to ignore the images coming in from the wandering eye.

Bilateral amblyopia is a term used when both eyes don't see well, and glasses don't improve the acuity much or at all. This condition is typically deemed to be irreversible in adults. In the case of children, glasses are usually prescribed anyway and are supposed to be worn all day so the child can learn to see through them. Although the acuity with glasses may improve after a year or more, the prescription is likely to get stronger during that time.[1]

In Bates' time, amblyopia was supposed to be incurable after age six (nowadays age eight seems the arbitrary cut-off date, although one study from 2005 quotes age seventeen),[2] yet Bates felt that suppression, amblyopia and strabismus were functional problems that responded well to his visual relaxation methods, regardless of age.

Fears of going blind
I regularly get phone calls from parents who tell me their child has been diagnosed with suppression, amblyopia or strabismus, and the eye doctor has terrified them about the dire need to rectify this before the child reaches eight years of age, or else the affected eye will become functionally blind. This is a scary scenario, and I understand why the parents are fearful for their child's vision, but this fear is unfounded. Yes, if left untreated, the affected eye may have a lifelong visual impairment,[3] but it has been proven that the brain can learn to see through a previously suppressed or amblyopic eye *at any age*, not just until age eight! Susan Barry's[4] and my own experience prove this. (See Chapter 1 and my story

below.) Yet eye doctors continue to pass on the old perspective on suppression and thus scare parents needlessly.

My 2-D world

When one eye is suppressed, the three-dimensional world appears more like a postcard image. This was my world until my mid-thirties. My left eye didn't cooperate much with my right eye, although it moved along in sync and had fairly good vision. I was never diagnosed as having suppression or amblyopia, and I had no idea that something wasn't quite right, because I simply knew nothing better than the rather flat world I lived in. Estimating distances was hard for me; I would usually give wildly wrong answers if asked how far away something was.

Learning to drive a car was challenging too; it took a long time to master the rapid input of distances that I had to process in my 2-D brain. Car speeds are quite a step up from bicycling speeds! I was also nervous about not being able to properly judge the width of the car, causing a tendency to drive close to the center stripes in the road. My sister once remarked that it made her nervous that I drove so far from the side of the road. So the next day, I carefully parked my car alongside a long straight curb, until my wheels touched the curb, and I looked at where the curb-line ahead of me intersected the hood of my car. I memorized that spot on the hood and used it to better judge the car's width while driving.

It was during my Bates Method teacher training that I first realized that my left eye had suppression issues. A simple demonstration with a pencil, where I was instructed to look "through" the pencil at a blank wall behind it, was meant to show the illusion of two pencils, both of equal density. That is what you expect to see when both eyes are used equally by the brain. It is not what I saw. I saw one clear pencil, and a ghostly one to the right of it which had a gap in the middle and a weird tendency to come and go. That ghostly pencil to the right was what my left eye perceived. My left eye's central vision was suppressed, while its peripheral field was used only intermittently. Due to the left's poor performance, my brain tended to mostly ignore that eye, leaving me with a less than three-dimensional world.

I was told to cover my right eye with a patch to help "switch on" my left eye. Using the patch on my dominant right eye was annoying to me, as the left eye didn't seem to like being the only one in use, and the loss of peripheral vision to the right caused me to bump into things on that side. Another tool I was given was a "fusion halo," which was supposed to create a "gate" in front of my face that I was to look through. But it was a huge effort just to have the gate appear, never mind looking through it. The gate was often not there, and therefore this practice frustrated me tremendously.

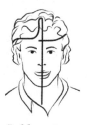

Bobby using a fusion halo

Overcoming suppression of my left eye

I soon gave up on trying to get my left eye to switch on fully; it was far too challenging. But I did become a vision teacher and ended up working with eyesight all the time, so I couldn't help but improve my own vision further as I helped others do the same. One day in my mid-thirties, driving to New Paltz on a New York freeway, my left eye unexpectedly "switched on" and the world in front of me opened into a world where there was suddenly S P A C E between the trees along the freeway and the mountains in the background. WOW!!! This was weird and exhilarating at the same time. I screamed with delight and I loved the experience of seeing this new 3-D world. At the same time, it was overwhelming. It seemed like a huge sensory overload to me to keep perceiving all these empty spaces. A few minutes later, the depth disappeared, and my "normal" flat world returned.

I thought about what just happened, and in re-experiencing the exhilaration, I found the 3-D world reappeared! Simply by tuning into the euphoric feeling it created for me, I could make this 3-D world come and go at will. So I played with that, but still found it exhausting to keep 3-D "on" for any length of time. There was far too much extra data to process that my brain clearly wasn't used to dealing with.

Solidifying depth perception in my forties

So, most of the time, I was quite happy in my familiar, 2-D world and enjoyed only brief excursions into my new way of seeing spaces between objects. That is, until I started using Jacob Liberman's new Eyeport (see Chapter 9). At first I used it sporadically; it wasn't until my mid-forties, when I started using the Eyeport regularly for a month, that the 3-D world started to appear at random – when I wasn't even thinking about it. Driving was still the most common time for it to show up; the strong effect of apparent motion while driving helped stimulate the left eye. But the more I used the Eyeport, the more depth I experienced, and I slowly realized that depth perception happens on a continuum. It isn't just ON or OFF; it has various levels.

At first I only saw big spaces, such as between trees in the foreground and mountains in the distance, but over time this effect was visible in smaller objects. I clearly remember one day walking along a road in Upper Ojai where I now live, looking at a tree – and for the first time ever, seeing the tree as a three-dimensional, round object, with spaces between the branches! It truly is a sweet experience when trees that have always appeared flat like a painting become objects that occupy space. The mountains in the distance suddenly showed their curves to me, and I finally got to see "the lay of the land" and came to understand that expression on a much deeper level.

The magic of a 3-D brain

This delight at seeing in 3-D is still with me, even though it has now become more normal for me to see in 3-D than in my old way of perceiving postcard-like images. I can now even see depth in 2-D images, which I used to think was impossible; but once a brain knows how to create 3-D, it can create it even from a 2-D image. The first time I ever perceived depth while watching a video, I presumed some new software had been invented that created a 3-D effect, or perhaps my computer had had a software update? It took a while to realize my own brain was now capable of converting 2-D into 3-D, and this amazed me! When I'm tired, stressed, or overwhelmed, the old 2-D world still returns, so I now use this as a message that it is time for some personal relaxation.

 How to achieve 3-D vision

There are five steps to achieving depth perception:

Step 1. Equalize visual acuity in both eyes.
Step 2. Switch on the suppressed or amblyopic eye.
Step 3. Align the eyes to track together.
Step 4. Achieve fusion and basic depth perception.
Step 5. Increase depth perception.

The steps are provided in a natural order of progression. For example, if you have strabismus with single vision because one eye is suppressed, you won't be able to tackle Step 3 until Step 2 has been mastered and you have achieved double vision. Plus, your brain may refuse to take Step 2 unless the eyes have reasonably equal visual acuity, gained in Step 1. From personal experience, I know that Step 4 is not the end; it is only the beginning of gaining depth perception, which continues in Step 5.

Depending on what you are dealing with, you may be able to skip a step or two. For example, if you have suppression issues but not strabismus, skip Step 3. If you have strabismus with double vision you won't need Step 2, yet you won't be able to tackle Step 4 until Step 3 has been achieved.

The five steps are described below, along with suggested practices to help you toward each goal. Give each practice a chance to produce results for you, and regularly repeat the ones you enjoy most. There are more ways to improve depth perception than just the few practices I suggest for each step, so if you want more options, I recommend you work with an experienced teacher.

Remember: Learning to see depth takes time! Neural pathways in the brain can be slow to build or re-build, so during this process the work put into achieving depth perception can be overwhelming and tiring. Take plenty of breaks from these practices and be extra gentle with yourself or your child during this time. With each practice session you take a small step in the right direction. Each and every step counts; they accumulate over time until the day when suddenly things fall into place and your first exciting moments of depth perception can be celebrated. Even then, the old ways of seeing may return and the 3-D world may come and go for a while. Keep working with it for the beautiful reward of more consistent depth perception and the joy of becoming more and more comfortable in the 3-D world.

Step 1. Equalize visual acuity in both eyes

A. Choose a better label

When you see best with one eye you may call that your "good eye," while the other eye has probably picked up the label of "my bad eye" or "the weak eye." Yet the truth is that you do not have a bad, weak or lazy eye. The eye with worse vision or the eye out of alignment is typically under more strain than the other eye. There is nothing bad, weak or lazy about muscles under chronic strain! This eye simply needs more relaxation. I invite you to change the labels – you could call the more strained eye your "strong eye," which is more accurate and also sounds more positive. For children it is more fun to let them choose actual names for each eye. This not only helps them let go of any negative labels given to one eye but can also affect how they think of themselves; now disassociating their own abilities from the eye's abilities.

B. Cover the basics

All the basics of Parts II and III of this book apply to achieving Step 1. Unless your better eye already has excellent acuity, you will be working on relaxation for both eyes. Sometimes the more strained "strong" eye will catch up quickly with the better eye; other times it won't budge until the better eye has achieved clear vision. You obviously can't force a strained eye to be the first to relax, so go with the flow, rest often with closed eyes or palming, practice shifting and swinging, enjoy sunning, etc.

> **The best treatment for squint is mental rest. Many patients with squint suffer very much from eyestrain. By closing the eyes and resting them, or by palming for a few minutes or longer, about ten times a day, most of these cases are cured without other treatment.**
> William H. Bates, M.D.[5]

When one eye sees less clearly, check for neck tension and any other tension on that side of the body and work on releasing those muscles too. Perhaps you clench your jaw, scrunch up a cheek, or raise a shoulder? Amy had an acuity of 20/20 in her right eye, while her left saw 20/40. When I pointed out that she also had tension in her left hand, she let her fingers relax and her left eye experienced sudden soreness of muscle tension releasing there too. This soreness lasted a few minutes, and then her left eye's acuity caught up one line, improving from 20/40 to 20/30 as a result.

C. Patch the better eye

When your better eye has normal sight, you can begin to cover it with an eye-patch and help the other eye regain clarity too. Patching the better eye provides an opportunity for you to work with the other eye on its own so you can better tune into its needs. Not only will it be easier to release that eye's strain, but you will also learn to make more use of this eye, re-paving its neural pathways to the brain.

The eye-patch has its uses but also has its disadvantages. One disadvantage is that it completely puts the dominant eye "out of the picture," which feels unnatural. Also, a large part of the peripheral field is lost, which is a handicap. Besides, it can be very frustrating to use a patch for long periods of time. I distinctly remember my own intense frustration with the patch, so I kept my eyes open for an alternative, which was provided some years later by my colleague Carol Gallup, whom I visited in Port Townsend, Washington. With scissors, she cut a hole in a regular patch to open the side away from the nose. Using this "half-patch" was much more tolerable because the entire peripheral field was now visible, which made it easier to relax and thus get better results. I always prefer a half-patch over a full one, while others, especially those with alternate exophoria (when the eyes take turns pointing outward), may find a full patch more useful.

Patches are available at drugstores, and you'll find links to sellers on my website.[6] To create a half-patch, fold it in half over its horizontal axis then cut from the center straight along its vertical axis. Curve around to create a hole in the side away from the nose, leaving enough of the edge to keep its shape and leaving the half nearest the nose intact.

How long to use a patch

You may find you tire quickly while using a patch, so start with just a few minutes of using it and build up slowly as your tolerance for it increases. The more you use it, the sooner you'll see results. You may want to use a patch for several hours per day, yet I suggest taking a break whenever it becomes stressful.

What to do while wearing the patch

To ensure that you make the most of your patching time, pick something you enjoy doing and that really captivates your interest. The more movement is involved, the better it is. Ball games are good even if a little challenging at first, but you can also read something of interest. As long as you keep your mind engaged, your non-dominant eye will get the stimulation it needs.

It will also help to look at a chart at a distance where most lines can be read easily while keeping your better eye covered with a patch. Spend a minute or two (longer if you like) per day on chart-reading, but never to the point of frustration. Do any of the suggested chart practices from Chapter 17 while using the patch.

For children who do not know the alphabet yet, use a Tumbling E or Rolling C chart (charts with "E's" or "C's" pointing in different directions). Alternatively, use toy animals of various sizes and colors and teach the child to name the colors and animals at a distance where they see best. Once they are familiar with the toys, patch the better eye and repeat as needed. Gradually increase the distance of the letters or animals and start using smaller letters and toys to be recognized.

D. Balance the eyes with mental pictures
When one eye sees distinctly better than the other, it will be useful to practice flashing with one eye at a time. You may find that vision photographs taken with your better eye create a clearer mental picture than photographs taken by the other eye. This can be used to your advantage: the clearer mental picture remembered after using the better eye can be a tool to help your strained "strong" eye get to the same level.

You can use details of any favorite object for this practice; I will use a chart as an example. Cover your better eye and establish the optimal practice distance for the eye that sees less clearly. At what distance can this eye make out the 15 line but not yet the 10 line on the largest chart? Place the chart there.

Now cover the eye that sees less clearly. With the better eye, pick a letter that you enjoy looking at on the 15 line. Check the details of this letter and memorize how it looks. After creating a good mental picture with the better eye, close both eyes, cover the better eye, uncover the other, and then start taking flash photographs of this letter with your "strong" eye, while remembering the clearer image of the letter you just saw with your better eye. Imagine this eye can see it just as clearly! This practice will help your "strong" eye to relax further, until that eye too is able to provide a similarly good mental picture.

 Step 2. Switch on the suppressed or amblyopic eye
Once both eyes are fairly balanced in acuity, the brain is likely to start using both images, yet it may need a little encouragement to do so. The practices in this section will help you to use both eyes.

In cases of strabismus when the brain uses both eyes, the result is double vision. That sounds undesirable, but this double vision is a prerequisite to straightening the eye. The brain needs the visual feedback of where the eye is pointing in order to align it with the dominant eye, thereby regaining binocular vision. As soon as double vision is achieved, you have reason to celebrate; you can then proceed to step 3 and learn to align both eyes.

In many cases of squint, double vision can be demonstrated. These cases are more readily cured than those cases of squint which do not see double. This fact suggests that all cases of squint should be taught how to produce double vision.

William. H. Bates, M.D.[7]

A. Limit the dominant eye's view

A method that works for many people is to limit the dominant eye's view to half of what the suppressed eye can see. Here's how: Stand 5 to 10 feet from a chart that is placed at eye-level. Cover your suppressed eye. Hold a blank piece of paper in your hand, hold it up in front of your dominant eye and position the piece of paper so that only half of the chart is visible with this eye. If your left eye is dominant, hide the left half of the chart with the paper in your hand. If the right eye is dominant, you cover the right half of the chart.

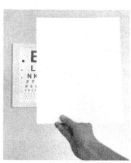

Obscuring half the chart in case of right eye dominance.

Next, cover the dominant eye and open the other eye without moving the white paper from its position. You should be able to see the entire chart with this eye. Now open both eyes and notice what happens.

If you lose the image of the complete chart when both eyes are open, then alternately cover and uncover the dominant eye, so the suppressed eye gets a clear picture of what it is supposed to see, even when the dominant eye is open.

You may feel discomfort when viewing the letter chart like this. Elizabeth, a student in New York, experienced distinct nausea when practicing with a chart in this manner, but she was excited to keep at it because this was the only way she had ever experienced her non-dominant eye switching on.

Tips:
- Instead of a blank piece of paper you can use your hand to block half the view for the better eye.

- Feel free to replace the chart with any object you love to look at.

- Make sure the chart or object which you encourage your suppressed eye to see is better lit or more brightly colored than the paper or hand you use to conceal half its view from the better eye.

- It may help to massage or lightly tap your fingers on the temple next to your suppressed eye.

B. Blur the dominant eye's vision

To encourage use of the suppressed eye, it can help to temporarily blur the vision of the dominant eye, for example by using a translucent eye patch or holding a colored sheet of see-through plastic in front of that eye. This will help you see through the unobstructed eye, as the brain will be more tempted to use its better images. You can also use the chart in the same way as above, either with or without the paper to conceal half the chart, and check if diminishing the quality of the image from your better eye improves your ability to see the chart through your suppressed eye.

In case of strabismus, instead of a chart to look at, use a small, bright object such as a small lamp, when you blur the dominant eye's vision. When you look at a small light with both eyes open, you may be able to see two lights instead of one, because the light seen by the better eye is very much blurred. If not, palming frequently helps – while resting the eyes imagine that you see the lamp with both eyes. Imagine these lights to be moving gently, then open your eyes (blur the better eye's vision with a filter again) and continue to imagine that you see the lamp with each eye, thus producing two lamp images some distance apart. Imagine you receive (and mentally accept) these two images. With the help of the swing, the two images may gradually approach each other and merge into one light.

C. Use the Eyeport

I've mentioned the Eyeport a few times already. Besides its value when learning to shift your eyes with ease (see Chapter 9), this machine is also a great tool for switching on a suppressed eye. A pair of red/blue glasses is worn during the first eight minutes of every ten-minute Eyeport session, which causes one eye to only see the blue lights flash on, while the other eye sees only the red lights. Thus, in order to see all lights, the brain is invited to alternate its use of the dominant eye with momentary use of the suppressed eye. As the speed of the alternating red and blue lights gradually increases, the brain learns to switch between the two eyes faster, and eventually learns to keep both eyes switched on. This happens effortlessly and was highly effective on my own journey to having both eyes work together.

D. Bar Reading

No, I'll not ask you to visit your local pub with a book in hand… Bar reading, in this case, refers to a very simple technique that you can use any time you have either a pen, pencil, ruler, or something similar available while you read. If no such item is "on hand," you can even hold up your thumb and create the same effect!

While reading this paragraph, hold a ruler flat between the page and your eyes (as shown in the image), about 4 inches from the nose. Hold the ruler in that place. With your attention on the text, first close one eye, then open it and close the other, and notice that each eye sees the ruler in a different location in front of the text. The ruler blocks part of the right side of the text when only the left eye is open, and blocks part of the left side of the text when only the right eye is open. The distance between the two ruler images increases if you hold the ruler closer to your nose and vice versa.

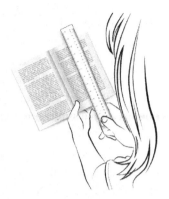

Experiment to find the best distance to hold the ruler, so both its images block part of the page you want to read. Once you've found a good position for the ruler, hold it there and start reading with both eyes open. When your dominant eye reaches the area where its view of the text is barred by the ruler, the suppressed eye gets an opportunity to jump in and help read. Both eyes take turns and cooperate to see the entire line. Avoid staring! Continue bar reading for as long as you can be relaxed with it.

E. View through a colored corridor

You'll need two different-colored 3x5-index cards held together, or two different colored sticky notes, or you can color each side of a 3x5 piece of white cardboard with a different color. Bright green, yellow, orange, red, pink or blue tend to be good colors to use. Hold this card in front of your face with one end touching your nose and the far end extending away from you, so each eye sees a different color.

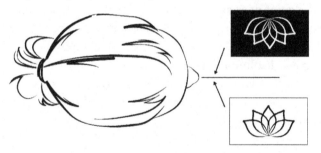

1 USE 2 DIFFERENT IMAGES
  OR 2 DIFFERENT COLOR CARDS

2 PLACE IMAGES FACING OUT

3 HOLD CARD AGAINST YOUR NOSE

4 LOOK AT A BLANK WALL
  NOTICE IF A HALLWAY APPEARS
  WITH ONE IMAGE/COLOR ON EITHER SIDE

When you look at the card, you may see the two different colors possibly alternating with each other at first, or perhaps only one side is noticed. If you only see one side of the card, one color, shine a light on the opposite side to help that eye switch on and see the other color. It helps to use the brighter of the two colors on the side of the suppressed eye, and if you angle the card slightly toward that eye it can help trigger it into action and make that color appear too. It may also help to stimulate peripheral vision of the suppressed eye by waving your hand on that side. Ask someone to gently push against the back of your shoulder on the same side as the suppressed eye, as such sensory input can also help activate this eye.

Once you notice both sides of the card, even if only intermittently, look directly ahead into the distance and the two colors will separate, creating a space in the middle, thus resembling a corridor. It is likely that one side of the corridor will seem more solid, while the other side may disappear at times. You can then choose to notice the side of the corridor that wants to disappear while keeping your primary attention on any distant objects. Your interest in the colored "wall" will help it reappear. Extra light on that side of the card will too. Be careful not to lose the opposite side of the corridor. Can you stay aware of both sides at the same time while looking at the distance? Can you move the card away from you and back while continuing the illusion of the corridor? Can you walk around with it and keep your awareness of the corridor?

Experiment with a variety of colors and see how that affects the corridor illusion. Sometimes a bright orange, red or pink will stimulate a suppressed eye while a blue or green will relax a dominant eye.

Take breaks!
Stimulating a suppressed eye can be very tiring at first, so intersperse your practices with palming!

 Step 3. Align the eyes to track together
The typical response of eye doctors to a strabismic eye is to suggest surgery to straighten it. Having read most of this book, you already know enough about eye muscles that you can picture how an eye that, for example, points in toward the nose has tension in the rectus muscle nearest the nose. When an eye doctor does surgery to straighten that eye, he cuts and shortens the muscle on the opposite side, resulting in an eye that may look straight but still has one tense muscle near the nose – and now also a surgically shortened muscle on the temple side. Does this sound like a good solution? What if you could just release the tension on that muscle near the nose? If you can do that, you achieve the same result of a straight eye; but now it has a full set of healthy muscles, no undue tension, and no surgically shortened muscle to balance out the tension.

Alignment of a wandering eye doesn't necessarily take a long time, as the case history of Zoe in the previous chapter shows. Zoe's mother did try to tell the eye doctor that relaxation had helped so much, but the doctor didn't show any real interest in how this was achieved. The reason it was so easy is that this was a young child, yet old enough to understand and apply my instructions, and the strabismus had become severe only a few months earlier. Zoe had already used palming for a month or two to overcome her blurry vision, plus her brain had not yet begun to suppress the image from the wandering eye, which made my job a lot simpler. You could say she and I were lucky to get to work together at the right time. I agree. We were lucky, yet I also believe that similar positive results can be achieved in cases that are more challenging, and I think eye doctors are far too quick to suggest surgery while being tremendously ignorant about the option and effectiveness of releasing muscle strain. I hope this book will help change that.

Having double vision is a prerequisite to eye alignment, yet double vision is typically an annoying experience, so the sooner alignment is achieved, the better. Sometimes relaxing the tense muscle(s) is fast and easy; sometimes it takes longer and requires more persistence, but it is always worth doing alignment practices before you agree to surgery.

The following practices do not have to be done in order. I suggest you test each one to find how well it works for you. If you feel stuck, get help from an experienced vision educator. This tends to be exhausting work, so take plenty of breaks!

A. Release stressful memories
Some cases of strabismus have a stressful incident at their core, like the roofer who had fallen down a ladder, down to his left, whose left eye was stuck in a down-to-the-left position. Or stress can build over time, which happened for Diana, a woman in New York whose left eye turned in toward her nose and couldn't be teased out of its corner.

Diana's left eye was not suppressed, so she had double vision all the time. As I got to know her, I learned that she had an abusive husband whom she was taking to court over custody of their child. They were still living together, and due to Diana's double-vision issues, her husband drove while she was always the passenger, her husband to her left. At their dinner table, her husband sat to her left. He also slept to her left. He seemed to be "on her left" much of the time, and when I pointed this out to her it made some sense that her left eye turned to the nose – she preferred not to look at him. It wasn't until their day in court, when their legal battle was finalized and Diana was awarded custody of their child, that, for the first time, she glanced over at her husband (who happened to be standing to her left) and she saw only one of him. The mental tension was released in that moment, and her eye came back to center.

If you can pinpoint a mental strain that is linked to your wandering eye, it pays to work toward releasing it. Chapter 11 has suggestions to help release mental strain.

B. Make your double vision worse
This is easier said than done, but if, through effort, you learn how to make a wandering eye deviate further off-center, or turn it in a different direction, you will also gain the ability to lessen its turn by relaxing out of that strain.

This practice can be done with eyes open but is usually easier to accomplish first with eyes closed. Look at any bright and easy to recognize object and notice where its twin image hangs out. Now close your eyes and remember both images, then imagine increasing the distance between them. Go back and forth between increasing and decreasing the gap between the double images.

Can you gain some sense of control?
Can you move the twin image around?
Do you find that imagining them closer together is easier and more relaxing than imagining them further apart?
If you lightly touch your closed eyelids with the tips of your fingers, can you feel your eyes move along with the imagination?

You can repeat this with eyes open, perhaps using the same bright object or a small lamp, a lit candle, or a laser beam shining its bright dot on a blank wall. I'll use a candle in this example. Place it on a table and sit a comfortable distance from it. When you look at the candle flame, notice where its twin flame shows up. Now look directly toward the point where you saw the twin image. This will place the flame fairly centrally in front of the wandering eye, while the dominant eye is pointed away from the candle.

Can you still see two candle flames?
And can you imagine you see the flame best with your wandering eye?
Can you then look further away from the candle with your dominant eye while you keep looking at the flame with your other eye?

Keep your head in this position but let your full attention return to the candle, so your dominant eye will want to look at the candle again too and thus point in the same direction as the wandering eye.
Did you notice a (perhaps temporary) reduction in distance between the two flames?
Can you release neck tension and let your head turn toward the candle too, while you keep the flame images closer together?

Feel free to attempt other angles of vision too, but take plenty of breaks, palm or close your eyes often, do some rapid blinking, practice a few swings – and then have another go at this gap-changing game. You may learn to control your eye muscles with this practice.

If it is too difficult to do this with your eyes open, close them and use your imagination to do the same practice. Eyes-closed practice will help you do the same later with eyes open. You can alternate imagining the two flames moving with eyes closed and then watch the two flames move into different positions with your eyes open. When both ways become easy, your wandering eye will be straight more often.

C. Release the tense muscle(s)

Establish which of the six extraocular muscles is tenser than the others. This can also be two muscles. If the eye turns toward the nose, the medial rectus muscle is likely the most strained muscle. If the eye rolls straight up, the superior rectus muscle is probably tense. If the eye goes up and out, then either the inferior oblique or both the superior and lateral recti carry undue tension. If the deviation is down and inward, the superior oblique or both the inferior and medial recti may be involved. If you aren't sure which muscle to focus on, it is okay to imagine one tense muscle attached where your eye turns most, and work toward releasing that imaginary muscle; you'll find this works just as well.

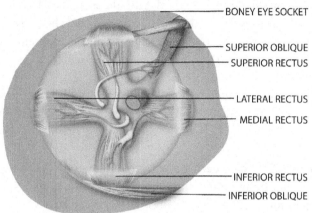

A view of the six extraocular muscles in the right eye socket

To release the tense muscle(s), practice the gentle eye rotations from Chapter 6. Do these rotations with eyes closed first, and feel free to palm while doing so. Then repeat this practice with your better eye covered, the wandering eye open. Alternate with palming, swinging, rapid blinking, or anything else that you find enjoyable and relaxing.

D. Let your eyes swing into alignment

Three-year-old Leah in Kentucky loved shaking her head to realign her eyes. It worked every time, even if only temporary. Happily shaking your head in the direction your wandering eye turns is a great way to release tension from recti muscles.

A baby can be held in a parent's arms and swayed from side to side, up and down, or turned in circles. A small child can be held by the hands to sway together with the parent or can be swung around fast enough that their feet come off the ground. Older children and adults can use the long swing or a head swing. Dancing can also have a positive influence, so play your favorite music and dance!

Tip: Looking toward a blank wall or ceiling while swaying can reduce tension to a minimum and make it easier to straighten the eyes.

E. Patch the dominant eye

If you enjoy sways and swings, cover your better eye with a patch while you move around. Imagine that stationary objects are moving. Begin with large motions like the long swing and gradually reduce them down to the following letter-swing.

Look at the large letter chart from a comfortable distance and look a few inches to the right of the big "B." Notice this top letter is to the left of where you are looking. When you look a few inches or further to the left of the "B" it appears to the right of where you are looking. By alternately looking from right to left of the "B" you can imagine the letter to be moving in the opposite direction. By shortening the distance of your shift, the swing also diminishes. Practicing swings in a relaxed, easy way will help your eyes align. Check Chapter 10 for further instructions and suggestions on apparent motion, and practice your favorite sways and swings with your dominant eye covered.

In Step 1C, I explained using a patch to help balance acuity for both eyes. Dr. Bates mentioned using the patch in some cases of strabismus (called "squint" at that time). He wrote:

> Some cases are benefited by wearing a patch over the good eye, so that the patient is compelled to use the squinting eye for vision. After several weeks or months, the vision of the squinting eye may become normal by constantly wearing a patch over the good eye. Many cases of squint are cured in this way.[5]

Emily (Lierman) Bates wrote the following about the use of the patch for thirteen-year-old Rose, whose left eye turned in:[8]

> She was directed to wear a cloth patch over her good eye all day long and to do her usual duties for her mother as well as she could, with her squint eye. What a faithful child she was, and how she did hate that patch. I asked her every time she came how she got along with it. 'Well, Mrs. Lierman' she said, 'I don't like that black patch at all. I want to take it off many times every day. I don't like to have my good eye covered, but I know I must wear it if I want to be cured; and I do want to, so I just think of you and how much better my eye looks and then I don't mind a bit.'

> On her second visit her left eye improved to 10/20 and her right eye became normal, 10/10. […] Rose continued her visits and in two months her sight became normal, and her eyes were perfectly straight continuously. She practiced faithfully and the result was that, one week before school started, she was able to remove the patch permanently, without any return of the squint.

Notice that Bates wrote that he used the patch in "some" cases of squint, not all, so if you find it too frustrating to wear a patch, don't let this discourage you. I left this choice to last for a reason! Try the half-patch or simply stick with any of the first four options in this section. Also, aim to use a patch for two hours per day, not all day long.

Tip: When you finish using a patch, enjoy a few head swings or long swings to help both eyes stay aligned without effort.

When strabismus is intermittent.

A wandering eye isn't necessarily always out of alignment. Recently sixteen-year-old Josie came to see me. Ever since age eight she experienced double vision, but only when reading. At age nine she had tried glasses for a few months, but those had not helped at all. She had also tried eye exercises, with the result that her eyes hurt; they hadn't helped either. So she had learned to "force her eyes to focus" while reading, resulting in staring eyes that tired easily, as well as headaches and motion sickness. She wasn't sure which eye wandered, but she could easily alternate between her forced-focus single vision and letting the images become double. So I observed her read while she alternated in and out of double vision.

I noticed her left eye moved out a bit each time she reported seeing double. Her acuity was fine both near and far, which meant my job was simple. Her chronic eyestrain affected only one muscle – the lateral rectus of her left eye – and she had trained her medial rectus muscle to fight against that strain, which enabled her to pull the eye into alignment. In effect she had doubled her strain. This "focusing" as she called it, clearly took a lot of effort, but it worked for her, so she had stuck with that solution for eight years.

I explained that she had another option; Instead of straining the medial rectus muscle, she could learn to release the tension on the lateral rectus. I let her play the game of making the double vision worse by widening the gap between the doubled images (as per Step 3B above). She was able to do so, and easily released back out of it too, thereby gaining some sense of what her muscles were doing. We then released her muscle tension through palming followed by flashing, which provided a first experience of effortless single vision at the near point. Then we added blinking and natural shifting to her repertoire. Her ability to keep her near vision single without effort steadily increased.

If your strabismus is intermittent like Josie's or alternates from one eye to the other, you may need to adapt the techniques to your specific situation. An experienced teacher can help you do this.

Step 4. Achieve fusion and basic depth perception

Once the eyes are aligned and balanced in acuity, the brain can start to fuse both images into one and create depth perception. This may happen automatically in cases where depth perception existed in the past and the brain already knows what to do, while for others some extra stimulation is required.

A. The white blindfold

During a group meditation I took part in, it was suggested that participants cover their eyes with a white cloth blindfold, so that those who had trouble keeping their eyes closed during the meditation would not get distracted by anything if they opened their eyes. I used the blindfold, and when I opened my eyes during that meditation, I noticed that this blindfold could be a good vision education tool. Needless to say, I did get distracted and did not follow the rest of the meditation, as I began contemplating how this white blindfold might be useful to improve vision. What struck me about the white blindfold is that it promotes relaxation similar to palming, yet, contrary to palming, the white cloth allows sufficient light to come through to activate the eyes. While during palming you practice visual relaxation with eyes closed, a white blindfold can be used for practicing visual relaxation with eyes open. For people who have habitual eyestrain, the experience of having both eyes open AND relaxed while wearing a white blindfold can trigger clearer vision after the blindfold is taken off.

In addition to this 'eyes open' relaxed seeing practice, the two small open spaces between the cloth and the nose allow each eye to see down along the nose to the floor. As each eye sees a different side of the nose and a different part of the floor and your lap, the two fractions of sight are very different from each other, and when the brain fuses them, a white triangular shape forms which points down to your chest. This is where the white blindfold becomes useful to people with eye suppression issues.

So get a strip of white cloth (cotton, silk, or anything similar will be great) and tie it loosely around your head; covering the area from the tip of your nose to the middle of your forehead. Ensure that there is no pressure on the eyelids. (If you don't have a piece of white cloth, a blank sheet of white paper can create the same effect when you hold it up against your face, bending it around toward both ears.)

Close your eyes a while to rest them, then open them and observe the white in front of your eyes. It may be blurry white, and it can at first be a challenge to have something so close to the eyes. Simply keep your breathing and blinking relaxed and allow your attention to wander around the white for a while, noticing areas of shade and areas of brighter white. Then look down past the nose and notice what you can see in your lap or on the floor. By alternately closing one eye, it will become obvious which eye sees what, and by opening both eyes you can observe your brain fusing the two images to some extent, which creates a downward-pointing white triangle where the white cloth or paper touches the tip of the nose.

It may take a couple of minutes before your brain will want to play the game of fusion, so be patient and relax into this practice as much as you can.

B. Point your ghostly finger

When the non-dominant eye is switched on to some extent, but not yet enough to provide two equally solid images, the following practice will help solidify the image from the non-dominant eye and thus improve your fusion.

Hold your index finger up in front of your face and look past it at anything of interest a foot or more beyond your finger. You'll become aware of two fingers, possibly one solid finger and one ghostly. This ghostly finger can be put to good use. Although the solid finger will be more obvious, notice what the ghostly finger is pointing at. (You may want to move your finger sideways a bit toward your non-dominant eye, until you find the place where you get the best image of the ghostly finger while looking beyond it.) Point at any object of interest with the tip of the ghostly finger. The closer to the nose you hold the finger, the greater the distance between the two finger images, which may help the ghostly one become more prominent. The tricky part is to keep your attention on the details you point at, but your awareness is also partially with both finger images, especially the ghostly one. Practice letting your ghostly finger follow your attention. Remember that your main attention stays with distant objects, because when you look at your finger its two images will fuse into one single finger.

This awareness of the ghostly finger may be a little tricky and tiresome at first, but persist and use it on fun objects to look at to help you enjoy it. This practice will get easier and more natural over time; it helps repave neural pathways from the non-dominant eye to the brain, so that eventually both fingers appear similar.

C. Cord fusion

You'll need a 10-foot piece of cord for this fusion practice, and, optionally, three colored beads. Placing a few colorful beads along the cord gives your eyes easy targets to aim for and may make this process of developing fusion more fun. Slide one of the beads toward the end of the cord, place one near the center, and one about a foot from your nose. (If you don't have beads, you can tie a knot in the cord at three different distances.) Tie one end of the cord to a doorknob (or somewhere at least a foot lower than your eye level) and hold the other end near the tip of your nose, pulling the cord somewhat taut. Keep your neck loose by avoiding the temptation to get closer to the rope with your nose. Don't stare or hold your breath: blink and breathe with ease. Shift your attention to the nearest part of the cord and notice that the cord appears to split into two, forming a V with the bottom of the V closest to you. If you do not get a V but only see one single cord, check that the cord is centered in front of your nose, rather than to the side in front of your dominant eye. If you still see only one cord, go back to Step 2 to help switch on the non-dominant eye.

If you do see two cords, let your attention go to the nearest bead, and notice if the two cords now cross right at that bead. The V will begin to look like an X, with the center of the X exactly where your attention is on the cord. The center of the X shows where your brain fuses the two separate images of the cord into one. Also notice if the two cords cross at the same level or does one appear to cross above the other? If they are at different levels, your eyes are at different heights, which can be due to a habitual head tilt. Check the angle of your head and neck and aim to keep the images of the two cords level with each other.

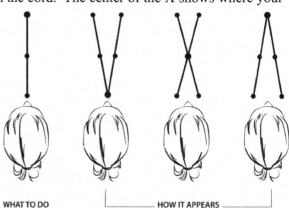

WHAT TO DO   HOW IT APPEARS

You can now let your attention glide along the cord toward the center bead and notice the center of the X move along with your point of attention. Continue to shift further out until your attention is on the doorknob, which creates an image of an upside-down V: Λ.

If at any point you lose the illusion of seeing two cords, go back to where you were able to see two, and use your memory and imagination of that image to help you create the same illusion at the point where it does not appear at first. Let it be easy though! There is no use forcing this, as any trying will negate the effort. A relaxed awareness of the entire room keeps your peripheral vision engaged and allows for ease in central vision.

Spend about a minute with the fusion cord and practice daily until seeing two cords becomes easy. You can then advance to a 20-foot cord with multiple beads.

D. Eyeport fusion

The Eyeport can also be used as a fusion cord, which is the last of its five standard positions recommended in each ten-minute session. You hold the device with one end near your nose, the other end pointing away and slightly down from your nose. Do not use the red/blue glasses for this practice. The white strip between the lights acts as the cord, the lights resemble the beads. The advantage of the Eyeport is that it will automatically draw your attention from one lit light to the next, and the speed and order in which these lights flash on can be adjusted to your current ability.

Step 5. Increase depth perception

Playing with any of the techniques in this chapter will stimulate your brain into seeing a three-dimensional world. It may take a while for that to happen, as the brain has to re-pave some neural pathways, so both patience and persistence are required. At first the 3-D world can feel overwhelming, but if you keep going and stay relaxed with it, this will pass. I no longer feel overwhelmed in the 3-D world, and the reward of a higher level of depth perception has been well worth the time I put into achieving it.

Here are two more suggestions to help you go beyond basic depth perception.

A. Continued practice

Daily use of fusion practices from Step 4 combined with the least use of glasses or contact lenses will provide the best results. For me, using the Eyeport at higher speeds and in its random-pattern program was a great help in my ability to solidify my depth perception. At times I still practice a few fusion techniques to keep and further develop my delightful 3-D world.

B. Doubling at the peripheries

This advanced fusion technique comes from Robert Hagmann's "Omnision" practices.[9] Hagmann recommended you practice this as often as possible, yet without effort. Stay within personal limits of comfort and intersperse it with palming as needed. You'll need two differently colored pencils and a blank wall, ceiling or bright sky for background. I will use a red and green pencil as examples.

Hold the red pencil pointed up in front of your face and look at the background so you notice two red pencil images in the foreground. Vary the distance you hold the red pencil from your face until you find where it is easiest to see two pencils. Hold the red pencil there. Now hold the green pencil alongside the red one. This green one should double too, resulting in seeing four pencil images. If you hold the pencils close together you will see a red, a green, a red and a green side by side. Continue to gaze at the background while you move the two doubled pencils apart, sideways into your periphery, but only to the point where you can keep them both doubled. The two red pencil images will move to one side, the greens move opposite. If either pair becomes one pencil, move that pencil slightly back toward center until it doubles again. Hold it there until it feels more solidly present before moving it slightly further out again. Gradually work on moving the two pencils further out into your peripheral field as far as you can keep them doubled.

You can progress to holding two or three pencils in each hand, each pencil a different color, so you can tell if you are doubling each color in each hand.

24. Dr. Bates' Perspective on Eye Diseases

I am not an eye doctor, so I do not advise anyone on how to overcome an eye disease. Interestingly, I learned that even Dr. Bates had been hesitant to use his methods for eye diseases. He thought it would only work for functional vision issues. In the January 1921 issue of *Better Eyesight,* Bates wrote:[1]

> I began to treat cataract by the operative method, because I did not know anything better to do. Then I learned from Dr. James E. Kelly of New York that incipient cases would yield to hygienic treatment. My first inkling of the value of central fixation in such conditions came to me through a patient who had incipient cataract in one eye and hypermetropia (farsight) in the other. By the time the error of refraction had been relieved the cataract had disappeared. After this I had many similar experiences, but it did not occur to me that a ripe cataract, or a congenital cataract, could be cured by this or any other treatment.
>
> In 1912, however, a young girl of seventeen came to my clinic with the left eye enucleated and a congenital cataract in the right. The left had been operated upon for the same condition, and, having become infected, was taken out to save the better eye. The latter having recently become worse, the patient had come to have it operated upon. Before performing the operation, I thought it best to treat her by the method of relaxation, for the purpose of improving the condition of the eye as much as possible so that the operation might have a better chance of success. To my surprise the vision improved and kept on improving, until in three months it was normal and the cataract had disappeared.

Soon after this experience Bates witnessed a mature cataract disappear as well, and to his astonishment, even a traumatic cataract yielded to his relaxation methods. Not only cataracts proved curable; Bates described similar surprises with glaucoma, corneal opacity, and even sympathetic ophthalmia. Here is another example of Bates' own surprise, this one with a case of conical cornea (keratoconus):[2]

> About ten years ago a girl, aged twenty, came to me with a diagnosis of conical cornea in the right eye, the left eye being nearly normal. The vision of the right eye was 10/200 not improved by glasses. I told the patient that I did not think I could improve the conical cornea but I might be able to relieve her of the pain and discomfort in her good eye. The palming after a half hour or longer relieved her discomfort temporarily and, much to my surprise, the vision of the eye with

conical cornea was improved from 10/200 to 10/50. The patient felt much better at this quick relief and improvement in the sight of the eye with conical cornea, as it was the first encouragement that she had had in a long time. Under the relaxation treatment this patient's vision continued steadily to improve until it became normal after some weeks. The conical cornea disappeared.

As Bates continued to use his relaxation methods for eye diseases, his confidence grew. He wrote:

I have never seen an eye so badly injured that its vision could not be improved.[3]

And...

Except in extraordinarily rare cases blindness is curable. In fact, unless the eyeball has been removed from the head, I should be unwilling to set any limits whatever to the possibility of relieving this greatest of human ills, for I have never seen a case or injury or disease of the eye which was sufficient to prevent improvement of vision. In all cases of blindness, whatever their cause, a mental strain has been demonstrated, and when this strain has been relieved perception of light has always been obtained.

The good news [is] that the eye is not a blunder of nature, as the textbooks teach, but an instrument as perfectly adapted to the needs of civilized man as to those of the savage.[4]

So, Bates' experiences show that using the eyes the way nature intended not only improves visual acuity but also improves overall performance and health of the eyes. Bates trained his assistant Emily, who had no medical training of her own, to achieve similar results in his clinic. For example, Emily wrote about Lewis, a blind boy aged 12 who had atrophy of the optic nerves:

After the examination, Dr. Bates came to my office and told me about the case and asked: "Wouldn't you like to see him? I think you could help him to see again." Oh! Wonderful faith. It is the faith Dr. Bates has in me that keeps me going. His encouragement has helped me to benefit cases that would otherwise have seemed hopeless to me.[5]

Emily helped Lewis see again simply by teaching him how to release eyestrain.

When I began to study Dr. Bates' written legacy in depth, I lived in Joshua Tree, a small town in Southern California. During the six months I was there, I had only one student: Albert, the owner of the local health food store. I briefly mentioned him in Chapter 21.

Albert was sixty-two, diabetic, and two years earlier he had experienced sudden blindness in his left eye. Doctors were unable to help him, so he did not have surgery. Albert turned to nutritional supplements and gradually recovered much of his sight. Then at age sixty-one, the same problem re-occurred; this time his right eye suddenly went blind. When I met Albert a year later, his right eye was slowly recovering its sight, yet both eyes had trouble seeing well. He was unable to drive at night because oncoming lights blinded him, bright lights in general hurt his eyes, and his handwriting was illegible.

With only a few lessons, his vision acuity with both eyes together went from 10/80 to 10/20, his right eye improved from 5/200 to 10/80 while the left went from 10/60 to 10/20. His gratitude was immense. He wrote this after his first lesson:

> I'm seeing things I haven't seen in two years! Becoming aware of my tendency to squint was key. Now I keep my eyes open. I regularly do the sunning and am no longer so sensitive to bright light. It's going really well. I look forward to more lessons.

A month and a couple of lessons later, Albert wrote:

> My eyesight is a thousand times better. I am even driving at night again, I haven't been able to do that in over a year! I don't know how I can ever repay you for what you've done for me. Yesterday I penned a letter and it was written on the lines and it was even legible. I haven't been able to do that in a year. That was a big deal for me. Thank you for all that you are doing for me.

Albert boosted my confidence in teaching the Bates Method to anyone, even if they have an eye disease. I simply work on the eyestrain with my student, and if the eye disease decides to respond to the changes in visual habits too, it's a very welcome bonus and "happy side-effect" of this work.

Here are three examples from students who experienced happy side-effects while releasing eyestrain.

Jay's floaters

Jay, a teenager from Idaho, had been prescribed glasses for mild myopia and astigmatism but they gave him a giant headache. After finding my website and learning how not to strain his eyes anymore, he wrote to share some good news because he had been "enjoying the fruits of relaxed and effortless vision." Besides gaining much clearer vision, he also got rid of floaters in his eyes. In his own words:

I am proud to announce that I can read the 15 line from 20-22 feet away (I measured). One day my right eye could even pick out a few letters on the 10 line! It is truly amazing how well you see when you don't try to see!! Thankfully the habit of trying not to see is already very strong within me, and only very rarely do I find myself trying to see (which I quickly correct).

I have also had a few more bonuses using this relaxed vision. I have several floaters in both eyes, which, as you can imagine, is very annoying. This new, relaxed vision gets rid of them virtually instantly, using blinking, shifting, and not trying to see. Now only very rarely do I see my floaters!! Let me tell you it's very nice to look up into that sapphire blue sky and see nothing but endless blue, minus those floaters!! I am also not as sensitive to sunlight as I used to be; sunning really helps.

Alex's keratoconus

In 2012, I worked with a young man who had keratoconus. Alex had 3 diopters of myopia with -6.25 and -5.25 diopters of astigmatism in his right and left eye, respectively. He felt embarrassed about how bad his vision was and tried to hide this fact from other people, which added to his stress. He took eight online video lessons with me in 2012 and followed that up with three days of private lessons in Oregon.

Alex greatly benefited from using a foundation memory – being a carpenter, he chose a hammer that had belonged to his grandfather. He could easily imagine the details of that hammer, could feel the weight of it in his hand, and with his eyes closed, he thought about using it, which helped relax his mind. Upon opening his eyes, his vision was much improved. Playing with a bounce ball was another useful trick for him. Overall, he discovered he had been trying too hard to see, and the Bates Method took the trying out of his seeing. By the end of the third day, Alex's visual acuity was 20/20 -4 (miscalling only 4 of the 12 letters on the 20 line from 20 feet) – a tremendous improvement.

Monika's cataracts

Monika from Switzerland had cataracts in both eyes and had fairly strong myopia with astigmatism when she first took my email course in 2012. Her prescription at the start was: right eye -3.00, -1.00 x 175, and left eye -6.00, -1.75 x 166. Besides the more pronounced cataract in her left eye, that eye also had double vision. She was dealing with frequent headaches and had tried eye exercises in the past, but said it was hard to find time to do them and she hadn't made any progress.

During the email course, both her eyes improved, and she found the relaxed vision habits much easier to incorporate than the previous eye exercises. Her headaches got better too. In June 2018, she contacted me again. Her prescription had changed dramatically, with the left eye now totally clear, while the right had -2.25, -1.00 x 158. A lesson via Skype at that point cleared up some wrong thoughts about "weakness" in her right eye and having to "try hard." She switched back to relaxation and receptive seeing. In February 2019 she passed her driver's test without glasses and was given an unrestricted driver's license in her new home of Canada. She now only uses glasses for driving at night or in rainy conditions to help the right eye participate better. Her left eye has completely clear vision – no more cataract.

Many eye diseases benefit from relaxation
Besides Dr. Bates' examples above of cataracts and conical cornea disappearing, his writings are full of examples of other eye diseases that benefited from his relaxation methods. Among them are glaucoma, nystagmus, corneal opacity, blindness, conjunctivitis, iritis, macular degeneration, optic nerve atrophy, retinal detachment, scar tissue, and sympathetic ophthalmia. I expect that any eye disease can benefit from, or may be prevented by, you learning and applying the relaxation techniques described in this book. It can take many months to heal the eyes, yet there is always hope that vision can improve, no matter what the problem is.

Get Dr. Bates' personal view
Dr. Bates found that some diseases had specifically good results with certain parts of the method. For example, in cases of inflammation and optic nerve atrophy, sunning was emphasized as an essential part of the treatment.

To get an overview of which techniques Dr. Bates used in a variety of eye diseases, I compiled a series of booklets called *The Bates Method View of…* with each one focusing on a different visual challenge and providing everything Dr. Bates wrote on that specific topic. See the Resources for a list of books available in this series.

Eye emergencies
Call an ophthalmologist immediately if you have worrisome symptoms, such as sudden loss of vision, severe eye pain, eye injuries, a bleeding eye, a sudden onset of flashes of light, a foreign object or chemicals in your eye, etc. These are acute eye emergencies that require urgent medical care.

 Give nature a chance
With mild or chronic eye diseases you have the luxury of time to give the relaxation practices in this book a chance to do their magic. Palming is a popular first choice for many visual issues, but don't forget to consider the influence of your diet, as visual challenges may be related to a nutrient deficiency or toxic excess. In Appendix F, you will find a list I compiled of links that doctors and researchers have found between visual challenges and possible causes.

For best results, start releasing your eyestrain right now.

> **If you focus on results, you will never change.**
> **If you focus on change, you will get results.**
> Jack Dixon, Welsh Rugby Union Player

Note: A few suggested books on how to treat eye diseases without drugs or surgery:[7]

- *Natural Eye Care: Your Guide to Healthy Vision and Healing* – Marc Grossman, O.D., L.Ac., and Michael Edson, M.S., L.Ac. (2018)
- *Healthy Vision* – Neal Adams, M.D. (2014)
- *Smart Medicine for your Eyes* – Jeffrey R. Anshel, O.D. (2011)
- *Cataract, Glaucoma and Other Eye Disorders* – John Tobe (1973)

Postscript

As you now know, optimal eyesight is not achieved by a daily regimen of standard eye exercises. Acuity of 20/20 and better is regained by letting your eyes be free from strain and by letting them do what they naturally do best: effortlessly following every little shift in your attention, and doing this without glasses, or with lower-diopter lenses if you cannot yet function completely lens-free. As the strain releases, sight improves, and you take the next step to greater dynamic relaxation and clarity.

All parts of the Bates Method are likely to help to some extent, although their usefulness will vary from one person to the next. Many love palming; for others swings are of more help. Almost everyone improves by using memory and imagination of perfect vision, yet again, those won't work for all, or perhaps not at first. The key is to test everything, discover which technique gives some benefit quickly, and use that often until other parts of the method begin to show results too.

> **The same method cannot be used with everyone. The ways in which people strain to see are infinite, and the methods used to relieve the strain must be almost equally varied. Whatever the method that brings most relief, however, the end is always the same, namely relaxation. By constant repetition and frequent demonstration and by all means possible, the fact must be impressed upon the patient that perfect sight can be obtained only by relaxation. Nothing else matters.**
> William H. Bates, M.D.[1]

Each time you catch a squint or stare, do not let such strain continue! Instead, respond to blurriness with extra blinking, motion awareness, or any other better vision habit that best counteracts your old habits of straining. This is how you change the direction that your eyesight is headed toward – from ever-worsening vision to ever-improving vision. Each step you take in the right direction brings you healthier and happier eyes that see with more and more clarity.

> **In essence, if we want to direct our lives, we must take control of our consistent actions. It's not what we do once in a while that shapes our lives, but what we do consistently.**
> Anthony Robbins[2]

To succeed, you do not need to apply the relaxation techniques 100% of the time. If you think success requires perfection, you set yourself up for failure and you may not try again. So, be kind to yourself when your old, strained vision habits kick in and seem hard to overcome. It is common for them to persist for some time. When you practice looking in a relaxed, receptive way at least 51% of the time, you halt that slippery slope toward worse vision and begin to make progress toward clarity. When you gradually increase this to 75 or 80% of the time, your vision will steadily improve and, sooner or later, you will reach your goal of optimal eyesight.

You can create your personalized daily relaxation reminders out of the If-Then List in Chapter 16. Decide which one or two habits you need to adopt most to overcome your biggest eyestrain issues. Find a way to remind yourself of these relaxed habits often, perhaps with a sticky note on your computer screen, phone, fridge, mirror, etc. After a few weeks, or when you notice you are establishing better habits, change the reminder for any other habit you need to adopt. Whenever you close your eyes, bring these habits to mind and check if any old habit of straining can be released further.

The Bates Method may continue to be ridiculed and disputed by eye doctors, yet its successes cannot be denied. The traditional Bates Method will therefore persist, as all truth persists, and will one day be considered common sense. All it requires is an open mind – your willingness to experiment in how you see and how you think about what you see. The resulting change in vision will prove Dr. Bates right or wrong. I will gladly let you decide.

Enjoy your path to clarity!

With Gratitude

This book rests on the extensive writings and legacy left by the famous ophthalmologist William H. Bates, who together with his assistant and later wife Emily (Lierman) Bates, proved to the world that eyesight can and will improve naturally when it is given a proper chance.

Many colleagues have influenced me in my work in this field of natural vision education. I'm grateful to Tom Quackenbush for getting me started on this vision path. I so very much appreciated Robert (Bobby) Lichtman's friendship, whose brilliant mind managed to drag me along in understanding Dr. Bates' extensive writings. Other colleagues whose understanding of the Bates Method influenced my work are Gloria Ginn, Margaret Montgomery, Ray Gottlieb, O.D., Ph.D., Amelia Salvador, M.D., and numerous others I met at holistic vision conferences both in Europe and the U.S.

When it came to the essential fact-checking and medical research, I had invaluable help from Bobby's delightful wife, Tamar Shinar, Ph.D. She located a multitude of research papers and saved me many hours and countless trips to a university library.

Richard Hobday, M.Sc, Ph.D., kindly provided links to useful references that helped shape the chapter on sunlight. His knowledgeable comments and probing questions regarding that chapter caused me to clarify several points which improved its flow.

Grateful hugs go to my "ancient" Ojai friend, Mark Latker, M.S., for "whipping" me into writing in the gorgeous setting of his vacation house in Port Royal, Roatan, when I had trouble focusing and sitting still long enough to get pen to paper. His countless follow-up phone calls always started with "How's the book going?" as he urged me onward.

Excellent advice on how to effectively write a book came from Penny Legg in the U.K., who talked me out of my constant self-editing habit and triggered my completion of a first draft of this book in mere months, not years.

No book ends up being readable without some dedicated editors: I thank Vivian D. Sudhalter of Ojai, California, who jettisoned the mixed grammatical influences of my tri-lingual mind's writings and converted my first draft into a uniformly American English text. Emma Ellis then went through what I thought was my final, "near-perfect" draft, and kept me surprisingly busy for a few months with her questions, comments and suggestions which tremendously improved the readability of this book! I didn't know editing could be so much fun and so educational at the same time. Thanks so much, dear Emma; I am delighted to have gained a new friend in you! A longtime supporter of my work and former journalist to boot, Jean-Noel Bassior then took on the task of taking the final draft to "mainstream-level" and polished it up in oh-so-many more places. Jean-Noel, you're an absolute treasure! And that was awesome teamwork, my dear ladies!

The many excellent illustrations and the striking book cover are a testimonial to the amazing talent of Jane Shanahan, my fabulous illustrator. Thanks Jane, for doing such a great job! Also thanks to Kevin Wooding of Bates Method International (www.seeing.org) for providing the high-quality images of Dr. Bates and his wife on pages *iv* and *v*. The back-cover photo credit goes to my wonderful friend and neighbor, Aubrie Woods.

Gratitude to my friend Irene Tirella, the first person to read the entire manuscript. She had not yet heard of the Bates Method, but began to enthusiastically tell her friends all about it, and she gave me greatly encouraging feedback. Sincere thanks also to my dear friends Malcolm J. McKeand and Dirk Schubert for proof-reading parts of this book and offering their sound advice!

I found that I like to write with some gentle music playing in the background, so thanks to a multitude of musicians whose peaceful music accompanied me throughout many hours of writing! Especially instrumental tracks from Paolo Ferro, Kitaro, Brûlé, the late Johnny Pearson, and my friends Ray Flores, Alan Thornhill and Martin Young on their acoustic guitars, were played over and over.

My heartfelt thanks go to my sweet parents, who love and support me in all I do – even though some of my wild adventures have been responsible for many of their gray or missing hairs. I'm so grateful they are both still alive and well, and that they get to see this book come into the world in lieu of a grandchild… ☺

Most of all, I thank the many students who placed their trust in me over the past nineteen years, whether they came with minor issues or serious vision challenges; whether they had never heard of the Bates Method before or came to me as colleagues needing a little extra help. I learned from each one of them, and I am grateful for the many questions asked and the useful feedback received that helped hone my skills. I would not be the experienced and confident Bates Method teacher I am now, if it hadn't been for all these students asking me to help them improve their eyesight.

Finally, to you, dear reader, I extend my gratitude. You are willing to think outside the box; you ask questions and want truthful answers; you know deep in your heart that there has to be a better way – an effective alternative to the glasses, contact lenses, drugs or laser surgery that you have been offered, and you are ready to act on the answers. I hope you will let me know your thoughts on the natural solutions this book provides, along with your experiences in applying the relaxation methods. And perhaps, one day, I'll get to look into your bright and beautiful, healthy eyes!

Appendix A

Find Your Optimal Practice Distance

The distance at which you are most comfortable with the chart and where you notice the most progress is your optimal practice distance. For most people with myopia, this is going to be relatively close, not 20 feet away. Looking at any chart at a distance where all letters look incredibly blurry is unlikely to help you relax. At that point it is much more likely that you'll get frustrated or feel like a failure, neither of which is of any use to you. I want you to find the distance at which the entire chart is easy to read and where the small letters on the last line appear blurry but are still readable. Whether you use the small or medium chart in your hand or the large chart hanging on the wall doesn't matter. What matters is your ease in reading the chart.

Start in your preferred light conditions, set up a chart close to you where you have your best vision, and slowly increase your distance from the chart until the last line is no longer perfectly clear but remains readable. Measure this distance (from your eyes to the chart) and make a note of it. I suggest you use this distance for initial chart practice. This distance will change, so don't think you need to practice at the same distance every day. Feel free to adjust it as needed each time you use the chart.

The advantage of using a chart at this distance is that it will seem so easy. That's good – you want it to be easy! Once you get to the point of comfortably reading the last line from this distance, you can increase the distance by small increments. Small, easy steps ensure steady progress, whereas if you take a step that's too big, you may slow progress down because it is harder to do.

On (date) _____ my optimal practice distances with the S/M/L chart are:
for both eyes together _____,
for right eye only _____,
for left eye only _____.

Which size chart you choose depends on your current level of myopia. At -6 or above the smallest chart held near your eyes is likely to be easiest, while someone between 3 and 6 diopters of myopia may prefer the medium chart, either held in the hand or hanging nearby on a wall. Those below -3 diopters probably prefer the largest chart taped to a wall.

Tip: If you tape the chart to a piece of cardboard and set it on a music-stand, you can easily adjust both the distance and height of the chart.

Appendix B

Measure Your Far Point

When you hold a chart in your area of best vision, it will appear perfectly clear; yet when you move the chart further away, at some point it blurs. The furthest clear point, just before your blur zone, is known as your "far point." It is checked one eye at a time. Regularly measuring your far point for each eye will help track your progress, and it can also help you decide what diopter lenses are best to use on your path to clarity. When you measure the distance in centimeters from your eye to the chart held at the far point, you can easily convert it to your diopter strength, as this is a mathematical equation:

$$\frac{100}{\text{far point in cm}} = \text{diopters}$$

So, someone whose clarity reaches 25 cm (9.8 inches) from one eye while beyond 25 cm things get blurry, has 100/25 = 4 diopters of myopia in that eye, which a doctor writes as -4.00 D. Measuring your far point allows you to check if your current lenses are right for you or whether it's time to change to a lower diopter.

If you already know your diopters, the equation shows where to look for your far point:

$$\frac{100}{\text{diopters}} = \text{far point in centimeters}$$

For example: someone with 2 diopters of myopia can see clearly up to 50 cm (19.7 inches).

If you have astigmatism as well as myopia, there will be two far points: one for the sphere and one for the cylinder. I'll show you on the next page how you can determine your own diopters for both.

How to measure your far point for a myopic eye

Use optimal light conditions for higher accuracy. Use text size appropriate for the distance; either one of the small charts (page 281) has the sizes you need. One chart lists distance in feet, the other in centimeters. The latter may be less confusing when you are measuring in centimeters. Check one eye at a time and cover the other with the palm of your hand rather than closing it. It's easiest when a friend measures the distance for you while you cover one eye with one hand and hold the chart in the other.

If you know your prescription, you can use the table on page 259 to find which line of the chart is probably best to use. If you don't know your prescription, hold either chart where the last line (1 ft or 35 cm line) can be read with total clarity. If this is within 1 ft/35 cm, check if you can still read this line with perfect clarity at 1 ft/35 cm from your eye. If so, shift to the line above it (2 ft/50 cm) and check how far away you can still read that before it begins to blur. If the 2 line is still perfectly clear at 2 feet, or the 50 cm line is still clear at 50 cm, shift up to line 3 or 75 cm respectively, and so forth, until you find the distance where letters begin to blur.

Once you find that edge between total clarity and slight blur, hold the chart at the furthest point of clarity and have someone use a tape-measure with the zero-end held at the side of your eye so they can read the distance at which you hold the chart. Either use the equation above or use the table below to convert this distance into diopters. If you don't have astigmatism, this diopter number represents the sphere of your prescription.

Two far points in astigmatism

If astigmatism is present in the eye, that eye will have two far points: one for the sphere, another for the cylinder that is added to the sphere. For example, someone with -4 myopia (the sphere) and -1 astigmatism (the cylinder) at 180 degrees (the axis) will have clarity up to 20 cm for all angles of print, while slightly beyond 20 cm horizontal lines (180 degrees) start to blur but vertical lines still appear perfectly clear. So 20 cm is the nearest far point, which represents the combination of cylinder and sphere (100÷20 cm = 5.00 diopters). Just beyond 25 cm vertical lines also start to blur, while right at 25 cm those vertical lines still appear clear. So 25 cm is the other far point, this one is for the sphere (100:25 cm = 4.00 diopters in this example). The difference between the two far-point diopters indicates the amount of astigmatism, in this case 1 diopter. The sphere has a 4-diopter curvature; the cylinder has an additional 1-diopter curvature, making a total of 5 diopters at the 180 axis.

As it can be challenging to tell when some lines become blurry when you use a letter-chart, it may be easier to use the astigmatism chart on page 285 to determine the first far point. The following illustration may help you along.

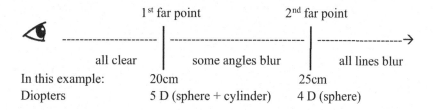

Not all cases of astigmatism are easy to measure, so this method does not work for everyone. If in doubt, let an eye doctor measure your prescription for you.

Monitor your progress with the help of the far point table

The table on the next page will help you monitor your own vision acuity and shows how close you are to seeing with total clarity with each eye.

When you start to improve your vision, your initial steps forward may seem small and insignificant, yet they are not. For example, someone who improves from -3.25 to -3.00 diopters gains "only" one inch in their range of clarity, as their far point increases from 12.1 to 13.1 inches. Yet when they continue to make quarter diopter improvements, their far point jumps out more and more! You will notice that a quarter diopter improvement from -1.25 equals nearly 8 inches, while the improvement from -0.50 to -0.25 diopters gives you a giant gain of 78.7 inches! And that final quarter, from -0.25 to zero, is the step into infinity.

So, every centimeter or inch gained and every quarter diopter counts and is a reason to celebrate! It proves that vision can and does get better.

The far point table from 0.25 to 20 diopters of myopia

Far Point (cm)	Far Point (inches)	Diopters	Use this line of the chart (centimeters)	(feet)
400	157.5	-0.25	500	15
200	78.8	-0.50	200	7
100	39.4	-1.00	100	4
80	31.5	-1.25	100	3
66.6	26.2	-1.50	75	3
57.1	22.5	-1.75	75	2
50	19.7	-2.00	50	2
44.4	17.5	-2.25	50	2
40	15.75	-2.50	50	2
36.4	14.3	-2.75	50	2
33.3	13.1	-3.00	35	2
30.8	12.1	-3.25	35	2
28.6	11.2	-3.50	35	1
26.7	10.5	-3.75	35	1
25	9.8	-4.00	35	1
23.5	9.25	-4.25	35	1
22.2	8.7	-4.50	35	1
21	8.3	-4.75	35	1
20	7.9	-5.00	35	1
19	7.5	-5.25	35	1
18.2	7.2	-5.50	35	1
17.4	6.9	-5.75	35	1
16.7	6.6	-6.00	35	1
15.4	6.1	-6.50	35	1
14.3	5.6	-7.00	35	1
13.3	5.2	-7.50	35	1
12.5	4.9	-8.00	35	1
11.8	4.6	-8.50	35	1
11.1	4.4	-9.00	35	1
10.5	4.1	-9.50	35	1
10	3.9	-10.00	35	1
8.3	3.3	-12.00	35	1
7.1	2.8	-14.00	35	1
6.25	2.5	-16.00	35	1
5.5	2.2	-18.00	35	1
5	2	-20.00	35	1

Appendix C

Measure Your Visual Acuity and Monitor Progress

With the help of a letter chart you will be able to check your own visual acuity on a regular basis. Hang the largest chart on a wall, with the center of the chart at eye level. While wearing your current glasses, check with each eye separately if you can read the letters on the 20 line from 20 feet. If so, these lenses are too strong for you. They will slow down your vision improvement progress. Start using lower diopter lenses as soon as possible, and regularly check your visual acuity while wearing them. Whenever you notice that you can read the 20 line from 20 feet with each eye with these glasses, it is time to progress to the next lower prescription.

When checking your acuity without glasses or contact lenses, begin at a distance where you can read the entire chart easily. Measure this distance and make a note of it. Then step back to the point where you experience some blurry vision but where you can still read the first seven lines with ease. (That's down to the 20-line on the large chart or down to the 10-line on the medium chart.)

After checking what the lowest line and letters are that you can read with both eyes open, write down the distance you read it from and the number next to the last line you were able to read. Then cover the left eye with your left hand and note the acuity for the right eye. Go back to using both eyes for a few moments before you cover the right eye with your right hand to check the acuity for the left eye. (It doesn't matter in which order you check your eyes.) Write your results in the table on page 262.

Visual acuity is written down as follows: write the distance in feet that you stood from the letter chart before the slash (/). After the slash write the number that you find next to the last line of letters that you were able to read, regardless of how blurry it appears. If you can distinguish what the letter is (without squinting or straining to see), it counts. Using readability as the standard of measurement eliminates a subjective judgment about your level of clarity.

When you can read all the letters on a line, for example the 20 line from 5 feet, you write it as 5/20. If you also recognize one letter on the 15 line, but not the rest of the 15 line, you can write 5/20 +1. If you recognize most of the letters on the 15 line, but miss two of them, you can write 5/15 -2.

Here's another example:

John stands 10 feet from the chart. With both eyes open he can read the line that has the number 20 next to it. He writes down his visual acuity for both eyes as 10/20. At that same distance, with his right eye covered, his left eye can only read the letters on the 30 line, but not those on the 20 line, so his left eye's acuity is written as 10/30. When he switches over and covers his left eye, (giving his right eye a few moments to re-adjust) he can read the 20 line, but not yet the 15 line, although he correctly identifies one letter on that 15 line. So his right eye on its own has an acuity of 10/20 +1.

Average "normal" vision is 20/20 (ability to read the 20 line from 20 feet), but this is still slightly myopic vision, and many people can improve to 20/15 or an even sharper 20/10 (reading the 10 line from 20 feet).

Record your progress

Once a week, record your progress in visual acuity, using the table on the next page. It is normal for acuity to be better with both eyes together than with one eye at a time. Also, your vision can be quite different at night under artificial light than in daytime in bright sunlight, so always make a note of the light conditions; then you can make a fair comparison from week to week. For example, if one week you check your vision at noon in bright sunlight, but the next week (also at noon), it's heavily overcast, you'll understand if the results for the second week are not as good as the week before.

When you see clear improvements happening – a line better on the chart from the same distance, or increased distance to read the same line – your enthusiasm and motivation to continue on this path to clear vision will get a nice boost! That's another great reason to keep track of your acuity on a regular basis.

You are likely to forget how blurry your vision was, so making a note of it now will guarantee that you know for sure if you're making progress.

Visual Acuity

Date	Time	Both Eyes	Left Eye	Right Eye	Light conditions
		/	/	/	
		/	/	/	
		/	/	/	
		/	/	/	
		/	/	/	
		/	/	/	
		/	/	/	
		/	/	/	
		/	/	/	
		/	/	/	
		/	/	/	
		/	/	/	
		/	/	/	
		/	/	/	
		/	/	/	
		/	/	/	
		/	/	/	
		/	/	/	
		/	/	/	
		/	/	/	
		/	/	/	
		/	/	/	
		/	/	/	
		/	/	/	
		/	/	/	
		/	/	/	
		/	/	/	
		/	/	/	
		/	/	/	
		/	/	/	
		/	/	/	
		/	/	/	
		/	/	/	
		/	/	/	

Appendix D

Conversion Table for Visual Acuity Values

This table is provided for easy comparison of visual acuity notations in fractions (feet and meters), decimal, percentage, LogMAR (Log of Minimum Angle of Resolution), and VAS (Vision Acuity Score, which is 100 – 50 x LogMAR).

Imperial	Metric	Decimal	%	LogMAR	VAS
20/10 *	6/3	2.0	200	-0.3	115
20/12.5	6/3.8	1.6	160	-0.2	110
20/16	6/4.8	1.25	125	-0.1	105
20/20 *	6/6	1.0	100	0	100
20/25	6/7.5	0.8	80	+0.1	95
20/32	6/9.5	0.63	63	+0.2	90
20/40 *	6/12	0.5	50	+0.3	85
20/50	6/15	0.4	40	+0.4	80
20/63	6/19	0.32	32	+0.5	75
20/80	6/24	0.25	25	+0.6	70
20/100	6/30	0.2	20	+0.7	65
20/125	6/38	0.16	16	+0.8	60
20/160	6/48	0.125	12.5	+0.9	55
20/200	6/60	0.1	10	+1.0	50
20/250	6/75	0.08	8	+1.1	45
20/320	6/95	0.06	6	+1.2	40
20/400	6/120	0.05	5	+1.3	35
20/500	6/150	0.04	4	+1.4	30
20/630	6/190	0.032	3.2	+1.5	25
20/800	6/240	0.025	2.5	+1.6	20
20/1000	6/300	0.02	2	+1.7	15
20/2000	6/600	0.01	1	+2.0	0

* Notes:
20/10 is what Dr. Bates considered to be the normal visual acuity of healthy eyes.[1]
20/20 is commonly considered to be normal visual acuity.
20/40 is the typical minimum acuity required for driving in most states in the U.S.

Appendix E

Your Guide to Buying Glasses Online

If you need lower diopter glasses to bridge a large gap between your current blurry vision and clarity, and if you don't want to spend a fortune, you can buy them online. But buying glasses on the internet can be daunting, especially the first time. To help you, here are some useful tips and explanations of terms that may ease the process, so you will hopefully get an affordable pair of glasses that turn out to actually fit when they arrive.

- An internet search for "cheap glasses" will provide a list of websites to buy from, or you can look at the list of such sites on my website.[1]

- Be sure to get the **right frame size**. The online store should ideally let you choose frames based on size by letting you select the overall frame width, lens height, and length of the temples or "arms" first, then show their available options within those parameters. Measure your current or most comfortable glasses for this (in millimeters) and use the same numbers or stay close to them.

- Some sites only give frame options of small/medium/large. If they are vague about actual size, you might prefer to shop elsewhere. A few sites allow you to send in an old pair of glasses and they will put in new lenses (re-lens or re-glaze). Some stores will even send frames to your home so you can try them on for free!

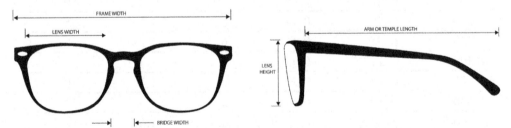

For each pair of glasses on sale there should be a frame size, as in this example:
Frame size: 47-20-140 mm. These three numbers indicate lens width, bridge (nose) width and temple length. All measurements are in millimeters.
Total frame width: 135 mm.
Lens height: 25 mm.
That's clear and useful. You may not find a frame with the exact same measurements as your current glasses, but if the numbers come close it will likely still be a good fit.

- To minimize neck tension, please **avoid bifocal/trifocal/progressive lenses**. These are guaranteed to add or increase the need for astigmatism cylinders. See Chapter 12. If you currently use such lenses, ask your eye doctor for help in determining how best to proceed on your path to clarity.

- **IMPORTANT**: **Be sure to include the minus symbol for sphere and cylinder!** Sphere and cylinder numbers always have either a plus or minus in front of them. Use the correct symbol! If, for example, you order 4.25 diopter glasses meant for myopia, you will instead receive strong reading glasses (+ lenses) if you forget to put the minus symbol (-) in front of the 4.25 sphere you ordered.

- **Avoid tinted, "transition" or photochromic lenses**. In general, it's best to get clear lenses that do not darken in bright light and that have no UV coating. See Chapter 15.

- You probably do want **anti-reflective (AR) coating**; it helps not to have those annoying light reflections.

- If your glasses tend to get some rough handling, **anti-scratch coating** is useful too.

- You need to know your **pupil distance.** See page 267 for how to measure it.

- **Astigmatism** is expressed as a combination of two numbers: the diopter of the cylinder and the degree of the axis. The axis number will be between 0 and 180. The diopters are often minus yet can also be plus, so make sure you copy the correct symbol. The cylinder diopter number can be as low as 0.25 for glasses. In contact lenses the lowest cylinder diopter that can be put in is 0.75. If you ask for a lower number, it will typically be left out.

- **High index** (or hi-index) glasses are thinner and weigh less than regular glasses. They are useful for those who need higher diopters. For further details about this topic and on the high index number you might want, you'll find a link on my website.[2]

- **Frame material**: Frames can be metal, plastic, titanium, half rims or rimless. Your choice depends on your preference. Stick with what has worked for you in the past or try something new; it's up to you.

What the abbreviations on your prescription mean:

DV	Distance Vision
NV/NVO	Near Vision/Near Vision Only
SV	Single Vision. Single vision glasses are used mainly for one distance, such as reading glasses, computer glasses or distance glasses (as opposed to bi-focal, tri-focal or progressive lenses).
OU	Both eyes (Oculus Uterque in Latin)
OD	Right eye (Oculus Dexter in Latin)
OS	Left eye (Oculus Sinister in Latin)
SPH	Sphere, the curve of the lens given in diopters. A minus number indicates nearsightedness, or myopia, while a plus number indicates farsightedness, or presbyopia (reading glasses). Diopters go by quarters. Some doctors write -50 or +225 without inserting the dot. In those cases your diopters are -0.50 and +2.25 respectively. If sphere is **left blank** or says "**plano**" you have no nearsightedness or farsightedness in that eye, although it may have astigmatism.
CYL	Cylinder (the level of any astigmatism for that eye, given in diopters). If it shows SPH or DS or is left blank, you leave it blank when ordering glasses.
X or AXIS	The angle of any astigmatism for that eye in degrees. If there is a cylinder number, there must also be an axis number. It will be between 0 and 180 degrees.
ADD	The number of diopters that bifocal or progressive lenses differ in the bottom portion from the rest of the glass. This is mainly used after age forty when nearsighted people find it harder to focus up close with their glasses on, so the bottom part of each lens has a lower prescription to allow for reading. If nothing is written in that part of your Rx, leave it blank.
PRISM	This is often left blank, unless there is strabismus or convergence/divergence insufficiency. You may not be able to get glasses online if you need a prism. Prisms are given in prism diopters, and they have a base (thickest edge) which can be in/out/up/down.
PL or P	Plano, which means zero, or no correction needed for that eye.
PD	Pupillary Distance (see below)

Pupillary distance measurement

To order glasses online you will need to provide the pupillary distance, or PD. This is the distance in millimeters between the centers of your two eyes. Sometimes this number is written on your prescription, but often it is not. If it is provided, it will usually have PD in front or above it, and it either shows a single number, such as 61, or sometimes you'll find two numbers, such as 32/32. If you have the latter, add the two together to get the "single" PD. In general, PD measurements fall in the range of 48 mm to 73 mm. The most common measurements are between 58 mm and 68 mm.

If no PD number is given, you can either ask your eye doctor what your PD is, as they will usually have it on file, or you can visit any eye doctor's office and ask them to measure it for you. It's quick and easy for them to do. Alternatively, you can measure your PD yourself. All you need is a millimeter ruler and a friend or a mirror.

Measure your own PD – with help from a friend

Ask your friend to hold a millimeter ruler just below the center of your eyes and measure the distance between the outside edge of one pupil to the inside edge of the other pupil.

Both of you should be at the same approximate height, seated opposite each other. The measurer holds the ruler in their left hand across your nose and closes their RIGHT eye to avoid any parallax error. With their LEFT eye open, they line up the ruler with the inside edge of your right pupil. Then without moving the ruler, they close their LEFT eye and with their RIGHT eye read off the measurement to the outside edge of your LEFT pupil.

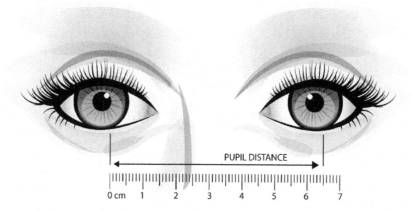

You should be looking directly in front of you at the open eye of your friend. This should ideally be about 16 inches away. If you have trouble with measuring this way, an alternative is to ask your friend to take a photo of your eyes with the ruler held as shown above while you look at the distance. You can then digitally enlarge it and read off the measurement more easily.

Measure your own PD – using a mirror

You can measure your PD using a mirror, either while wearing glasses, contacts, or with "bare eyes." Follow these steps:

1. Stand with your face about 20 cm (8 inches) from the mirror.
2. Close your right eye and look only with your left eye.
3. Place the ruler flat against the mirror and align it horizontally so the markings are near your eyes.
4. Look along the edge of the ruler and align the zero mark in the center or one side of your left pupil.
5. Open your right eye and close the left, but do not move your face or the ruler.
6. Read the millimeter measurement corresponding to the center or side of your right pupil.
7. Repeat the procedure several times to make sure you have a consistent measurement.

Excellent additional information can be found online.[3]

Appendix F

Visual Challenges and Nutrient Deficiencies

Visual Challenge	Possible Deficiency/Issue/Excess
Amblyopia (suppression of one eye)	A, B-complex
Bags under the eyes	General toxicity
Blepharitis (flaking and swelling of the eyelids)	B-complex
Blepharospasm (involuntary twitching of eyelids)	B-1, B-2, B-6, magnesium
Bloodshot eyes	B-complex, especially B-2
Blurred vision	A, B-1, B-2, B-6, E, chromium, GABA
Burning and/or itching of the eyes	B-2
Cataracts	A, beta carotene, B-complex, C, D, E, alpha lipoic acid, amino acids, calcium, chromium, copper, cysteine, glutathione, quercetin, rutin, selenium, zinc General toxicity (esp. high levels of lead, mercury, iron, cadmium), dehydration, lactose intolerance, excessive vitamin C or E, and steroid use contribute.
Color blindness	A, B-12
Conjunctivitis (inflammation/redness of the whites of the eyes)	A, B-2
Corneal ulcers	A, B-1, B-2, C
Crusting of the eyelids (granulated eyelids)	B-2
Dark circles under the eyes	B-12
Diabetic retinopathy	A, B-6, C, E, EFAs, bioflavonoids, magnesium, selenium, zinc
Double vision	A
Drooped eyelid	C, E, potassium
Dry cornea syndrome	A, B-7, B-9, C, amino acids High sugar consumption is dehydrating.
Dry eyes, xerophthalmia	A, B-6, B-7, B-9, B-12, C, E, CoQ10, EFAs, potassium. General toxicity and dehydration worsen it (as does staring or a low blink rate).
Excessive tearing of the eyes	A, B-2
Eye fatigue	A, B-2

Feeling of "sand" under the eyes	B-2, EFAs
Floaters, spots in visual field (also known as Muscae Volitantes)	A, beta carotene, C, D, E, calcium, copper, EFAs. General toxicity, smoking, alcohol, dehydration, medications, and vitamin C overdose can lead to floaters.
Glaucoma (damage to the optic nerve)	A, B-complex (B-1, B-3, B-12), C, E, alpha lipoic acid, bioflavonoids, choline, CoQ10, magnesium, EFAs, quercetin, zinc. Some medications, and high blood sugar can contribute to glaucoma.
Inflammation of the eye	A, D, E, quercetin. Lack of sunlight.
Keratoconus / conical cornea	A, C, E, antioxidants, beta carotene, lutein, magnesium, selenium, zeaxanthin
Macular degeneration (loss of central vision)	A, B-2, B-3, B-6, B-12, C, D, E, alpha lipoic acid, beta carotene, bioflavonoids, cysteine, chromium, copper, CoQ10, EFAs, lutein, manganese, quercetin, selenium, taurine, zeaxanthin, zinc General toxicity, vitamin C or E overdose and high blood sugar can contribute to macular degeneration.
Macular edema	C, E, bioflavonoids
Myopia (nearsightedness)	A, B-2, B-9, D, E, calcium, chromium A diet high in refined sugars can play a role in developing myopia. Lack of outdoor time (little use of distance vision) also contributes.
Night blindness	A, B-complex, lutein, zeaxanthin, zinc
Ocular rosacea (painful, burning, feels like foreign body in eyes)	B-complex, especially B-2, Enzymes
Photophobia (sensitivity of eyes to light)	B-2, magnesium, selenium, zinc
Presbyopia ("middle-age sight" farsighted, resulting in a need for reading glasses)	A, B-1, B-2, B-6, C, E, glutathione, iron, selenium, zinc Highly fluctuating or high blood sugar levels can contribute to presbyopia.
Retinal bleeding	B-1, E, zinc
Retinopathy	C, E, bioflavonoids
Retinal detachment or retinitis	A, B-2, zinc General toxicity and vitamin C overdose can lead to retinal detachment.
Retinitis pigmentosa (pigment clumps at the back of the eye)	A, B-complex, C, E, alpha lipoic acid, EFAs, CoQ10, cysteine, taurine, lutein, zeaxanthin, zinc
Styes on the eyelids	A, zinc

Strabismus / squint (misaligned eyes)	A, B-complex
Swelling of the eyelids or swelling under the eyes	Potassium, iodine (causing sluggish thyroid)
Unable to produce tears	A, EFAs
Uveitis (eye inflammation)	B-6, C, E, bioflavonoids, CoQ10, EFAs, zinc
Vitreous degeneration / detachment	C, lutein, zeaxanthin. Excess of vitamin C, zinc and vanadium can contribute.

See References for a list of sources used to compile the above table.

Appendix G

Food Sources of Eye-Essential Nutrients

Note: The following list of food sources is provided for your convenience, yet despite my best efforts, I cannot vouch for it to be 100% accurate, as some sources contradict each other. I therefore highly recommend that you consult with a health professional of your choice, and that you do your own research if you suspect you have a nutrient deficiency or imbalance.

I mainly list plant sources because those nutrients tend to be more bio-available, and a predominantly plant-based diet is more environmentally friendly; that's a win-win. Yet not all nutrients are available in plant foods, so for those I list animal-based sources. If you choose a strictly vegetarian or vegan diet, you can substitute these options with non-synthetic supplements.

Eye-essential nutrients and some of their best food sources

Beta Carotene (which converts into vitamin A)	Dark leafy greens (kale, turnip greens, mustard greens, spinach, dandelion greens, collard), sweet potatoes, carrots, goji berries, paprika, red pepper, chili peppers, butternut squash, lettuce, apricots, cantaloupe melon, parsley, basil
Vitamin A Retinol	(The body synthesizes vitamin A from carotenoids such as beta carotene.) Liver, egg yolk, fermented cod liver oil, butter from grass-fed cows
Vitamin B-1 Thiamin	Spinach, seeds (sunflower, flax, sesame, poppy, mustard), navy beans, black beans, soybeans, peas, lentils, barley, oats, asparagus, cremini mushrooms, Brussels sprouts, nuts (pine, pistachio, macadamia, pecan, hazelnuts)
Vitamin B-2 Riboflavin	Spinach, almonds, sesame seeds, sun-dried tomatoes, cremini mushrooms, asparagus, soybeans, grains, chili peppers, paprika, coriander, spearmint
Vitamin B-3 Niacin	Peanuts, mushrooms, green peas, sunflower seeds, avocados, paprika, sea vegetables, chia seeds, sprouted beans, soybeans, almonds
Vitamin B-5 Pantothenic Acid	Mushrooms, avocados, sunflower seeds, sweet potatoes
Vitamin B-6 Pyridoxine	Sunflower seeds, pistachios, prunes, raisins, avocados, spinach, banana, sweet potatoes, sesame seeds, chili peppers, paprika, garlic, hazelnuts/filberts, peanuts, pine nuts, walnuts, kidney beans, brown rice, soybeans, oats, wheat
Vitamin B-7 Biotin	Almonds, pecans, peanuts, walnuts, sunflower seeds, green peas, lentils, split peas, cauliflower, bananas, avocados, green leafy vegetables (spinach, kale), raspberries, carrots, tomatoes, mushrooms

Vitamin B-9 Folate	Chickpeas, lentils, soybeans, spinach, asparagus, lettuce, avocados, peanuts, broccoli, mangoes, papayas, pomegranates, guava, kiwi, bananas, oranges
Vitamin B-12 Cobalamin	Clams, liver, trout, salmon, tuna, crab, beef, eggs
Vitamin C Ascorbic acid	Hot chili peppers, sweet bell peppers, guava, kiwi, oranges, tangerines, strawberries, papayas, mangoes, broccoli, kale, mustard greens, garden cress, cauliflower, Brussels sprouts, thyme, parsley
Vitamin D-2 Ergocalciferol Vitamin D-3 Cholecalciferol	D-2: Maitake mushrooms (D-2 is not as easily absorbed by the body as D-3; you require 4 times the amount of D-2 to make the equivalent of 1 unit of D-3) D-3: Sunlight exposure on bare skin without sunscreen for 10-30 minutes daily D-3: Salmon, mackerel, swordfish, tuna, herring, cod liver oil, whale, egg yolk **Note**: Vitamin D from sunlight (UVB radiation) is far superior to vitamin D from food sources,[1] and vitamin D supplements are not an effective substitute for adequate sun exposure.[2]
Vitamin E (group)	Almonds, spinach, beet greens, peanuts, pumpkin, collard, muskmelons, sunflower seeds, paprika, tomatoes, red chili peppers, pine nuts, asparagus
Vitamin K (group)	Basil, kale, spinach, mustard greens, collard, beet greens, parsley, chard, turnip greens, dandelion greens, broccoli, spring onions, garden cress, endive, radicchio, lettuce, celery, Brussels sprouts, cabbage, bok choi, asparagus, leeks
Alpha Lipoic Acid	Spinach, broccoli, tomatoes, green peas, Brussels sprouts, rice bran
Bioflavonoids	Sweet bell pepper, strawberries, citrus fruit, broccoli, Brussels sprouts, garlic, mangoes, papayas, spinach, green tea, cacao (unsweetened), apples
Calcium	Watercress, collard, kale, spinach, dandelion greens, turnip greens, arugula, beet greens, okra, bok choi, almonds, soybeans, black-eyed peas, acorn squash
Choline	Shiitake mushrooms, lentils, fava beans, split peas, chickpeas, mustard seeds, flax seeds, coriander, parsley, peanuts, cashews
Chromium	Broccoli, sweet potatoes, corn, oats, green beans
Copper	Kale, mushrooms, avocados, nuts (cashews, hazelnuts, Brazil, walnuts, pine, pistachios, pecans, almonds, peanuts), seeds (sesame, sunflower, pumpkin, squash, flax), chickpeas, soybeans, prunes, apricots, currants, figs
CoQ10	Peanuts, pistachios, walnuts, sesame seeds, hazelnuts, almonds, green beans, spinach, parsley, avocados, broccoli, cauliflower, olives
Enzymes	Papayas, apricots, avocados, banana, pineapple, mangoes, kiwi, grapes (Enzymes are destroyed in cooking, so eat plenty of fresh foods and chew well to let your saliva enzymes do their work.)
Essential Amino Acids	All foods contain amino acids; they are the building blocks of protein. Some amino acids are considered to be essential, as we don't make them in the body.
- Leucine	Pumpkin seeds, peanuts, beans (white, pinto, kidney, yellow, navy, pink, black)
- Isoleucine	Spirulina, watercress, chard, bok choi, spinach, kidney beans, alfalfa sprouts, sunflower seeds, sesame seeds
- Lysine	Beans (white, yellow, pinto, kidney, black, chickpeas, lima, navy, lentils), peas, seeds, pistachios, pine nuts, cashews, peanuts, walnuts, almonds

- Methionine	Brazil nuts, walnuts, pistachios, pine nuts, cashews, beans (white, roman, pink, black, pinto, kidney), seeds (sesame, pumpkin, chia, sunflower, flax)
- Phenylalanine	Seeds (pumpkin, sunflower) peanuts, almonds, pistachios, beans (pinto, white, adzuki, kidney, roman, mung, black, chickpeas, lentils)
- Threonine	Beans (roman, yellow, kidney, black, pink, white, chickpeas, lentils), seeds (pumpkin, sunflower, sesame, flax, chia), pistachios, cashews, almonds
- Tryptophan	Seeds (pumpkin, squash, chia, sesame, sunflower), oats, buckwheat
- Valine	Pumpkin seeds, beans (navy, kidney, adzuki, roman, yellow, black, chickpeas), Portobello mushrooms, white mushrooms, wild rice
- Histidine	Beans (roman, yellow, kidney, pink, black, pinto, chickpeas, lentils), seeds (pumpkin, sunflower), peanuts, quinoa, wild rice
- Cysteine	Seeds (sunflower, sesame, chia, pumpkin), nuts (pistachios, Brazil, pine), oats, split peas, chickpeas, white beans, lentils
Essential Fatty Acids (EFAs)	We synthesize most of the fats we need in the body, however, there are two that must be obtained from food and are therefore essential fatty acids. Alpha linolenic acid is made into omega-3 fats while linoleic acid becomes omega-6 fats. They need to be taken in appropriate ratios for best results.
- Alpha Linolenic Acid	Seeds (camelina, flax, perilla, chia, hemp, pumpkin, mustard), soybeans, walnuts, pecans
- Linolenic Acid	Green leafy vegetables, flax seeds, grains, nuts
Gamma-amino butyric acid	Nuts, almonds, bananas, broccoli, brown rice, lentils, oats, oranges, spinach, fermented foods (unpasteurized sauerkraut, kefir)
Glucosamine	The body makes glucosamine using glucose and an amino acid called glutamine. Glutamine is found in raw parsley and spinach.
Glutathione	Asparagus, avocados, spinach, broccoli, potatoes, squash, cauliflower, walnuts, peppers, carrots, onion, garlic, tomatoes, grapefruit, peaches, oranges, melons
Inositol	Grapefruit, oranges, cantaloupe, cabbage, peaches, pears, bananas, bell peppers, tomatoes, potatoes, asparagus, green leafy vegetables, nuts, seeds
Iodine	Sea vegetables, cranberries, navy beans, strawberries, potatoes, prunes, bananas, green beans, pineapple, rhubarb
Iron	Spinach, chard, squash, pumpkin seeds, beans, lentils, pomegranates, sun-dried tomatoes, sesame seeds, cashews, pine nuts, hazelnuts, almonds, chestnuts
Lutein & Zeaxanthin	Dark leafy greens (kale, spinach, collard, parsley, salad greens), summer squash, broccoli, Brussels sprouts, asparagus, green peas, leeks, green beans
Lycopene	Guava, watermelon, tomato, papaya, grapefruit, sweet red peppers, asparagus, purple cabbage, mangoes, carrots
Magnesium	Nuts (almond, cashew, hazelnuts, peanuts, walnuts, pecan, pine), seeds (flax, pumpkin, sesame), spinach, chard, kale, collard, turnip greens, beans (white, black, lima, kidney, navy, green, soy, lentils)
Manganese	Nuts (hazelnuts, pine, pecan, walnuts, macadamia, almonds, cashew, pistachio, chestnuts), coconut, pineapple, seeds (pumpkin, chia, sesame, flax, sunflower), beans (soy, lima, adzuki, white, kidney, chickpeas), spinach, chard

Molybdenum	Beans (lentils, lima, kidney, black, pinto, chickpeas), peas, barley, oats, almonds, cashews, chestnuts, green leafy vegetables
PABA	Whole grains, rice, eggs. The body also makes its own by intestinal bacteria.
Phosphorus	Seeds (pumpkin, sunflower, chia, sesame, watermelon, flax), nuts (Brazil, pine, almonds, cashews, pistachios), beans, lentils
Potassium	Avocados, guavas, bananas, passion fruit, kiwi, persimmons, cantaloupe, apricots, pomegranates, figs, beans, lentils, potatoes, acorn squash, spinach
Quercetin	Lovage leaves, dock leaves, hot peppers, apples, onions (red, yellow), kale, okra, elderberries, cranberries, goji berries, carob, radicchio, asparagus
Rutin	Buckwheat, asparagus, apples (unpeeled), figs, citrus fruits, peaches, apricots
Selenium	Brazil nuts, walnuts, sunflower seeds, flax seeds, oats, legumes
Taurine	Sea vegetables, fish, meat, eggs
Vanadium	Parsley, dill, black pepper, buckwheat, oats, corn, green beans, carrots, cabbage, garlic, tomatoes, radishes, onions, lentils, navy beans
Zinc	Seeds (sesame, pumpkin, squash, watermelon, flax, hemp), beans (kidney, soy, lima, lentils, chickpeas), green peas, oats, wild rice, spinach, nuts (cashews, almonds, pine, pecans, walnuts, peanuts)

Appendix H

Medicines That Can Affect Vision

Medicine	Possible effects on vision
Alpha-blockers (for high blood pressure and enlarged prostate): Alfuzosin (Uroxatral and generic) and Tamsulosin (Flomax and generic)	Blurred vision and eye pain; may affect cataract surgery
Antibiotics: Ciprofloxacin (Cipro and generic)	Double vision
Atropine eye drops	Blurred near vision; itching, red, swollen or watery eyes; pink eye; conjunctivitis; increased light sensitivity; increased intraocular pressure (glaucoma)
Cholesterol drugs: Atorvastatin (Lipitor and generic), Lovastatin (Mevacor and generic), simvastatin (Zocor and generic)	Double vision; cataracts
Corticosteroids (for allergies and autoimmune disorders): Prednisone	Cataracts; eye infection; glaucoma (with prolonged use); possible permanent optic-nerve damage
Erectile dysfunction drugs: Sildenafil (Viagra), Tadalafil (Cialis), Vardenafil (Levitra)	Bluish tinted vision; blurred vision; light sensitivity
Osteoporosis drugs: Alendronate (Fosamax and generic), Risedronate (Actonel and generic)	Blurred vision; conjunctivitis; light sensitivity
Various medications used for depression, Parkinson's disease, seizures, ulcers, asthma, arrhythmia, and hemorrhoids	Acute angle-closure glaucoma (a rapid or sudden increase in intraocular pressure)
Steroids	80% Increased risk of cataracts

Charts

The following charts are included for you to practice the relaxation techniques:
- A large practice chart can be downloaded for free from the Optimal Eyesight website[1]
- Medium practice chart, page 279
- Small practice chart and far point measurement chart, page 281
- Optimal Eyesight card, page 283
- Astigmatism chart, page 285

Letter height and font size of the lines on the practice charts are provided below, so if you like, you can make your own charts with words that are easy to remember for you.

Someone with good vision can read the 20 line from 20 feet, but many people can do even better and read the 15 or 10 line from 20 feet.

Letter chart font sizes
(rounded to half and whole font sizes)

Line on chart (feet)	Letter height (inches)	Letter height (mm)	Arial Bold font size	Line on chart (meters)	Letter height (mm)	Arial Bold font size
200	3.49	88.7	355	60	87.3	349
150	2.62	66.5	266	50	72.7	291
100	1.75	44.3	177	40	58.2	233
80	1.4	35.5	142	30	43.6	174
60	1.05	26.6	106	20	29.1	116
50	0.87	22.2	89	18	26.2	105
40	0.7	17.7	71	15	21.8	87
30	0.52	13.3	53	12	17.5	70
25	0.44	11.1	44.5	10	14.5	58
20	0.35	8.9	35.5	8	11.6	46
15	0.26	6.6	26.5	6	8.7	35
10	0.17	4.4	17.5	5	7.3	29
7	0.12	3.1	12.5	4	5.8	23
5	0.09	2.2	9	3	4.4	17.5
4	0.07	1.8	7	2	2.9	11.5
3	0.05	1.3	5.5	1	1.5	6
2	0.035	0.9	4	0.5	0.7	3
1	0.02	0.4	2	0.35	0.5	2

Medium Practice Chart

FT

B

. ■

L I
60

. ■

40

. ■
N K O
30

. ■
F T E N
25

. ■
R E C E I
20

. ■
V E L I G H T
15

. ·
O P E N P E R I
10

. ·
P H E R Y E N J O Y
7

. ·
S M A L L D E T A I L S
5

. ·
© 2019 VISIONS OF JOY • OPTIMAL EYESIGHT PRACTICE CHART.
3

Optimal Eyesight
Medium Practice Chart
by Esther Joy van der Werf
www.optimaleyesight.com

Small Practice Chart

Far Point Measurement Chart

	FT
B	20
L I	15
N K O	10
F T E N	7
R E C E I	5
V E L I G H T	4
O P E N P E R I	3
P H E R Y E N J O Y	2
S M A L L D E T A I L S	1

© 2019 VISIONS OF JOY • OPTIMAL EYESIGHT PRACTICE CHART FOR NEAR VISION.

	CM
B	600
L I	450
N K O	300
F T E N	200
R E C E I	150
V E L I G H T	100
O P E N P E R I	75
P H E R Y E N J O Y	50
S M A L L D E T A I L S	35

© 2019 VISIONS OF JOY • FAR POINT MEASUREMENT CHART.

Optimal Eyesight
Far Point Measurement Chart
by Esther Joy van der Werf
www.optimaleyesight.com

Numbers on the right side represent distance in centimeters from where someone with good vision can read that line.

Optimal Eyesight
Small Practice Chart
by Esther Joy van der Werf
www.optimaleyesight.com

Numbers on the right side represent distance in feet from where someone with good vision can read that line.

Optimal Eyesight

by Esther Joy van der Werf ~ www.optimaleyesight.com

1. Use lower diopter glasses, and only when absolutely necessary.

2. **Blink** frequently and effortlessly. Blinking cleanses, lubricates and rests the eyes while giving them the opportunity to refocus.

3. **Central clarity** is seeing best where you are looking and allowing the eyes to continually **shift** to the next point of attention. Remain aware of peripheral vision, which is not seen as clearly as the small "crystal ball" of central vision.

4. **Close your eyes** whenever they are tired. When palming the eyes, feel any muscle strain disappear easily from your eyelids, eyes, face and neck; then imagine already seeing clearly at any distance, effortlessly.

5. **Sunshine** on closed eyelids will help build light tolerance and reduces dependency on sunglasses. Regular sunning is excellent for vision and health. Enjoy time outside each day.

6. Allow your head to **move** along with your eyes. A tall and balanced **posture** will aid this movement and will help release neck tension.

7. **Think positive**. Look for solutions and focus on the bright side of life. A happy mind creates happy eyes.

8. Practice **reading** small print, using all the good vision habits. Follow the thin bright white line right underneath the letters. This reduces strain and relaxes the eyes. Vary the reading distance and look up regularly to briefly focus afar.

9. Improve natural abdominal **breathing** by learning to gently extend the exhale. **Relaxation** is the key to both breathing and vision.

10. Forget about your eyes; **receive** images easily by letting your brain do the seeing. You can now let go of old habits of staring, squinting or trying to see.

11. Notice **apparent motion**. Due to continual shifting of the eyes, stationary objects appear to be moving. Imagine that you see this gentle swinging motion all day long.

12. Improving the **memory** of letters or other objects improves the vision for everything. Let your **imagination** provide even more details and clarity.

13. Gently **massage** around the eyes to stimulate acupressure points. This also improves circulation.

14. The best foods for your eyes are **green leafy vegetables**. Enjoy a salad or green smoothie daily.

Optimal Eyesight
Reading Practice Card
by Esther Joy van der Werf
www.optimaleyesight.com

Font sizes range from 16 at the top to 3 at the bottom.

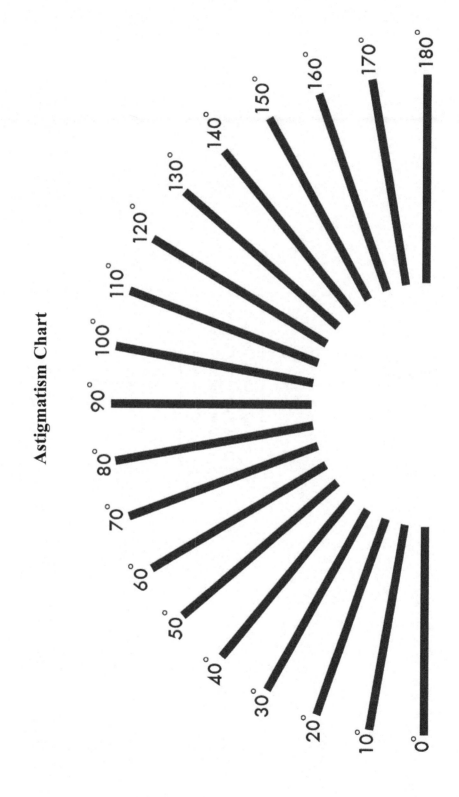

Astigmatism Chart

Optimal Eyesight
Astigmatism Chart
by Esther Joy van der Werf
www.optimaleyesight.com

Glossary

Accommodation: The automatic adjustment of the eye for focusing at different distances.

Amblyopia: Reduced vision in one eye that results from the brain suppressing input from the affected eye due to unequal visual signals from each eye (as in strabismus or anisometropia). Also termed lazy eye.

Anisometropia: A condition in which the two eyes have unequal refractive power.

Astigmatism: An irregularly shaped eye, lens or cornea, causing rays from a point to fail to meet in a focal point on the retina, resulting in a blurred and imperfect image.

Axial Length: The distance between the front of the cornea and the retina, measured in millimeters, which at birth tends to be approximately 17 mm, while for an adult human eye it's typically about 24 mm. It is often longer than 24 mm in myopic eyes and shorter than 24 mm in hyperopic eyes. Each millimeter of change in axial length of the human eye corresponds to approximately 2.50 diopters.

Central Fixation: "By 'central fixation' is meant a passive, receptive, or relaxed condition of the eyes and brain. When the mind is sufficiently at rest, the eye sees best the point fixed – in other words, the eye sees best what it is looking at." (Dr. Bates)[1]

Cornea: The transparent outer layer of the eyeball at the front; the area that covers the iris and pupil.

Ciliary Muscle: A circular muscle situated in the ciliary body and connected to the lens by zonular fibers (suspensory ligament). When the ciliary muscle contracts it relaxes the zonular fibers so that the lens is permitted to become more rounded for near vision. When it relaxes, the fibers are pulled taut and the lens flattens for distance vision.

Circadian Rhythm: The 24-hour cycle set by the sun, also known as your body clock. Solar rays trigger ganglion cells behind the rods and cones in the retina and thus influence various biological processes, such as sleep, wakefulness, and digestive activity. A chronic lack of exposure to natural light during the day, or an over-exposure to bright or predominantly blue light at night can disrupt this cycle, which can lead to sleep disorders and health issues.

Diopter: A unit of measurement of the refractive power of a lens; it relates to the capacity of the lens to bend rays of light. See Appendix B.

Eccentric Fixation: "By eccentric fixation is meant the ability of the eye partially or completely to suppress the vision of the center of the fovea and to see best with other parts of the retina." (Dr. Bates)[2]

Extraocular muscle: Any of the six muscles attached to the outside of the eye which control the movement of the eye within the eye socket.

Hyperopia/Hypermetropia/Farsightedness/Long Sight: A condition in which visual images come to a focus behind the retina of the eye and vision is better for distant than for near objects.

Iris: The opaque-colored diaphragm visible at the front of the eye with the pupil at its center.

Lazy Eye: See Amblyopia

Legal Blindness: Blindness as recognized by law, which in most states of the U.S. means that the better eye, using the best possible methods of correction, has a visual acuity of 20/200 or worse, or that the visual field is restricted to 20 degrees or less.

Minus Lens/Concave Lens: A lens that is ground thinner in the center to improve focus for people with myopia.

Motion Blur: When eyes are in non-stop motion, images received will have motion blur, resulting in an inability to resolve details. To avoid this, the eyes alternate between saccades (quick eye movements) and fixation (very briefly focusing on a single point).

Myopia/Nearsightedness/Short Sight: A condition in which the visual images come to a focus in front of the retina of the eye and vision is better for near than for distant objects.

Night Blindness: Difficulty seeing in low light or a slow adaptation to low light.

Optic Nerve: A cranial nerve that connects the retina at the back of each eye to the visual cortex in the back of the brain.

Phoropter: An instrument used by eye doctors to evaluate a person's refractive error. The unit has a variety of lenses placed on dials which are positioned in front of the eyes.

Prescription: A written formula for the grinding of compensating lenses for glasses and contacts. Often abbreviated to Rx.

Presbyopia/Middle Age Farsightedness: A visual condition which generally becomes apparent in middle age and which manifests in defective accommodation and inability to focus sharply for near vision.

Plus Lens/Convex Lens: A lens that is ground thinner at the edges to improve focus for people with hyperopia or presbyopia.

Refractive Error: An inability of the eye to focus accurately. Nearsightedness, farsightedness, presbyopia and astigmatism are examples of refractive errors.

Retina: The sensory membrane that lines the back of the eye. It's composed of several layers, including one containing the rods and cones (our light-receptor cells), which are triggered by light coming through the lens. This layer then converts that stimulus into chemical and nervous signals that reach the brain by way of the optic nerve.

Saccadic Motion/Saccades: Small, rapid, jerky movements of the eye, especially as it jumps from one fixation point to another.

Sclera: The white, opaque outer layer of the eye.

Strabismus: Inability of one eye to align with the other due to imbalanced tension of its extraocular muscles. Strabismus can be intermittent and can alternate between the eyes. Cross-eyes and wall-eye are forms of strabismus.

Visual Acuity: The ability of the eyes to distinguish one detail from another relative to distance and size.

Visual Angle: The visual angle of an object is the angle formed by two imaginary lines projecting from the eye to the top and bottom (or left and right sides) of an object. Visual angles are used to indicate the size of the retinal image of the object – the larger the visual angle, the larger the retinal image. The visual angle is influenced by the size of the object and the distance of the object from the eye. The larger the object is, or the closer it is to the observer, the larger its visual angle will be. Visual angle is usually reported in degrees, minutes and seconds of the subtended angle. One minute of arc is 1/60th of one degree of arc.

Vitreous Humor: The transparent jelly-like fluid that fills the eyeball behind the lens. Also known as Vitreous Body.

Resources

Website links: For a list of links to the various internet pages listed in this book, please visit www.optimaleyesight.com.

Classes: I offer a variety of classes on eyesight improvement: private lessons and group classes, lessons via Skype, an email course and a video course, as well as teacher training seminars. Details are on my website at www.visionsofjoy.org.

Books: Various compilations of the best of Dr. Bates' writings have been published by Visions of Joy. These books are useful to anyone who is going through the process of improving vision naturally. All are available at www.visionsofjoy.org.

Paperback and E-book:
- *Read Without Glasses at Any Age: The Natural Method to Near Vision Clarity.*
- *Bates Method Nuggets: The Fundamentals of Natural Vision Improvement by William H. Bates, M.D.* Compiled by Esther Joy van der Werf.

E-books:
- *Better Eyesight: The original magazines as published by Dr. William H. Bates.* Compiled by Esther Joy van der Werf. The complete, unedited and searchable collection of all 132 of Dr. Bates' monthly magazines: July 1919 to June 1930.
- *Medical Articles by William H. Bates, M.D.* The complete collection of thirty medical articles written by Dr. Bates and published in various medical journals from 1886 to 1923.
- *The Bates Method View series.* E-books in this series are collections of Dr. Bates' writings on specific vision challenges. Each e-book also includes a summary of the methods used by Dr. Bates in overcoming that challenge. All are compiled by Esther Joy van der Werf.
  - *The Bates Method View of Cataracts*
  - *The Bates Method View of Conical Cornea*
  - *The Bates Method View of Floating Specks*
  - *The Bates Method View of Glaucoma*
  - *The Bates Method View of Nystagmus*
  - *The Bates Method View of Presbyopia*
  - *The Bates Method View of Retinitis Pigmentosa*
  - *The Bates Method View of Strabismus / Squint*
  - *The Bates Method View of Eye Education in our Schools*

References

Who this Book is For and How to Use It
1. A list of vision educators world-wide: Follow the link at optimaleyesight.com
2. Van der Werf, E. J. (2013). *Read Without Glasses at Any Age: The Natural Method to Near Vision Clarity*. Ojai, CA: Visions of Joy.

Preface
1. Atchison, D. A., Fisher, S. W., Pedersen, C. A. and Ridall, P. G. (2005). Noticeable, troublesome and objectionable limits of blur. *Vision Research*, 45(15), 1967-1974. "Optometrists are familiar with comments from patients that vision seems to improve after a period of time without refractive corrections."
2. Collection of Dr. Bates' 30 medical articles (1886-1923): Follow the link at optimaleyesight.com
3. Bates, W. H. (1918). *Better Eyesight Without Glasses*, NY: Henry Holt & Co. Inc.
4. MacFadden, B. & Bates, W. H. (1918). *Strengthening the Eyes – A New Course in Scientific Eye Training in 28 Lessons*. New York: Physical Culture Publishing Company.
5. Bates, W. H. (1919-1930). *Better Eyesight*, New York, NY: Central Fixation Publishing Company.
6. Bates, W. H. (1920). *The Cure of Imperfect Sight by Treatment without Glasses*. New York: Central Fixation Publishing. (Also known as: *Perfect Sight Without Glasses*)
7. Bates, W. H. (1923). Common Sense. *Better Eyesight*, June
8. Bates, W. H. (1940). *The Cure of Imperfect Sight by Treatment without Glasses*. New York: Burr.
9. Corbett, M. (1938). *How to Improve Your Eyes*. Los Angeles, CA: Willing Pub. Co.
10. Corbett, M. (1949). *Help Yourself to Better Sight*. New York: Prentice-Hall.
11. Corbett, M. (1957). *A Quick Guide to Better Vision*. Englewood Cliffs, NJ: Prentice-Hall.

Introduction
1. Quackenbush, T. R. (1997). *Relearning to See*, Berkeley, CA: Frog.
2. Quackenbush, T. R. (2001). *Better Eyesight, The Complete Magazines of William H. Bates*. Berkeley, CA, North Atlantic Books.
3. Proust, M., Scott-Moncrieff, C. K., Kilmartin, T., & Enright, D. J. (2005). *In Search of lost Time*. London: Vintage Books.

1. Your Eyes are Not Weak
1. North American Association of Vision Educators. http://naturalvisionteachers.com
2. Barry, S. R. (2009). *Fixing my Gaze*, New York, NY: Basic Books.
3. Horton, R. (2015). Offline: What is medicine's 5 sigma? *The Lancet, 385*(9976), 1380. doi:10.1016/S0140-6736(15)60696-1
4. Relman, A. S., Angell, M. (2002, December 16). America's other drug problem: how the drug industry distorts medicine and politics. *New Republic*. Retrieved from: https://facultystaff.richmond.edu/~bmayes/pdf/relmanangell_Rxdrugs.pdf
5. Ioannidis, J. P. A. (2005). Why Most Published Research Findings Are False, *PLoS Medicine, 2*(8). doi:10.1371/journal.pmed.0020124
6. Walia, A. (2015, December 11). Neuroscientist shows what fasting does to your brain & why big pharma won't study it. Retrieved from: https://www.collective-evolution.com/2015/12/11/neuroscientist-shows-what-fasting-does-to-your-brain-why-big-pharma-wont-study-it/

2. The Old View Turns a Blind Eye

1. French, A. N., Ashby, R. S., Morgan, I. G., & Rose, K. A. (2013). Time outdoors and the prevention of myopia, *Experimental Eye Research 114*, 58-68. doi:10.1016/j.exer.2013.04.018
2. Fleiszig, S. M. J., Evans, D. J. (2010). The Pathogenesis of Contact Lens-Associated Microbial Keratitis. *Optometry and Vision Science 87* (4) 225–232. doi:10.1097/OPX.0b013e3181d408ee
3. Zuckerman, D. M., Brown, P., & Nissen, S. E. (2011). Medical Device Recalls and the FDA Approval Process. *Archives of Internal Medicine, 171*(11). doi:10.1001/archinternmed.2011.30
4. Eydelman, M., Hilmantel, G., Tarver, M. E., Hofmeister, E. M., May, J., Hammel, K., Ferris, F. (2017). Symptoms and Satisfaction of Patients in the Patient-Reported Outcomes with Laser In Situ Keratomileusis (PROWL) Studies. *JAMA Ophthalmology, 135*(1), 13. doi:10.1001/jamaophthalmol.2016.4587
5. Information on laser surgery: Follow the link at optimaleyesight.com
6. MedicineNet, (no date). *Phakic Intraocular Lenses.* Retrieved from: https://www.medicinenet.com/phakic_intraocular_lenses/article.htm#what_you_should_know_and_do_before_during_and_after_surgery
7. Walline, J. J., Greiner, K. L., McVey, M. E., & Jones-Jordan, L. A. (2013). Multifocal Contact Lens Myopia Control. *Optometry and Vision Science, 90*(11), 1207-1214. doi:10.1097/opx.0000000000000036
8. Brooks Simpkins, R. (1958). *New Light on the Eyes*, Stuart, 77

3. Insights into the Root Cause of Blur

1. Young, F. A., Leary, G. A., Baldwin, W. R., West, D. C., Box, R. A., Harris, E., & Johnson, C. (1969). The Transmission of Refractive Errors Within Eskimo Families. *Optometry and Vision Science, 46*(9), 676-685. doi:10.1097/00006324-196909000-00005
2. Jones, L. A., Sinnott, L. T., Mutti, D. O., Mitchell, G. L., Moeschberger, M. L., & Zadnik, K. (2007). Parental History of Myopia, Sports and Outdoor Activities, and Future Myopia. *Investigative Ophthalmology & Visual Science 48*(8) 3524-3532. doi:10.1167/iovs.06-1118
3. Rose, K. A., Morgan, I. G., Ip, J., Kifley, A., Huynh, S., Smith, W., & Mitchell, P. (2008). Outdoor Activity Reduces the Prevalence of Myopia in Children. *Ophthalmology, 115*(8), 1279-1285. doi:10.1016/j.ophtha.2007.12.019
4. Bates, W. H. (1926). Eyestrain. *Better Eyesight*, February

4. What Eyestrain Does to Your Sight

1. Brooks, M. & Reiner, C., (1967). *The 2000 Year Old Man in the Year 2000.* [video].
2. Bates, W.H., (1920). Chapter X, Strain. *Perfect Sight Without Glasses,* 106
3. Bates, W. H. (1927). Fundamental Facts. *Better Eyesight*, April

5. What's Good About Blur?

1. Vasudevan, B., Esposito, C., Peterson, C., Coronado, C., & Ciuffreda, K. J. (2014). Under-correction of human myopia – Is it myopigenic?: A retrospective analysis of clinical refraction data. *Journal of Optometry, 7*(3), 147-152. doi:10.1016/j.optom.2013.12.007
2. List of behavioral optometrists: Follow the link at optimaleyesight.com
3. Affordable glasses online: Follow the link at optimaleyesight.com
4. EyeQue Corporation. (n.d.). Retrieved from http://www.eyeque.com/
5. Pinhole glasses: Follow the link at optimaleyesight.com

6. You May Close Your Eyes

1. Bates, W. H. (1919). The Effect of Light Upon the Eyes. *Better Eyesight*, November
2. Nightingale, F. (1909). *Notes on Nursing: What It Is, and What It Is Not.* London: Harrison.
3. Palming support and meditation: Follow the link at optimaleyesight.com
4. Body Slant mattress: Follow the link at optimaleyesight.com

5. Kiesling, D. https://www.iblindness.org
6. Mindfold: Follow the link at optimaleyesight.com
7. Bates, W. H. (1920). Palming. *Perfect Sight Without Glasses*, Chapter XII, 134-135

7. To Blink or Not to Blink

1. Caine, M. (1992). *What's it all about?: An autobiography*. New York: Turtle Bay Books.
2. Bates, W. H. (1926). Eyestrain. *Better Eyesight*, February
3. *Seven Signs That You Are Being Lied To*. Retrieved from http://www.contactomagazine.com/articles/liarsigns0808.htm#.V6IewrgrL4Y
4. Leal, S., & Vrij, A. (2008). Blinking During and After Lying. *Journal of Nonverbal Behavior, 32*(4), 187-194. doi:10.1007/s10919-008-0051-0
5. Martinez, V. (2015, January 24). How To Read Someone's Eyes, According To Science. Retrieved from https://www.medicaldaily.com/lying-eyes-or-something-else-how-blink-rate-pupil-dilation-give-insight-honesty-and-319164
6. Mann, S., Vrij, A., & Bull, R. (2002). Suspects, lies, and videotape: An analysis of authentic high-stake liars. *Law and Human Behavior, 26*(3), 365-376. doi:10.1023/a:1015332606792
7. *Just the Bat of an Eye*. (n.d.). Retrieved from https://www.psychologytoday.com/us/blog/let-their-words-do-the-talking/201405/just-the-bat-eye
8. Hurty, K. E. (1923). Teachers Question Dr. Bates. *Better Eyesight*, May
9. Bates, W. H. (1924). Blinking and Resting the Eyes. *Better Eyesight*, March
10. Doughty, M. J. (2001). Consideration of Three Types of Spontaneous Eyeblink Activity in Normal Humans: During Reading and Video Display Terminal Use, in Primary Gaze, and while in Conversation. *Optometry and Vision Science, 78*(10), 712-725. doi:10.1097/00006324-200110000-00011
11. Bacher, L. F., & Allen, K. J. (2008). Sensitivity of the rate of spontaneous eye blinking to type of stimuli in young infants. *Wiley InterScience, 51*(2), 186-197. doi:10.1002/dev.20357
12. Lee, J. (2009). OD shares drug-free approach to treating meibomian gland dysfunction. *Primary Care Optometry News,* November. Retrieved from https://www.healio.com/optometry/cornea-external-disease/news/print/primary-care-optometry-news/{f72f71ed-ec25-421a-8731-97cdafd0766c}/od-shares-drug-free-approach-to-treating-meibomian-gland-dysfunction
13. Bates, E. (1929). Amblyopia. *Better Eyesight*, November

8. The Surprising Reality About Clarity

1. Bates, W. H. (1917). Blindness relieved by a new method of treatment. *New York Medical Journal, 105*(5) 200-202.
2. Liberman, J. (1995). *Take Off Your Glasses and See: How to heal your eyesight and expand your insight*. New York: Crown, Chapter 4
3. Rūmī, J. A., & Barks, C. (2004). *The Essential Rumi: New expanded edition*. San Francisco, CA: Harper.
4. Jonas, J. B., Schneider, U., & Naumann, G. O. (1992). Count and density of human retinal photoreceptors. *Graefes Archive for Clinical and Experimental Ophthalmology, 230*(6), 505-510. doi:10.1007/bf00181769
5. Curcio, C. A., & Allen, K. A. (1990). Topography of ganglion cells in human retina. *The Journal of Comparative Neurology, 300*(1), 5-25. doi:10.1002/cne.903000103
6. Bates, W. H. (1927). Central Fixation. *Better Eyesight*, February
7. Bates, W. H. (1919). The Menace of Large Print. *Better Eyesight*, December
8. Liberman (1995).
9. Wide Angle Vision as taught by Tom Brown, Jr. in classes taken by the author at "Tracker School" in 1998. www.trackerschool.com

10. Courtois, F. (1986). *An Experience of Enlightenment.* Wheaton, IL: Theosophical Pub. House.

9. Set Your Eyes Free
1. Yarbus, A. L. (1967). *Eye Movements and Vision.* New York: Plenum Press.
2. Goodrich, J. (1987). *Natural Vision Improvement.* Newton Abbot, U.K.: Brunel House, 50
3. Corbett, M. (1938). *How to Improve Your Eyes*, 39

10. Getting into the Swing of Things
1. Bates, W. H. (1921). Fundamentals of Treatment – Shifting an Swinging. *Better Eyesight,* June
2. Bates, W. H. (1925). Swaying. *Better Eyesight,* July
3. Bates, W. H. (1927). Demonstrate. *Better Eyesight,* January
4. Bates, W. H. (1924). Swinging. *Better Eyesight,* March

11. Think Right for Your Sight
1. Bates, W. H. (1920). Presbyopia, Its Cause and Cure. *Perfect Sight Without Glasses,* 217
2. Bates, W. H. (1922). Reading without Glasses. *Better Eyesight,* February
3. Bates, W. H. (1920). Mental Strain Reflected in the Eye. *Perfect Sight Without Glasses,* 109
4. Corbett, M. (1938). *How to Improve Your Eyes,* 26
5. Lichtman, R. M. (2010). Myopia as an Adaptation. Follow the link at optimaleyesight.com
6. Stanton, L. M. (1927). Temperamental Strain. *Better Eyesight,* January
7. Bates, W. H. (1920). As Quick as Thought. *Perfect Sight Without Glasses,* 113
8. Bates, W. H. (1919). The Doctor's Story. *Better Eyesight,* September
9. Bates, W. H. (1925). Mental Strain. *Better Eyesight,* January
10. Bates, W. H. (1923). A study of imagination. *Reprints*
11. Bates, W. H. (1919). Memory as an aid to vision. *New York Medical Journal, 109*(21) 890-893
12. Bates, W. H. (1928). The Period. *Better Eyesight,* March
13. Bates, W. H. (1919). Memory as an aid to vision.
14. Bates, W. H. (1926). Memory. *Better Eyesight,* February
15. Bates, W. H. (1929). Mental Pictures. *Better Eyesight,* July
16. Bates, W. H. (1922). The Truth about Fatigue. *Better Eyesight,* March
17. Bates, W. H. (1929). Treatment. *Better Eyesight,* July
18. Langer, E., Djikic, M., Pirson, M., Madenci, A., & Donohue, R. (2010). Believing Is Seeing. *Psychological Science, 21*(5), 661-666. doi:10.1177/0956797610366543
19. Twain, M. (n.d.). *A Connecticut Yankee in King Arthur's Court.*
20. Berk, J. (1981). *The Down Comforter: How to beat depression and pull yourself out of the blues.* New York: Avon Books, 209
21. Lipton, B. (2005). *The Biology of Belief: Unleashing the power of consciousness, matter and miracles.* Mountain of Love/Elite books.
22. Lipton, B. (2016). *Mind Over Genes: The New Biology.* Retrieved from https://vimeo.com/146714061
23. Bates, W. H. (1923). A Talk to the League. *Better Eyesight,* September

12. Looking at Posture, Sleep and Massage
1. Forrest, E. B. (1988). *Stress and Vision.* Santa Ana, CA: Optometric Extension Program Foundation, 217-223
2. Tea, Y. C. (2008, February 15). Back to the Basics, Part 1: Prime Yourself to Prescribe Prism. Retrieved from https://www.reviewofoptometry.com/article/back-to-the-basics-part-1-prime-yourself-to-prescribe-prism
3. Brown, O. L. (1967). *Your Innate Power: To Achieve Integration, Health, Freedom.* London: George Allen & Unwin, 35

4. Bates, W. H. (1922). The Truth about Fatigue. *Better Eyesight*, March
5. Agranove, E. E. (1920). Progressive Myopia Relieved. *Better Eyesight*, March
6. Bates, W. H. (1923). Eye Strain when Sleeping. *Better Eyesight*, February
7. Quinn, G. E., Shin, C. H., Maguire, M. G., & Stone, R. A. (1999). Myopia and ambient lighting at night. *Nature, 399*(6732), 113-114. doi:10.1038/20094
8. Huxley, L. A. (1969). *This Timeless Moment; A personal view of Aldous Huxley.* London: Chatto & Windus.

13. Breathe Freely

1. Wangsa-Wirawan, N. D. (2003). Retinal Oxygen. *Archives of Ophthalmology, 121*(4), 547. doi:10.1001/archopht.121.4.547
2. Bates, W. H. (1923). Breathing. *Better Eyesight*, January
3. Corbett, M. (1938). *How to Improve Your Eyes,* 19
4. Stough, C., & Stough, R. (1981). *Dr. Breath: The story of breathing coordination.* New York: Stough Institute.
5. Douillard, J. (2001). *Body, Mind, and Sport: The mind-body guide to lifelong health, fitness, and your personal best.* New York: Three Rivers Press.
6. Lewis, D. (2004). *Free your breath, free your life: How conscious breathing can relieve stress, increase vitality, and help you live more fully.* Boston, MA: Shambhala.
7. Campaign for Safe Cosmetics-working for safer cosmetics. Retrieved from http://www.safecosmetics.org/

14. A Carrot a Day Keeps the Eye Doctor Away?

1. Bates, W. H. (1926). Eyestrain. *Better Eyesight*, February
2. Bates, W. H. (1927). Stories from the Clinic – Four Boys and a Girl. *Better Eyesight*, March
3. Bates, E. (1929). Itching of the Eyelids. *Better Eyesight*, June
4. Adams, P., & Mylander, M. (1998). *Gesundheit!: Bringing good health to you, the medical system, and society through physician service, complementary therapies, humor, and joy.* Rochester, VT: Healing Arts Press.
5. Eyesight experts issue warning on diet which can lead to blindness. (2016, October 15). Retrieved from https://www.theage.com.au/healthcare/eyesight-experts-issue-warning-on-diet-which-can-lead-to-blindness-20161012-gs0twl.html
6. Fuhrman, J. (2012). *Super Immunity: The essential nutrition guide for boosting our body's defenses to live longer, stronger, and disease free.* New York: HarperOne, 147
7. Too Much Vitamin C – Increased Risk for Blindness. Retrieved from http://www.nutrioptom.com/VITAMIN%20C.htm
8. Oranges improve eye health and guard against macular disease. (2018, July 13). Retrieved from https://www.wddty.com/news/2018/07/oranges-improve-eye-health-and-guard-against-macular-disease.html
9. Gopinath, B., et al. (2018). Dietary flavonoids and the prevalence and 15-y incidence of age-related macular degeneration. *The American Journal of Clinical Nutrition, 108*(2), 381-387. doi:10.1093/ajcn/nqy114
10. Nutritional Optometry. Benjamin Clarence Lane, O.D. Retrieved from https://www.nutrioptom.com
11. Your Vitamins May Be Doing More Harm Than Good, We'll Show You How You Can Check. (2018, December 09). Retrieved from http://worldtruth.tv/your-vitamins-may-be-doing-more-harm-than-good-well-show-you-how-you-can-check/
12. Gala, D., Gala, D. R., Gala, S. (n.d.). *Dr. Gala's Vision Training Programme.* Mumbai: Navneet, 116

13. Other Names for MSG. (n.d.). Retrieved from https://www.glutathionediseasecure.com/other-names-for-MSG.html
14. Health Concerns About Dairy. (n.d.). Physicians Committee for Responsible Medicine. Retrieved from https://www.pcrm.org/good-nutrition/nutrition-information/health-concerns-about-dairy
15. Lam, B. L., & Lee, D. J. (2015, February 01). Smoking Causes Blindness: Time for Eye Care Professionals to Join the Fight Against Tobacco. Retrieved from https://iovs.arvojournals.org/article.aspx?articleid=2212874
16. The Health Consequences of Smoking - 50 Years of Progress: A Report of the Surgeon General, 2014. Retrieved from https://www.surgeongeneral.gov/library/reports/50-years-of-progress/index.html
17. Kang, J. H., et al (2016). Contribution of the Nurses' Health Study to the Epidemiology of Cataract, Age-Related Macular Degeneration, and Glaucoma. *American Journal of Public Health, 106*(9), 1684-1689. doi:10.2105/ajph.2016.303317
18. Solberg, Y., Rosner, M., & Belkin, M. (1998). The Association Between Cigarette Smoking and Ocular Diseases. *Survey of Ophthalmology, 42*(6), 535-547. doi:10.1016/s0039-6257(98)00002-2
19. Fuhrman, J. (2013). The End of Diabetes: The Eat to Live Plan to Prevent and Reverse Diabetes. New York, NY: Harper One.

15. Sunlight: Friend or Foe?

1. Bates, W. H. (1921). Think Right. *Better Eyesight*, December
2. Ott, J. N. (1990). *Light, Radiation and You - How to Stay Healthy.* Greenwich, CT: Devin-Adair, 174. (Revised and updated edition; includes five new appendices)
3. Ott, J. N. (1973). *Health & Light: The effects of natural & artificial light on man & other living things.* Greenwich, CT: Devin-Adair, 30-31
4. Ott, J. N. (1973). *Health & Light*
5. John Ott: The Light Side of Health. (1986). *Mother Earth News,* January/February. Ogden Publications. Retrieved from https://www.motherearthnews.com/nature-and-environment/john-ott-zm0z86zhun
6. Ott, J. N. (1973). *Health & Light*
7. Ott, J. N. (1990). *Light, Radiation and You*
8. Ott, J. N. (1990). *Light, Radiation and You,* 134
9. Jones, L. A., Sinnott, L. T., Mutti, D. O., Mitchell, G. L., Moeschberger, M. L., & Zadnik, K. (2007). Parental History of Myopia, Sports and Outdoor Activities, and Future Myopia. *Investigative Opthalmology & Visual Science, 48*(8), 3524. doi:10.1167/iovs.06-1118
10. French, A. N., Ashby, R. S., Morgan, I. G., & Rose, K. A. (2013). Time outdoors and the prevention of myopia. *Experimental Eye Research, 114*, 58-68. doi:10.1016/j.exer.2013.04.018
11. Jones-Jordan, L. A., Sinnott, L. T., Cotter, S. A., Kleinstein, R. N., Manny, R. E., Mutti, D. O., Zadnik, K. (2012). Time Outdoors, Visual Activity, and Myopia Progression in Juvenile-Onset Myopes. *Investigative Ophthalmology & Visual Science, 53*(11), 7169. doi:10.1167/iovs.11-8336
12. Cohn, H. (1886). *Hygiene of the Eye in Schools.* London: Simpkin, Marshall and Co. As quoted in Hobday R. (2015). Myopia and daylight in schools: a neglected aspect of public health? *Perspectives in Public Health, 136*(1), 50-55. doi:10.1177/1757913915576679
13. Rona, Z. (2010). *Vitamin D The Sunshine Vitamin.* Summertown, TN: Books Alive.
14. Harding, J. J. (1995). The untenability of the sunlight hypothesis of cataractogenesis. *Documenta Ophthalmologica, 88*(3-4), 345-349. doi:10.1007/bf01203687

15. Harding, J. J. (1996). Testing time for the sunlight hypothesis of cataract. *Current Opinion in Ophthalmology, 7*(1), 59-62. doi:10.1097/00055735-199602000-00012
16. Collman, G. W., Shore, D. L., Shy, C. M., Checkoway, H., & Luria, A. S. (1988). Sunlight and other risk factors for cataracts: An epidemiologic study. *American Journal of Public Health, 78*(11), 1459-1462. doi:10.2105/ajph.78.11.1459
17. Klein, B. E., Cruickshanks, K. J., & Klein, R. (1995). Leisure time, sunlight exposure and cataracts. *Documenta Ophthalmologica, 88*(3-4), 295-305. doi:10.1007/bf01203683
18. Whitaker, T. (2010). Light and human health: LED risks highlighted. *LEDs Magazine*. Retrieved from https://www.ledsmagazine.com/articles/2010/11/light-and-human-health-led-risks-highlighted.html
19. Mayberry, S. A. (2017). Are Blue Eyes Sensitive to Light? Retrieved from https://www.axonoptics.com/2017/05/are-blue-eyes-sensitive-to-light/
20. Hoel, D. G., Berwick, M., Gruijl, F. R., & Holick, M. F. (2016). The risks and benefits of sun exposure 2016. *Dermato-Endocrinology, 8*(1). doi:10.1080/19381980.2016.1248325
21. Kime, Z. R. (1980). *Sunlight Could Save Your Life,* 225-226
22. Solomon, S., Ivy, D. J., Kinnison, D., Mills, M. J., Neely, R. R., & Schmidt, A. (2016). Emergence of healing in the Antarctic ozone layer. *Science, 353*(6296), 269-274. doi:10.1126/science.aae0061
23. Scientific Assessment of Ozone Depletion: 2018, Executive Summary. World Meteorological Organization, Global Ozone Research and Monitoring Project – Report No. 58, 67 pp., Geneva, Switzerland, 2018.
24. Bates, W. H. (1920). *Perfect Sight Without Glasses,* Chapter XVII, 186
25. Ott, J. N. (1990). *Light, Radiation and You,* 23
26. Sunning lamps: Follow the link at optimaleyesight.com
27. Traditional Bates Method teachers are listed on my website; look for TBM annotation next to their name. Follow the link at optimaleyesight.com
28. Anonymous nursery rhyme set to the tune of "Yankee Doodle", quoted in "The Health Club" in *School Life*, Vol. IV (January - June 1920), p. 17

16. Seeing Effortlessly All Day Long

1. Bates, W. H. (1920). Strain. *Perfect Sight Without Glasses*, 112
2. Bates, W. H. (1929). Time for Practice. *Better Eyesight*, January
3. Bates, W. H. (1928). Practice Methods. *Better Eyesight*, December
4. Bates, W. H. (1929). Questions and Answers. *Better Eyesight*, September
5. Bates, W. H. (1928). Practice Time. *Better Eyesight*, November
6. Bates, W. H. (1927). Blinking and Shifting. *Better Eyesight*, March

17. A Bold View of Letter Charts and Small Print

1. Bates, W. H. (1922). Glasses Keep up the Eye Strain. *Better Eyesight*, September
2. Bates, W. H. (1911). The Prevention of Myopia in School Children. *New York Medical Journal, 94*(30) 237-238.
3. Bates, W. H. (1919). Home Treatment. *Better Eyesight*, December
4. Bates, W. H. (1919). A Method that Succeeded. *Better Eyesight*, August
5. Boomerang ball: Follow the link at optimaleyesight.com
6. Letter charts: Follow the link at optimaleyesight.com
7. Bates, W. H. (1920). Fine Print a Benefit to the Eye. *Better Eyesight*, May
8. Lierman, E. C. (1928). Test Card Practice. *Better Eyesight*, September
9. Bates, W. H. (1924). Fine Print. *Better Eyesight*, May
10. Bates, W. H. (1926). Lord Macaulay. *Better Eyesight*, October

18. Clarifying Astigmatism
1. Bates, W. H. (1926). Simple Hypermetropic Astigmatism. *Better Eyesight*, December
2. Email correspondence between the author and Anna Bambridge, 6 May 2018
3. Forrest, E. B. (1980). Astigmatism as a Function of Visual Scan, Head Scan, and Head Posture. *Optometry and Vision Science, 57*(11), 844-860. doi:10.1097/00006324-198011000-00011
4. Harris, P. (1988). Visual conditions of symphony musicians. *Journal of the American Optometric Association 59*(12) 952-959
5. Forrest, E. B. (1980). Astigmatism as a Function of Visual Scan, Head Scan, and Head Posture. *Optometry and Vision Science, 57*(11), 845

19. Computer Screens: Look Beyond the 20/20/20 Rule
1. The Common Sense Census: Plugged-In Parents of Tweens and Teens 2016 | Common Sense Media. (2016, December 06). Retrieved from https://www.commonsensemedia.org/research/the-common-sense-census-plugged-in-parents-of-tweens-and-teens-2016
2. Screen projectors: Follow the link at www.optimaleyesight.com
3. EyeLeo software: www.eyeleo.com
4. Time Out software: http://www.dejal.com/timeout/
5. f.lux software: https://justgetflux.com
6. Iris software: https://iristech.co/
7. Redshift software: http://jonls.dk/redshift/
8. Sunset Screen software: http://www.skytopia.com/software/sunsetscreen/
9. Dark Reader: https://darkreader.org/
10. Laptop stand: Follow the link at www.optimaleyesight.com

20. Peering into the Night
1. Brooks Simpkins, R. (1968). *Improve Your Eyes at Home.* London: Fowler.
2. Gilbert, G. (1997 Unpublished manuscript). *Pagan Awakening*, Chapter XII
3. Dark-Sky Association: www.darksky.org
4. Bates, W. H. (1925). Night Blindness. *Better Eyesight*, March
5. Bates, W. H. (1920). A Lesson from the Greeks. *Better Eyesight*, June
6. Zink, N. and Parks, S. (Fall 1991). Nightwalking – Exploring the Dark with Peripheral Vision, *Whole Earth Review*
7. Hagmann, R. B. (1968). *"2-Brain" Calisthenics* (revised edition). Daly City, CA: Hagmann System
8. Hagmann, R. B. (n.d.). *Natural Eyesight Reclamation, 22*

22. Help a Child to Better Sight
1. Bates, W. H. (1920). What Glasses Do to Us. *Better Eyesight*, July
2. Bates, W. H. (1923). Hypermetropia in School Children. *Better Eyesight*, August
3. Leat, S. J. (2011). To prescribe or not to prescribe? Guidelines for spectacle prescribing in infants and children. *Clinical and Experimental Optometry, 94*(6), 514-527. doi:10.1111/j.1444-0938.2011.00600.x
4. Bates, W. H. (1920). Cures at All Ages. *Perfect Sight Without Glasses*, Chapter IX, 105
5. Hotson, P. (1925). An Optometrist's Experience. *Better Eyesight*, December
6. Naber, S. (2010). *Natuurlijk Zien en de Bates Methode.* The Netherlands: Natuurlijk Zien
7. Bates, W. H. (1919). The Story of Emily. *Better Eyesight*, August
8. Bates, W.H. (1923). Throw Away Your Glasses. *Hearst's International, 44*(3), 42-43 & 128-132
9. Bates, W.H. (1920). Save the Children's Eyes. *Better Eyesight*, August

10. Quinn, G. E., Shin, C. H., Maguire, M. G., & Stone, R. A. (1999). Myopia and ambient lighting at night. *Nature, 399*(6732), 113-114. doi:10.1038/20094
11. *Fairy Tales for Better Eyesight.* Follow the link at optimaleyesight.com

23. Two Points of View for 3-D
1. Friedman, K. K. (2012). Why can't my child see even WITH glasses? American Optometric Association. Retrieved from https://www.aoa.org/Documents/optometric-staff/Articles/Why-Can't-My-Child-See.pdf
2. Randomized Trial of Treatment of Amblyopia in Children Aged 7 to 17 Years. (2005). *Archives of Ophthalmology, 123*(4), 437. doi:10.1001/archopht.123.4.437
3. Attebo, K., Mitchell, P., Cumming, R., Smith, W., Jolly, N., & Sparkes, R. (1998). Prevalence and causes of amblyopia in an adult population. *Ophthalmology, 105*(1), 154-159. doi:10.1016/s0161-6420(98)91862-0
4. Barry, S. R. (2009). *Fixing my Gaze*
5. Bates, W. H. (1927). Squint. *Better Eyesight,* February
6. Eye patches. Follow the link at optimaleyesight.com
7. Bates, W. H. (1927). Squint. *Better Eyesight,* October
8. Lierman, E. C. (1923). Stories from the Clinic – 45: The Story of Rose. *Better Eyesight,* November
9. Hagmann, R. B. (n.d.). *How to Do the Omnision Practices.*

24. Dr. Bates' Perspective on Eye Diseases
1. Bates, W. H. (1921). Cataract, Its Cause and Cure. *Better Eyesight,* January
2. Bates, W. H. (1924). Conical Cornea. *Better Eyesight,* May
3. Bates, W. H. (1921). Blindness: Its Cause and Cure. *Better Eyesight,* March
4. Bates, W. H. (1920). The Mission of "Better Eyesight." *Better Eyesight,* July
5. Lierman, E. C. (1924). Stories from the Clinic ~ 52: A Blind Boy. *Better Eyesight,* June
6. The Bates Method View series of e-books: Follow the link at optimaleyesight.com
7. For a list of books on how to treat eye diseases naturally, visit optimaleyesight.com

Postscript
1. Bates, W. H. (1920). Relaxation Cures. *Perfect Sight Without Glasses*, Chapter IX, 101
2. Robbins, A. (2013). *Awaken the Giant Within: How to Take Immediate Control of Your Mental, Emotional, Physical & Financial Destiny!* NY, NY: Simon & Schuster Paperbacks.

Appendix D
1. Bates, W. H. (1919). Home Treatment. *Better Eyesight,* December

Appendix E
1. A list of websites that sell affordable glasses is at optimaleyesight.com
2. Information on high-index glasses: Follow the link at optimaleyesight.com
3. Guide to buying glasses online: Follow the link at optimaleyesight.com

Appendix F
Sources used in alphabetic order:
Adams, N. (2014). *Healthy Vision: Prevent and reverse eye disease through better nutrition.* Guilford, CT: Lyons Press, an imprint of Globe Pequot Press.
Anshel, J. (1999). *Smart Medicine for Your Eyes.* Garden City Park, NY: Avery Publishing Group.
Evans, S. C. (1978). *Nutrition in Eye Health and Disease.* London: Roberts Publications.
Fuhrman, J. (2011). *Super Immunity.* New York: HarperOne.
Grossman, M. & Swartwout, G. (1999). *Natural Eye Care: An encyclopedia.* Los Angeles, CA: Keats.
Igram, C., & Gray, J. K. (1994). *The Self Test Nutrition Guide.* Hiawatha, IA: Knowledge House.

Johnson, G. J., Minassian, D. C., Weale, R. (1998). *The Epidemiology of Eye Disease*. Philadelphia, PA: Lippincott-Raven.

Kaplan, R. (1995). *The power behind your eyes*. Rochester, VT: Healing Arts Press.

Kime, Z. R. (1980). *Sunlight Could Save Your Life,*

Office of Dietary Supplements - Vitamin A. (n.d.). Retrieved from http://ods.od.nih.gov/factsheets/VitaminA-HealthProfessional/

Sardi, B. (1994). *Nutrition and the Eyes: How to keep your eyes healthy naturally*. Montclair, CA: Health Spectrum.

Appendix G

1. Kime, Z. R. (1980). *Sunlight Could Save Your Life,* 152
2. Moan, J. Grigalavicius, M., Dahlback, A., Baturaite, Z., Juzeniene, A. (2014). Ultraviolet-radiation and health: optimal time for sun exposure. *Advances in Experimental Medicine and Biology, 810*:423-428

The list of eye-essential nutrients was compiled through many web searches, using sites such as: https://www.myfooddata.com and https://nutritiondata.self.com

Appendix H

Sources used in alphabetic order:

Atropine eye drops package leaflet – user information

Fowler, P. (n.d.). Medications: Eye Problems and Vision Changes. Retrieved from https://www.webmd.com/eye-health/features/medications-cause-vision-problems#2

Harding, J. J. (1995). The untenability of the sunlight hypothesis of cataractogenesis. *Documenta Ophthalmologica, 88*(3-4), 345-349. doi:10.1007/bf01203687

McCarthy, K. (n.d.). Meds That Cause Blurred Vision, Hearing Loss, and More. Retrieved from https://www.consumerreports.org/drugs/meds-that-cause-blurred-vision-hearing-loss-and-more/

Charts

1. Practice charts are available via optimaleyesight.com

Glossary

1. Bates, W. H. (1917). Blindness relieved by a new method of treatment. *New York Medical Journal, 105*(5) 200-202.
2. Bates, W. H. (1915). The radical cure of errors of refraction by means of central fixation. *New York Medical Journal, 101*(19) 925-933.

Index

Made in the USA
Columbia, SC
14 August 2020